Community Medicine
Practical Workbook

Complete practical workbook in

- **Community Medicine**
- **Preventive and Social Medicine | Social and Preventive Medicine**
- **Community and Family Medicine**
- **Public Health in India**

Presenting all aspects of the subject

- **Epidemiology**
- **Biostatistics**
- **Museum**
- **Laboratory**
- **Case Discussion**
- **National Health Programs**
- **Public Health Updates**
- **Public Health Management**
- **Sociology and Other Topics**

Community Medicine
Practical Workbook

Arti Gupta

MBBS (Gold Medalist), MD, DNB, PGDCR, PGDHHM

Assistant Professor
Department of Community Medicine
Veer Chandra Singh Garhwali Government
Medical Sciences and Research Institute
Srinagar, Uttarakhand

Sidharth Sekhar Mishra

MBBS, MD, DNB

Faculty
Delhi Academy of Medical Sciences
New Delhi

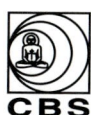

CBS

CBS Publishers & Distributors Pvt Ltd

New Delhi • Bengaluru • Chennai • Kochi • Kolkata • Mumbai

Bhopal • Bhubaneswar • Hyderabad • Jharkhand • Nagpur • Patna • Pune • Uttarakhand • Dhaka (Bangladesh)

Community Medicine
Practical Workbook

ISBN: 978-93-88108-38-6

Copyright © Authors and Publisher

First Edition: 2019

Published by Satish Kumar Jain and Produced by Varun Jain for

CBS Publishers & Distributors Pvt Ltd
4819/XI Prahlad Street, 24 Ansari Road, Daryaganj, New Delhi 110 002, India.
Ph: 23289259, 23266861, 23266867   Fax: 011-23243014   Website: www.cbspd.com
e-mail: delhi@cbspd.com; cbspubs@airtelmail.in.
Corporate Office: 204 FIE, Industrial Area, Patparganj, Delhi 110 092
Ph: 4934 4934   Fax: 4934 4935   e-mail: publishing@cbspd.com; publicity@cbspd.com

Branches

- **Bengaluru:** Seema House 2975, 17th Cross, K.R. Road,
  Banasankari 2nd Stage, Bengaluru 560 070, Karnataka
  Ph: +91-80-26771678/79   Fax: +91-80-26771680   e-mail: bangalore@cbspd.com
- **Chennai:** 7, Subbaraya Street, Shenoy Nagar, Chennai 600 030, Tamil Nadu
  Ph: +91-44-26680620, 26681266   Fax: +91-44-42032115   e-mail: chennai@cbspd.com
- **Kochi:** 42/1325, 1326, Power House Road, Opp. KSEB Power House
  Ernakulam 682 018, Kochi, Kerala
  Ph: +91-484-4059061-65   Fax: +91-484-4059065   e-mail: kochi@cbspd.com
- **Kolkata:** 6/B, Ground Floor, Rameswar Shaw Road, Kolkata-700 014, West Bengal
  Ph: +91-33-22891126, 22891127, 22891128   e-mail: kolkata@cbspd.com
- **Mumbai:** 83-C, Dr E Moses Road, Worli, Mumbai-400018, Maharashtra
  Ph: +91-22-24902340/41   Fax: +91-22-24902342   e-mail: mumbai@cbspd.com

Representatives

• Bhopal	0-8319310552	• Bhubaneswar 0-9911037372	• Hyderabad 0-9885175004	• Jharkhand	0-9811541605
• Nagpur	0-9021734563	• Patna 0-9334159340	• Pune 0-9623451994	• Uttarakhand	0-9716462459
• Dhaka (Bangladesh)	01912-003485				

Printed at Nutech Print Services, Faridabad, Haryana, India

Contributors

1. **Dr Arti Gupta** MBBS, MD, DNB, PGDCR, PGDHHM
   Assistant Professor, Department of Community Medicine, Veer Chandra Singh Garhwali Government Medical Sciences and Research Institute, Uttarakhand, India.

2. **Dr Arun Padmanandan** MBBS
   Junior Resident, Department of Community Medicine, Vardhman Mahavir Medical College and Safdarjung Hospital, New Delhi, India.

3. **Dr Ashish Pundhir** MBBS, MD
   Senior Resident, Department of Community and Family Medicine, All India Institute of Medical Sciences, Jodhpur, Rajasthan, India.

4. **Dr D Surendra Babu** MBBS, MD
   Assistant Professor, Department of Community Medicine, Apollo Institute of Medical Sciences & Research, Chittoor, Andhra Pradesh, India

5. **Dr Manish Taywade** MBBS, MD
   Assistant Professor, Department of Community and Family Medicine, All India Institute of Medical Sciences, Bhubaneswar, Orissa, India.

6. **Dr Munesh Kumar Gupta** MBBS, MD
   Assistant Professor, Department of Microbiology, Institute of Medical Sciences, Banaras Hindu University, Varanasi, India.

7. **Dr Nitika** MBBS, MD
   Senior Resident, Postgraduate Institute of Medical Education and Research, Chandigarh, India.

8. **Dr Pallavi Lohani** MBBS
   Junior Resident, Department of Community Medicine, Patna Medical College and Hospital, Patna, Bihar, India.

9. **Dr Puja Dudeja** MBBS, MD, PhD
   Associate Professor, Department of Community Medicine, Armed Forces Medical College, Pune, Maharashtra, India.

10. **Dr Sahil Goyal** MBBS, MD
    Surveillance Medical Officer, World Health Organization, Uttar Pradesh, India.

11. **Dr Sidharth Sekhar Mishra** MBBS, MD, DNB
    Community Medicine faculty at Delhi Academy of Medical Sciences (DAMS), New Delhi, India.

12. **Dr Sudip Bhattacharya** MBBS, MD
    Senior Resident, Postgraduate Institute of Medical Education and Research, Chandigarh, India.

13. **Dr Swagata Mandal** MBBS
    Junior Resident, Department of Community Medicine, R. G. Kar Medical College and Hospital, Kolkata, India.

14. **Dr Venkatashiva Reddy B** MBBS, MD, DNB, PGDCR, PGDHHM
    Assistant Professor, Department of Community Medicine, Veer Chandra Singh Garhwali Government Medical Sciences and Research Institute, Uttarakhand, India.

Preface

This book provides a comprehensive body of community medicine subject. It is the book for students and faculty. Community medicine is a vast base subject covering epidemiology, biostatistics, nutrition, communicable diseases, non-communicable diseases, sociology, mental health, demography, national health programmes, research, maternal and child health, geriatric health, adolescent health, environment, and others. Owing to this huge curriculum and the time constraints associated with other subjects, it is difficult for the students to read and comprehend the entire subject. The advances in electronic communication and its effects on entrance examinations are a growing challenge to the students. At times the questions asked in entrance examinations are not the part of standard reading. This book is an effort to bridge the gap between the community medicine academic curriculum and various entrance examinations. The book is not the surrogate for in detail reading for the subject, but provides important information in various heads.

The book aims to cover the important aspects of community medicine with respect to professional and entrance examinations. Selecting the appropriate information was challenging because of rapid growth of preventive medicine and public health. The basic principles of epidemiology are presented with emphasis on its importance in community medicine. It presents the biostatistics together with its applications. It demonstrates various aspects of public health laboratory. The book offers numerous images in museum section to make student understand the community and hospital level working in community medicine. It provides a broad context and perspective to different clinical cases. It focuses on the critical appraisal approach to national health programmes. Public health update is the highlight of the book. Every chapter was scrutinized for updates and modified accordingly. The book addresses the various aspects of research and publication frequently asked. A student often encounters problems in applying the knowledge, which is usual to our discipline. The book is directed towards the true gain in knowledge and its application. This book stores vast knowledge and experience for faculty across India. On behalf of the team, we wish the students a brilliant and successful career in life.

Arti Gupta
Sidharth Sekhar Mishra

Acknowledgments

We wish to acknowledge the following reviewers

1. **Dr Bhawana Pant**, Professor, Department of Community Medicine, Subharti Medical College, Meerut, Uttar Pradesh, India.

2. **Dr Parul Sharma,** Associate Professor, Department of Community Medicine, Dr DY Patil Medical College, Pune, Maharashtra, India.

3. **Dr Akhil Goel,** Assistant Professor, Department of Community and Family Medicine, All India Institute of Medical Sciences Jodhpur, Rajasthan, India.

4. **Dr Anindo Majumdar,** Assistant Professor, Department of Community & Family Medicine, All India Institute of Medical Sciences Bhopal, Madhya Pradesh, India.

5. **Dr Amarveer Singh Mehta**, Assistant Professor, Department of Community Medicine, FH Medical College, Tundla, Uttar Pradesh, India.

6. **Dr Amrita N Shamanewadi,** Assistant Professor, Department of Community Medicine, MVJ Medical College and Research Hospital, Hoskote, Karnataka, India.

7. **Dr Arti Gupta,** Assistant Professor, Department of Community Medicine, Veer Chandra Singh Garhwali Government Medical Sciences and Research Institute, Uttarakhand, India.

8. **Dr Dewesh Kumar,** Assistant Professor, Department of Preventive and Social Medicine, Rajendra Institute of Medical Sciences, Ranchi, Jharkhand, India.

9. **Dr Hariom Kumar Solanki,** Assistant Professor, Department of Community Medicine, Government Medical College, Haldwani, Uttarakhand, India.

10. **Dr Jyoti Landge,** Epidemiologist, Assistant Professor, Department of Community Medicine, Dr DY Patil Medical College, Pune, Maharashtra, India.

11. **Dr Khushboo Juneja,** Assistant Professor, Department of Community Medicine, School of Medical Sciences and Research, Sharda University, Greater Noida, Uttar Pradesh, India.

12. **Dr L Karthik Balajee,** Assistant Professor, Department of Community Medicine, Jawaharlal Institute of Postgraduate Medical Education & Research (JIPMER), Karaikal, Puducherry, India.

13. **Dr Mini Sharma,** Assistant Professor, Department of Preventive and Social Medicine, Pt. Jawahar Lal Nehru Memorial Medical College, Raipur, Chhattisgarh, India.

14. **Dr Nilanjana Ghosh,** Assistant Professor, Department of Community Medicine, North Bengal Medical College, Siliguri, West Bengal, India.

15. **Dr Nripendra Singh,** Assistant Professor, Department of Community Medicine, TSM Medical College and Hospital, Lucknow, Uttar Pradesh, India.

16. **Dr Saba Mohammed Manssor,** Assistant Professor, Department of Community Medicine, Kanachur Institue of Medical Sciences, Mangalore, Karnataka, India.

17. **Dr Shubha Davalgi,** Assistant Professor, Department of Community Medicine, JJM Medical College, Davangere, Karnataka, India.

18. **Dr Sidharth Sekhar Mishra,** Community Medicine faculty at Delhi Academy of Medical Sciences (DAMS), New Delhi, India.

19. **Dr Varun Gaiki,** Assistant Professor, Department of Community Medicine, Malla Reddy Institute of Medical Sciences, Hyderabad, Telangana, India.

20. **Dr Venkatashiva Reddy B,** Assistant Professor, Department of Community Medicine, Veer Chandra Singh Garhwali Government Medical Sciences and Research Institute, Uttarakhand, India.

21. **Dr Vijay Kumar Silan,** Assistant Professor, Department of Community Medicine, BPS Government Medical College, Khanpur Kalan, Sonepat, Haryana, India.

22. **Dr Amit Mohan,** Lecturer, Department of Community Medicine, Maharani Laxmi Bai Medical College, Jhansi, Uttar Pradesh, India.

23. **Dr Pradip Kharya,** Lecturer, Department of Community Medicine, Government Medical College, Kannauj, Uttar Pradesh, India.

24. **Dr Sudip Bhattacharya,** Senior Resident, Postgraduate Institute of Medical Education and Research, Chandigarh, India.

25. **Dr S Lena Charlette,** Junior Resident, Department of Community Medicine, Andaman Nicobar Islands Institute of Medical Sciences, Port Blair, India.

26. **Dr Pallavi Lohani,** Junior Resident, Department of Community medicine, Patna Medical College and Hospital, Patna, Bihar, India.

27. **Mr. Pandurang Vithal Thatkar,** Statistician, Andaman Nicobar Islands Institute of Medical Sciences, Port Blair, India.

28. **Dr Shubhanshu Gupta,** Junior Resident, Department of Community Medicine, Maharani Laxmi Bai Medical College, Jhansi, Uttar Pradesh, India.

29. **Dr Swagata Mandal,** Junior Resident, Department of Community Medicine, R. G. Kar Medical College and Hospital, Kolkata, India.

30. **Dr Vinod Rathod,** Junior Resident, Department of Community Medicine, Darbhanga Medical College, Darbhanga, Bihar, India.

Contents

Preface *vii*

1. Public Health Epi-Laboratory 1
Sidharth Sekhar Mishra, Venkatashiva Reddy B

Biostatistics 1
Measures of central tendency 1
Measures of variability/dispersion 1
Tests of significance 6
Epidemiology 13
Epidemic curves 13
Measuring disease frequency 15
Probability proportion to size (pps) sampling 19
Sample size calculation in epidemiological studies 24
Measures of association 26
Kappa statistic 29
Survival analysis 31
Sensitivity, specificity and predictive values 36
Likelihood ratios 39
Others 42
Family welfare 42
Immunization 45
Nutrition 48

2. Public Health Laboratory 53
Venkatashiva Reddy B, Munesh Kumar Gupta

Nutrition 53
Milk quality 53
Milk borne diseases 54
Food quality testing 55
Water 59
Water quality testing 59
Safe water/wholesome water 60
Environment instruments 63
Public health microbiology 67

3. Public Health Museum

78

Arti Gupta

Family welfare 78
Immunization 84
Nutrition 90
Drugs 99
Disinfectants/antiseptics 104
Entomology 108
Symbols 112

4. Family/Case

113

Introductory family/case viva 113

Nitika

Under-five children 123

Arun Padmanandan

Malnutrition 123
Pneumonia 134
Diarrhoea 138
Sick neonate 145

Adolescent 155

Ashish Pundhir

Anaemia 155
Mental retardation (intellectual disability) 161
Rheumatic fever and rheumatic heart disease 164
Epilepsy and seizures 166
Fever (pyrexia) 168

Antenatal and postnatal 176

D Surendra Babu

Adult 189

Puja Dudeja

Acquired Immuno Deficiency Syndrome (AIDS) 189
Leprosy 203
Tuberculosis (TB) 209

Elderly 215

Swagata Mandal, Sahil Goyal, Arti Gupta

Hypertension 215
Diabetes mellitus 222

Chronic obstructive pulmonary disease 229

Arti Gupta

Annexures 232

5. Evolution and Critical Appraisal of National Health Programs   245
Arti Gupta

6. Public Health Update   253
Sidharth Sekhar Mishra

Tuberculosis 253
Depression 253
Vaccination 254
Statistics: India 255
Maternal and child health 256
Family planning 257
Nutrition 257
Infectious disease 260

7. Miscellaneous   263
Manish Taywade, Sudip Bhattacharya, Pallavi Lohani, Arti Gupta

Public health literature 263
Management 265
Sociology 274
Others 279

8. Model Performa   284
Sidharth Sekhar Mishra

Index   289

Public Health Epi-Laboratory

Sidharth Sekhar Mishra, Venkatashiva Reddy B

BIOSTATISTICS

MEASURES OF CENTRAL TENDENCY

Mean: Average or sum of all observations divided by the total number of observations.
  a. Merits: Easy to calculate, based on all observations, it has sampling stability, important for majority of statistical tests.
  b. Demerits: Too sensitive to extreme observations, and not appropriate for skewed distributions.

Median: Middle or central value of distribution with arrangement. It divides the series into 2 equal groups.
  a. Merits: More representative of central value, not affected by extreme values/outliers.
  b. Demerits: Not based on all observations, cannot be calculated if data is not arranged in order.

Mode: Most frequently occurring value
  a. Merits: Easy to obtain, not affected by extreme values
  b. Demerits: May not be the central value, not based on all observations, not useful for further statistical analysis.

MEASURES OF VARIABILITY/DISPERSION

Standard deviation: It is the most common measure of dispersion. It is the square root of variance. It is also defined as the positive square root of average of squares of deviations taken from the mean. It is an absolute measure of dispersion.

Standard error: It is the measure of difference between sample and population values due to chance (due to sampling).

Coefficient of variation (CV): It is a relative measure of dispersion and hence a unit free measure which is useful to compare variability between variables. Less value of

CV indicates more consistency and larger value of CV indicates less consistency. Hence, consistency of data and CV are inversely proportional.

Range: Simplest way to describe spread of data by quoting lowest and highest values.

Disadvantage: It takes into account the extreme values and information about intermediate values cannot be gathered.

Interpretation:
1. Distribution:
   a. Normal: Mean = Median = Mode
   b. Skewed:
      i. Right/Positive: Mean > Median > Mode
      ii. Left/Negative: Mean < Median < Mode
   c. Unimodal/Bimodal:
      Bimodal distribution: Mode = 3 (Median) – 2 (Mean)
2. Mean and SD:

SD	Mean ± SD	Coverage
1	Mean ± 1 SD	68.3%
2	Mean ± 2 SD	95.4%
3	Mean ± 3 SD	99.7%

Practical Overview 1

Calculation of central tendency for discrete values:
1. Calculation of mean:
   Step 1: Adding all individual values
   Step 2: Dividing sum of individual values by actual number of observations
2. Calculation of median:
   Step 1: Arranging the data in ascending/descending order
   Step 2: Location of middle value:
      a. If the number of observations is odd numbered, then the middle value is taken.
      b. If the number of observations is even numbered, then the two values in the middle are taken, added and divided by 2 to obtain the median.
3. Calculation of mode:
   Step 1: Arranging the data in ascending/descending order.
   Step 2: The value occurring the maximum number of times is taken as the mode.

Calculation of mean for grouped series:

$$\text{Mean} = \frac{\text{Summation of [frequencies} \times \text{middle point]}}{\text{Summation of frequencies}} = \frac{\Sigma (f \times m)}{\Sigma f}$$

Calculation of mean deviation:
Step 1: Arithmetic mean ($\bar{X}$) is written against each individual value in column (a)
Step 2: Deviation of each value from the arithmetic mean ($X - \bar{X}$) is calculated in column (b)

Step 3: Summation (adding) of all deviations ignoring the sign

Step 4: Dividing the number of observations

$$\text{Mean deviation} = \frac{\Sigma (X - \bar{X})}{N}$$

Calculation of standard deviation:

Step 1: Arithmetic mean ($\bar{X}$) is written against each individual value in column (a)

Step 2: Deviation of each value from arithmetic mean ($X - \bar{X}$) is calculated in column (b)

Step 3: Each of the deviations calculated in step 3 is squared and written in column (c)

Step 4: Summation (adding) of all squared deviations

Step 5: Dividing the number of observations by n and if the sample size is less than 30, then dividing it by ($n - 1$)

Step 6: Formula of standard deviation

$$\sigma = \sqrt{\frac{\Sigma (X - \bar{X})^2}{n - 1}}$$

Calculation of coefficient of variation (CV):

Step 1: Calculate the mean

Step 2: Calculate the standard deviation

Step 3: CV = Standard deviation × 100

$$\text{Calculation of Standard Error: SE} = \frac{\text{SD}}{\sqrt{n}}$$

Practical Example

Q 1. Haemoglobin of 15 children aged 10 years in a school was estimated. Calculate the different central values (mean, median, and mode).

Given: 13, 11, 11, 12, 12, 10, 10, 13, 13, 12, 11, 14, 10, 13, 15

Calculate the mean deviation, standard deviation, and CV.

Answer:

1. Calculation of mean:

    Step 1: Adding all individual values

    $13 + 11 + 11 + 12 + 12 + 10 + 10 + 13 + 13 + 12 + 11 + 14 + 10 + 13 + 15 = 180$

    Step 2: Dividing the sum of individual values by the actual number of observations

    $180/15 = 12$

2. Calculation of median:

    Step 1: Arranging the data in ascending/descending order

    10, 10, 10, 11, 11, 11, 12, 12, 12, 13, 13, 13, 13, 14, 15

    Step 2: Location of middle value

    If the number of observations is odd numbered, then the middle value is median = 12

3. Calculation of mode:
   Step 1: Arranging the data in ascending/descending order
   Step 2: The value occurring the maximum number of times is the mode, mode = 13

4. Calculation of mean deviation:
   Step 1: Arithmetic mean ($\bar{X}$) is written against each individual value in column (a)
   Step 2: Deviation of each value from arithmetic mean ($X - \bar{X}$) is in column (b)
   Step 3: Summation (adding) of all deviation ignoring the sign
   Step 4: Dividing the number of observations, mean deviation = 18/10 = 1.8

Sl number	Haemoglobin (X)	Column (a) Arithmetic mean ($\bar{X}$)	Column (b) Deviation from mean ($X - \bar{X}$)	Column (c) $(X - \bar{X})^2$
1	13	12	1	1
2	11	12	−1	1
3	11	12	−1	1
4	12	12	0	0
5	12	12	0	0
6	10	12	−2	4
7	10	12	−2	4
8	13	12	1	1
9	13	12	1	1
10	12	12	0	0
11	11	12	−1	1
12	14	12	2	4
13	10	12	−2	4
14	13	12	1	1
15	15	12	3	9
	Total (ignoring the sign)		18	32

5. Calculation of standard deviation:
   Step 1: Arithmetic mean ($\bar{X}$) is written against each individual value in column (a)
   Step 2: Deviation of each value from arithmetic mean ($X - \bar{X}$) is calculated in column (b)
   Step 3: Each of the deviation calculated in step 3 is squared and written in column (c)
   Step 4: Summation (adding) of all squared deviations
   Step 5: Dividing the number of observations by n and if the sample size is less than 30, then dividing it by $n - 1$

Step 6: SD = $\sqrt{\dfrac{32}{14}}$ = 0.404

6. Calculation of coefficient of variation (CV):

$$CV = \frac{\text{Standard deviation} \times 100}{\text{Mean}}$$

$$CV = \frac{0.404 \times 100}{12} = 3.36\%$$

Q 2. Haemoglobin of 15 children aged 10 years in a school was estimated. Calculate the mean.

Hb level	Number of children/frequency (f)
10–11	6
12–13	7
14–15	2
Total	15

Answer:

Mean in grouped series has to be calculated.

Hb level	Midpoint of class interval (m)	Number of children/ frequency (f)	$m \times f$
10–11	10.5	6	63.0
12–13	12.5	7	87.5
14–15	14.5	2	29.0
Total		15	179.5

$$\text{Mean} = \frac{\text{Summation of [frequencies} \times \text{middle point]}}{\text{Summation of frequencies}} = \frac{\Sigma\,(f \times m)}{\Sigma f}$$

$$= 179.5/15 = 11.97$$

Confidence level: 95% means range of values which contain true population mean with probability of 0.95

Confidence limits: Upper and lower boundaries of a CI.

A. If confidence limits touch the null/neutral value, it becomes insignificant.
B. More the point estimate, better it is.
C. Narrow CI is better
   • Larger sample size
   • Smaller SD

Study	OR	95% CI	Inference
A	0.9	0.6–1.0	Useless
B	1.0	0.9–1.4	
C	1.2	1.1–1.5	Less useful
D	1.4	1.1–1.6	Useful
E	1.5	1.2–1.8	Most useful

TESTS OF SIGNIFICANCE

Overview

Test	Parametric	Nonparametric
Distribution	Normal	Nonnormal
Type of data	Quantitative	Quantitative
Sample size	Large	Small
Compares	Mean (SD)	%, proportions and fraction

1. Categorical vs Categorical Data

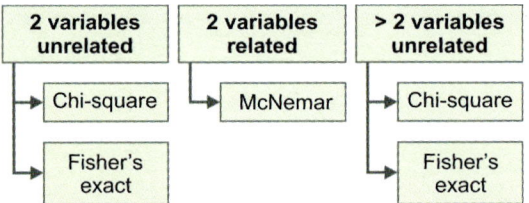

2. Categorical vs Quantitative
   a. *2 variables*

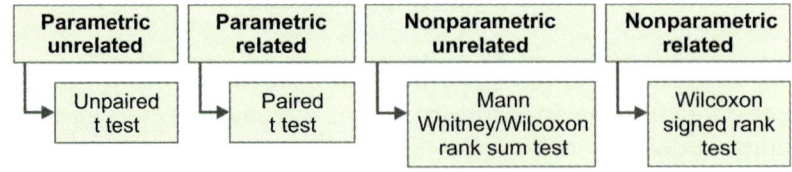

  b. *More than 2 variables*

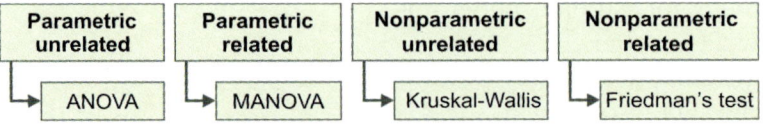

Practical Overview 2

Chi-Square Test

Step 1: Formulation of hypothesis

Null hypothesis (H_0): No difference in efficacy of 2 interventions

Alternate hypothesis (H_1): Difference exists between the 2 interventions

Step 2: Check for the number and nature of variables

If all the conditions mentioned above are satisfied, then we apply the Chi-square test.

Step 3: 2 × 2 table is constructed using the observed data (O)

Outcome	Intervention				Total
	1		**2**		
1	Cell a	O a	Cell b	O b	O a + O b
2	Cell c	O c	Cell d	O d	O c + O d
		O a + O c		O b + O d	O a + O b + O c + O d

Step 4: Expected value is calculated for each of the 4 cells and entered into each cell

Expected value = (Row total × column total)/grand total of all 4 cells

Step 5: Expected value is written under the observed value

Outcome	Treatment provided				Total
	Homemade ORS		**ORS**		
Not recovered	Cell a	O a E a	Cell b	O b E b	
Recovered	Cell c	O c E c	Cell d	O d E d	
				Total	O a + O b + O c + O d

Self-check for correct calculation of expected values:

$$O\,a + O\,b + O\,c + O\,d = E\,a + E\,b + E\,c + E\,d$$

Step 6: Calculation of Chi-square (χ^2)

$$\chi^2 = \frac{\text{Summation of (Observed} - \text{Expected)}^2}{\text{Expected}} = \frac{\Sigma\,(O - E)^2}{E}$$

Step 7: Calculation of degree of freedom (df)

df = (Number of rows −1) × (Number of columns −1)

Step 8: Interpretation:

- If calculated $\chi^2 < \chi^2$ table value at the particular df at 0.05, i.e. 5% level of significance then alternated hypothesis is accepted and failure to reject null hypothesis and that there is no association between exposure and outcome or both the interventions are equal.

- If calculated $\chi^2 > \chi^2$ table value at the particular df at 0.05, i.e. 5% level of significance then null hypothesis is rejected and that is association between exposure and outcome or both the interventions are not equal

Alternate formula of Chi-square for 2 by 2 contingency tables

Outcome	Intervention		Total
	1	**2**	
1	a	b	$a + b$
2	c	d	$c + d$
Total	$a + c$	$b + d$	

$$\chi^2 = \frac{N\,(ad - bc)^2}{(a + b)\,(c + d)\,(a + c)\,(c + d)}$$

Practical Example

Q 3. Out of 2500 diarrhoea cases with mild dehydration, 1500 were treated with homemade ORS and rest 1000 were treated with ORS. 300 did not recover from each group. Find out if there is any difference between the treatment outcomes in the two interventions.

Answer:

Step 1: Formulation of hypothesis:
- Null hypothesis (H_0): No difference in efficacy of 2 interventions (ORS and homemade ORS)
- Alternate hypothesis (H_1): Difference exists between the 2 interventions (ORS and homemade ORS)

Step 2: Check for the number and nature of variables
Test of significance to be applied:
- o 2 groups
- o Unrelated
- o Categorical variable [intervention given (yes/no) vs categorical variable recovered (yes/no)]: Chi-square test

Step 3: 2 × 2 table is constructed using the observed data

Outcome	Treatment provided				Total
	Homemade ORS		**ORS**		
Not recovered	Cell a	300	Cell b	300	600
Recovered	Cell c	1200	Cell d	700	1900
Total		1500		1000	2500

Step 4: Expected value is calculated for each of the 4 cells and entered into each cell

$$\text{Expected value} = \frac{\text{Row total} \times \text{column total}}{\text{Grand total of all 4 cells}}$$

For example, for cell A

Outcome	Treatment Provided				Total
	Homemade ORS		**ORS**		
Not recovered	Cell a	300	Cell b	300	600 (*i*)
Recovered	Cell c	1200	Cell d	700	1900
Total		1500 (*ii*)		1000	2500 (*x*)

$$\text{Expected value} = \frac{(i) \times (ii)}{(x)} = \frac{600 \times 1500}{2500} = 360$$

Similarly, calculating for other cells,

Outcome	Treatment provided				Total
	Homemade ORS		**ORS**		
Not recovered	Cell a	O = 300 E = 360	Cell b	O = 300 E = 240	600 (*i*)
Recovered	Cell c	O = 1200 E = 1140	Cell d	O = 700 E = 760	1900
Total		1500 (*ii*)		1000	2500 (*x*)

Step 5: Calculation of Chi-square (χ^2)

$$\chi^2 = \frac{\Sigma\,(\text{Observed} - \text{Expected})^2}{\text{Expected}} = \frac{\Sigma\,(O - E)^2}{E}$$

$$\text{or } \chi^2 = \frac{(300 - 360)^2}{360} + \frac{(300 - 240)^2}{240} + \frac{(1200 - 1140)^2}{1140} + \frac{(700 - 760)^2}{760}$$

Step 6: Calculation of degree of freedom (df)

df = [(Number of rows –1) × (Number of columns –1)]
df = (2 – 1) × (2 – 1) = 1

Step 7: Interpretation

Calculated χ^2 is more than the χ^2 table value (3.84) at 1 df at 0.05, i.e. 5% level of significance. Thus, null hypothesis is rejected.

Practical Overview 3

Student *t* Test

Step 1: Formulation of hypothesis

Null hypothesis (H_0): No difference in efficacy of 2 interventions

Alternate hypothesis (H_1): Difference exists between the 2 interventions

Step 2: Check for the number and nature of variables

If all the conditions mentioned above are satisfied, then we apply the *t* test

Step 3: Arithmetic mean is calculated for each of the two groups

Step 4: Arithmetic mean is written against each value against the two groups of the table

Step 5: Standard deviations of the two groups are calculated as explained in the earlier half of the chapter

Step 6: Summary table is written

Particulars	Group A without intervention	Group B with intervention
Number (n)	n_1	n_2
Mean (X)	$\bar{X}_1$	$\bar{X}_2$
Standard deviation (SD)	SD_1	SD_2

Step 7: Standard error of difference (SED) is calculated

$$SED = \sqrt{\frac{SD_1^2}{n_1}} + \sqrt{\frac{SD_2^2}{n_2}}$$

Step 8: *t* test is applied

$$t = \frac{\bar{X}_1 - \bar{X}_2}{SED}$$

Step 9: Degree of freedom is calculated as explained earlier

Step 10: *t* value table is referred

Interpretation:

- If calculated *t*< *t* table value at the particular df at 0.05, i.e. 5% level of significance, then null hypothesis is accepted and that there is no association between exposure and outcome or both the interventions are equal.
- If calculated *t*>*t* table value at the particular df at 0.05, i.e. 5% level of significance, then null hypothesis is rejected and that is association between exposure and outcome or both the interventions are not equal.

Practical Example

Q 4. Among the newly diagnosed patients with impaired glucose tolerance nine were put on lifestyle modifications and 9 were given metformin. Reduction of fasting blood sugar (mg/dl) is given.

With lifestyle modification	With metformin
2	4
3	5
4	6
5	7
6	8
7	9
8	10
9	11
10	12

Answer:

Step 1: Formulation of hypothesis

Null hypothesis (H_0): No difference in efficacy of 2 interventions

Alternate hypothesis (H_1): Difference exists between the 2 interventions

Step 2: Check for the number and nature of variables

If all the conditions mentioned above are satisfied, then we apply the *t* test.

Test of significance to be applied:

o 2 groups

o Unrelated

o Categorical variable [intervention given (yes/no) vs continuous variable (fall in blood sugar in mg/dl)]: Unpaired *t* test

Step 3: Arithmetic mean is calculated for each of the two groups

Group	With lifestyle modification	With metformin
Frequency	2	4
	3	5
	4	6
	5	7
	6	8
	7	9
	8	10
	9	11
	10	12
Total	54	72
N	9	9
Mean	6	8

Step 4: Arithmetic mean is written against each value against the two groups of the table.

With lifestyle modification				With metformin			
X_1	$\bar{X}$ (mean)	$X_1 - \bar{X}$	$(X_1 - \bar{X})^2$	X_2	$\bar{X}$ (mean)	$X_2 - \bar{X}$	$(X_2 - \bar{X})^2$
2	6	−4	16	4	8	−4	16
3	6	−3	9	5	8	−3	9
4	6	−2	4	6	8	−2	4
5	6	−1	1	7	8	−1	1
6	6	0	0	8	8	0	0
7	6	1	1	9	8	1	1
8	6	2	4	10	8	2	4
9	6	3	9	11	8	3	9
10	6	4	16	12	8	4	16
Total			60	Total			60

Step 5: Standard deviation of the two groups are calculated as explained in the earlier half of the chapter

$$SD = \sqrt{\frac{\Sigma (X_1 - \bar{X})^2}{n}}$$

If $n \geq 30$ then in the formula n is taken

If $n < 30$ then in the formula $n - 1$ is taken

SD_1 (with lifestyle intervention) $= \sqrt{(60/8)} = 2.7$

SD_2 (with metformin) $= \sqrt{(60/8)} = 2.7$

Step 6: Summary table is written

Particulars	Group A Without intervention	Group B With intervention
Number (n)	$n_1 = 9$	$n_2 = 9$
Mean ($\bar{X}$)	$\bar{X}_1 = 6$	$\bar{X}_2 = 8$
Standard deviation (SD)	$SD_1 = 2.7$	$SD_2 = 2.7$

Step 7: Standard error of difference (SED) is calculated

$$SED = \sqrt{\frac{SD_1^2}{n_1}} + \sqrt{\frac{SD_2^2}{n_2}}$$

$SED = \sqrt{(2.7)^2/9} + \sqrt{(2.7)^2/9}$

$SED = 0.9 + 0.9 = 1.8$

Step 8: *t* test is applied

$$t = \frac{\bar{X}_1 - \bar{X}_2}{\text{SED}}$$

$$t = \frac{6 - 8}{1.8} = 1.1 \text{ (ignoring the sign)}$$

Step 9: Degree of freedom is calculated as explained earlier
df = $n_1 + n_2 - 2 = 9 + 9 - 2 = 16$

Step 10: *t* value table is referred

Interpretation: Calculated *t*-value is less than the table value. Hence, do not reject H_0. Hence, it can be concluded that the difference is not significant.

EPIDEMIOLOGY

EPIDEMIC CURVES

Theoretical Overview

Common exposure point source	Propagated
• Rapid rise and rapid fall (explosive)	• Slow rise and slow fall (only when Number of susceptible is depleted/ there is no more exposure)
• No secondary wave	• Secondary wave present
• All cases in one incubation period (IP) as there is brief exposure	• More than one IP
• Clustering of cases	• Herd immunity plays an important role in such type of epidemic
• For example, Bhopal gas tragedy, Minamata disease, Chernobyl gas disaster, food poisoning	• For example, hepatitis A, polio

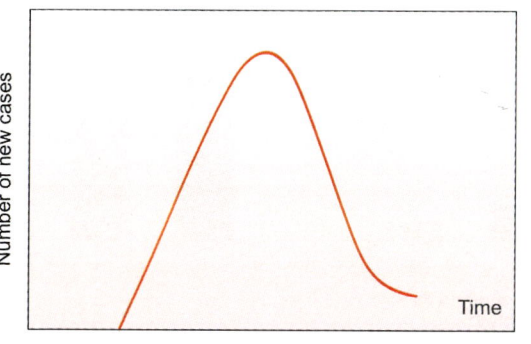

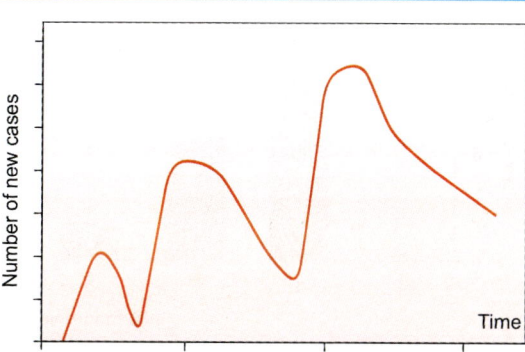

Practical Overview 4

Steps of calculating mortality rates:

1. Plot the number of cases of disease reported during an outbreak on the y-axis
2. Plot the time or date of illness onset on the x-axis
   a. Choice of time unit for x-axis depends upon the incubation period
   b. Begin with a unit approximately one quarter the length of the incubation period
   c. If the incubation period is not known, graph several epi curves with different time units
   d. Usually the day of onset of disease can be used as x-axis variable with date as the unit.
   e. If the incubation period is very short, hour of onset may be more appropriate
   f. If the incubation period is very long, week or month may be more appropriate
3. Epi curves are histograms:
   There should not be any space between the x-axis categories
4. Label each axis
5. Provide a descriptive title
6. Include the pre-epidemic period to show the baseline number of cases

Practical Example

Q 1. There were seven cases of hepatitis A reported in South Extension, New Delhi. Construct the epi curve from the line list below.

Date of onset	Date of diagnosis	Number of cases
Jan 4	Jan 10	10
Jan 5	Jan 12	7
Jan 6	Jan 8	2
Jan 7	Jan 12	2
Jan 8	Jan 16	1
Jan 9	Jan 12	0
Jan 10	Jan 13	17
Jan 11	Jan 20	12

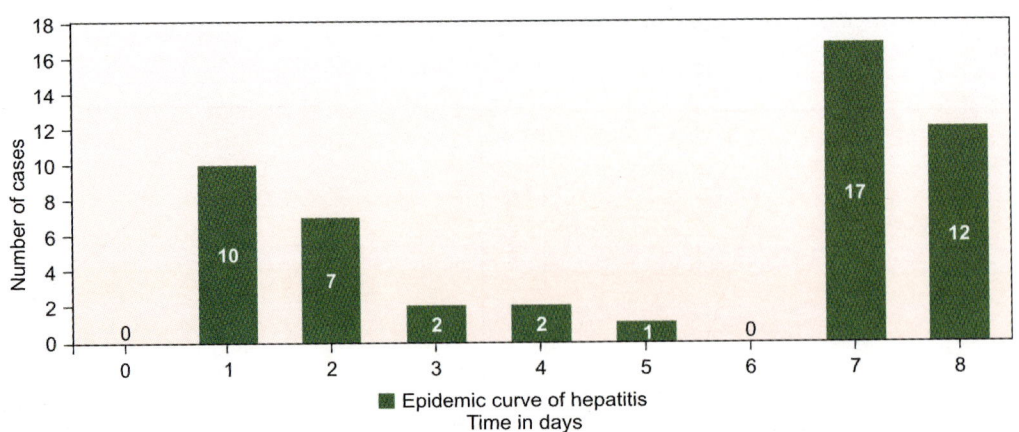

Epidemic curve of hepatitis
Time in days

MEASURING DISEASE FREQUENCY

Theoretical Overview

Mortality indicators	Morbidity indicators
1. Mortality rates	1. Incidence
a. Crude	
b. Specific	
2. Case fatality	2. Prevalence
3. Proportionate mortality	3. Attack rates

Mortality Indicators

Definitions

Crude death rate (CDR): Crude death rate is defined as the total number of deaths in a population residing in a defined geographical area in a given time frame (usually a year) divided by its mid-year population.

$$\text{Crude death rate} = \frac{\text{Total number of deaths in a population in a defined geographical area in a year} \times 1000}{\text{Total mid-year population}}$$

Specific death rate: It is the total number of deaths due to a specific cause/disease/age/sex in a particular geographical area divided by the total mid-year population.

$$\text{Specific death rate due to A} = \frac{\text{Total number of deaths in a population in a defined geographical area in a year due to A} \times 1000}{\text{Total mid-year population}}$$

Case fatality rate (CFR): It represents the killing power of a disease and actually is a proportion.

$$\text{Case fatality rate} = \frac{\text{Total number of deaths due to a particular disease} \times 100}{\text{Total number of cases due to the same disease}}$$

Proportional mortality rate: Deaths due to a specific cause/disease or deaths occurring in specified age/sex/per 100/per 1000 of total deaths.

$$\text{Proportional death rate due to disease A} = \frac{\text{Total number of deaths in an area in a year due to A} \times 1000}{\text{Total number of deaths}}$$

Practical Overview 5

Steps of calculating mortality rates:
1. Read the question carefully and note which indicator is being asked to be calculated.
2. Write separately:
   a. Total number of deaths
   b. Deaths due to specific diseases or deaths occurring in specified age groups/sex
   c. Total number of cases
   d. Total mid-year population
3. Apply the formula

Practical Example

Q 2. Assume that in a population of 1 lakh people, 20 are sick with disease X, and in 1 year 18 of the 20 die. In the same population 40 are sick with disease Y, and in 1 year 30 of the 40 die.
1. What is crude mortality rate/crude death rate (per 1 lakh population)?
2. What is case fatality fraction of disease X?
3. What is oproportionate mortality fraction for disease Y?

Answer:

Step 1:
   1. Crude mortality rate (per 1 lakh population)
   2. Case fatality fraction of disease X
   3. Proportionate mortality fraction for disease Y

Step 2:
   1. Total number of deaths = 48
   2. Total number of specific deaths due to disease = 18 (due to X) + 30 (due to Y) = 48
   3. Total number of cases = 20 (due to X), 40 (due to Y)
   4. Total mid-year population = 1,00,000

Step 3:
   1. CDR = Total number of deaths/mid-year population = 48/100000
   2. CFR = Total number of deaths due to a disease/total number of cases due to the same disease
      a. For disease X, 18/20
      b. For disease Y, 30/40
   3. Proportionate Mortality rate = Total number of deaths due to a disease/Total Number of deaths
      a. For disease X, it is 18/48
      b. For disease Y, it is 30/48

Morbidity Indicators

Definitions:

1. *Incidence:* The number of new cases occurring in a defined population at risk of the disease in a given time period and geographical area.
   a. Cumulative incidence:
      i. When all of the individuals in the population are considered to be at risk for the outcome for the entire time period
      ii. Measure of risk
   b. Incidence density/incidence rate: When different individuals are observed for different lengths of time (denoted by person time), incidence rate/density is calculated. The denominator consists of the sum of the units of time that each individual was at risk and was observed.
2. *Prevalence:* Prevalence denotes that what proportion of the population is affected by the disease at a specified time. It is the total number of cases (both old and new) divided by the population in a given time period in a given geographical area.

$$\text{Prevalence per 1000} = \frac{\text{Number of cases of a disease present in the population at a specified time} \times 1000}{\text{Number of persons in the population at a specified time}}$$

3. *Attack rates:*
   a. Number of people at risk in whom a certain illness develops/total number of people at risk
   b. Proportion (even though named as rate, time not taken into account explicitly as time is too short)
      • Secondary attack rates (SAR): Attack rate in the susceptible contacts of a primary case within one incubation period time.

$$\text{SAR} = \frac{\text{Number of exposed persons developing the disease within the range of the incubation period} \times 100}{\text{Total number of exposed susceptible contacts}}$$

Practical Overview 6

Incidence and Prevalence

Steps of calculating morbidity rates:

1. Read the question carefully and note which indicator is being asked to be calculated.
2. Write separately:
   a. New cases
   b. Total number of cases (new + old)
   c. Population at risk
   d. Time frame
3. Apply the formula

Practical Example

Q 3. In Delhi there are 100 females in an area, out of which 10 developed uterine cancer in 2015. In 2014, already 50 had undergone hysterectomy. What is the incidence of uterine cancer? It is assumed that no hysterectomy was done in 2013 and more in previous years and there were no cases of migration in or out.

Answer

Step 1: Incidence has been asked to be calculated.

Step 2:

1. Total number of new cases = 10
2. Population at risk = 50 (as out of 100 females 50 have undergone hysterectomy so they are no more susceptible for endometrial cancer)

Step 3: Incidence = 10/50

Q 4. Total population of an area = 1,83,000 (all are susceptible). The

- Number of new cases are 26
- Total number of cases = 264

What is incidence and prevalence in 1,00,000 population?

Answer:

1. Incidence:
   a. For a population of 1,83,000 incidence is 26
   b. For a population of 1,00,000 incidence is 14
      i. (26 × 1,00,000)/(1,83,000)
2. Prevalence:
   a. For a population of 1,83,000 prevalence is 264
   b. For a population of 1,00,000 prevalence is 144
      i. (264 × 1,00,000)/(1,83,000)

Practical Overview 7

Attack Rates

Steps of calculating attack rates:

1. Read the question carefully and note which type of attack rate is being asked to be calculated.
2. Write separately:
   a. Number of index cases
   b. Number of susceptible individuals (see for those who are immunized and those who have been diseased after the given incubation period)
   c. Numbers infected
3. Apply the formula

Practical Example

Attack Rates

Q 5. In a village of 100 children, 59% are immunized against measles. Two children travelled outside and returned with measles and infected other 26 children. What is the secondary attack rate (SAR)?

Answer:

Step 1: SAR has been asked to be calculated

Step 2:

1. Number of index cases = 2
2. Number of immunized children = 59
3. Susceptible individuals = 100 – 59 – 2 = 39
4. Cases = 26

Step 3: SAR = 26/39 = 0.67 or 67%

PROBABILITY PROPORTION TO SIZE (PPS) SAMPLING

Theoretical Overview

The sampling frame is the list of ultimate sampling units, which may be people, households, organizations, or other units of analysis. This is usually a list, arranged in any order, which shows all the units from which the sample is to be selected.

Random sampling is a type of sampling in which every person in the population has a known and equal chance of being selected. Random samples are always strongly preferred, as only random samples permit statistical inference.

Probability proportion to size is a sampling procedure under which the probability of a unit being selected is proportional to the size of the ultimate unit (giving larger clusters a greater probability of selection and smaller clusters a lower probability).

In order to ensure that all units (e.g. individuals) in the population have the same probability of being selected irrespective of the size of their cluster, each of the hierarchical levels prior to the ultimate level has to be sampled according to the size of ultimate units it contains, but the same number of units has to be sampled from each cluster at the last hierarchical level.

This method also facilitates planning for field work because a pre-determined number of individuals are interviewed in each unit selected, and staff can be allocated accordingly.

It is most useful when the sampling units vary considerably in size because it assures that those in larger sites have the same probability of getting into the sample as those in smaller sites, and vice versa.

First stage: PPS sampling larger clusters have bigger portability of being sampled

Second stage: Sampling exactly the same number of individuals per cluster.

Overall: Second stage compensates first stage, so that each individual in the population has the same probability of being sampled.

Practical Overview 8

1. List the primary sampling units (column A) and their population sizes (column B). Each cluster has its own *cluster population size (a)*.

2. Calculate the cumulative sum of the population sizes (column C). The *Total population (b)* will be the last figure in column C.

3. Determine the *number of clusters (d)* that will be sampled in each strata randomly.

4. Determine the *Number of Individuals to be sampled from each cluster (c)*. In order to ensure that all individuals in the population have the same probability of selection irrespective of the size of their cluster, the same number of individuals has to be sampled from each cluster.

5. Divide the total population by the number of clusters to be sampled, to get the *sampling interval* (SI).

6. Choose a random number between 1 and the SI. This is the *random start* (RS). The first cluster sampled contains this cumulative population (column D).

7. Calculate the following series: $RS; RS + SI; RS + 2SI; …. RS + (d – 1) \times SI$.

8. The clusters selected are those for which the cumulative population (column C) contains one of the serial numbers calculated in item 7. Depending on the population size of the cluster, it is possible that big clusters will be sampled more than once. Mark the sampled clusters in another column (column D).

9. Calculate for each of the sampled clusters the *probability of each cluster sampled (Prob 1)* (column E).

   Prob 1 $= (a \times d) \div b$

       $a =$ Cluster population

       $b =$ Total population

       $d =$ Number of clusters

10. Calculate for each of the sampled clusters the *probability of each individual being sampled in each cluster (Prob 2)* (column G).

    Prob 2 $= c/a$

        $a =$ Cluster population

        $c =$ Number of individuals to be sampled in each cluster

11. Calculate the overall basic weight of an individual being sampled in the population. The basic weight (BW) is the inverse of the probability of selection.

BW $= 1/(\text{prob } 1 \times \text{prob } 2)$

Check for correct calculation: BW obtained from all the individuals being sampled in the population should be approximately same.

PPS Master Table

A Cluster	B Size (a)	C Cumulative sum	D Clusters sampled	E Probability 1	F Individuals per cluster (c)	G Probability 2	H Overall weight
1							
2							
3							
4							
5							
6							
7							
8							
9							
10		(b)					

Practical Example

Q 6. Population 7,394 in 10 clusters. Sample 300 from 3 clusters using PPS and calculate overall weight.

A Cluster	B Size (a)	C Cumulative sum	D Clusters sampled	E Probability 1	F Individuals per cluster (c)	G Probability 2	H Overall weight
1	1028						
2	555						
3	390						
4	1309						
5	698						
6	907						
7	432						
8	897						
9	677						
10	501						

Answer:

1. List the primary sampling units (column A) and their population sizes (column B). Each cluster has its own *cluster population size (a)*. (Given a prior in the question)
2. Calculate the cumulative sum of the population sizes (column C). The *total population (b)* will be the last figure in Column C.

A Cluster	B Size (a)	C Cumulative sum	D Clusters sampled	E Probability 1	F Individuals per cluster (c)	G Probability 2	H Overall weight
1	1028	1028					
2	555	1583					
3	390	1973					
4	1309	3282					
5	698	3980					
6	907	4887					
7	432	5319					
8	897	6216					
9	677	6893					
10	501	7394					
		7394(b)					

3. Determine the *number of clusters (d)* that will be sampled in each strata randomly. Given a prior in the question = 3
4. Determine the *Number of Individuals to be sampled from each cluster (c)*. In order to ensure that all individuals in the population have the same probability of selection irrespective of the size of their cluster, the same number of individuals has to be sampled from each cluster.
   - Total sample to be selected = 300
   - Number of clusters = 3
   - Number of individuals to be sampled from each cluster (c) = 100
5. Divide the total population by the number of clusters to be sampled, to get the *sampling interval* (SI).

$$SI = 7934/3 = 2465$$

6. Choose a random number between 1 and the SI. This is the *random start* (RS). The first cluster to be sampled contains this cumulative population (column D). Suppose we get number 500.

7. Calculate the following series: $RS; RS + SI; RS + 2SI; .... RS + (d – 1) \times SI$.

$$500, 500 + 2465 = 2965, 2965 + 2465 = 5430$$

8. The clusters selected are those for which the cumulative population (column C) contains one of the serial numbers calculated in item 7. Depending on the population size of the cluster, it is possible that big clusters will be sampled more than once. Mark the sampled clusters in another column (column D).

A Cluster	B Size (a)	C Cumulative sum	D Clusters sampled	E Probability 1	F Individuals per cluster (c)	G Probability 2	H Overall weight
1	1028	1028	500		100		
2	555	1583					
3	390	1973					
4	1309	3282	2965		100		
5	698	3980					
6	907	4887					
7	432	5319					
8	897	6216	5430		100		
9	677	6893					
10	502	7394(b)					
		7394(b)			300		

9. Calculate for each of the sampled clusters the *probability of each cluster being sampled (probability 1)* (Column E).

   Probability 1 = $(a \times d) \div b$

   a = Cluster population, b = Total population, d = Number of clusters

10. Calculate for each of the sampled clusters the *probability of each individual being sampled in each cluster (Probability 2)* (Column G).

    Probability 2 = c/a

    a = Cluster population, c = Number of individuals to be sampled in each cluster

11. Calculate the overall basic weight of an individual being sampled in the population. The basic weight is the inverse of the probability of selection.

    BW = $1/(\text{prob } 1 \times \text{prob } 2)$

A Cluster	B Size (a)	C Cumulative sum	D Clusters sampled	E Probability 1	F Individuals per cluster (c)	G Probability 2	H Overall weight
1	1028	1028	500	41.7%	100	9.7%	24.7
2	555	1583					
3	390	1973					
4	1309	3282	2965	53.1%	100	7.6%	24.7
5	698	3980					
6	907	4887					
7	432	5319					
8	897	6216	5430	36.4%	100	11.2%	24.5
9	677	6893					
10	502	7394					
	7394(b)				300		

Since BW obtained from the entire individual, being sampled in the population should be approximately same (24.7) so the calculation performed is correct.

SAMPLE SIZE CALCULATION IN EPIDEMIOLOGICAL STUDIES

Theoretical Overview

Sample size in descriptive studies:

1. For proportions

$$n = \frac{Z^2 pq}{d^2}$$

where, n = sample size
Z^2 = abscissa of normal curve (1 – desired confidence interval)
p = estimated proportion of an attribute that is present in the population
q = complement of $p = 1 - p$
d = absolute precision

2. For mean

$$n = \frac{Z^2 \sigma^2}{d^2}$$

where, n = sample size
Z^2 = abscissa of normal curve (1 – desired confidence interval)
σ^2 = variance (square of standard deviation) of an attribute in population
d = absolute precision

Practical Example

Q 7. Calculate sample size for a descriptive study to find the prevalence of anaemia in school children 5 to 15 years for a 95% power with 5% precision. Earlier studies have indicated that prevalence is approximately 40%. In addition, if the non-response rate is 10%, then what is the final sample size?

Answer:

For proportions

$$n = \frac{Z^2 pq}{d^2}$$

where, n = sample size

Z^2 = abscissa of normal curve (1 – desired confidence interval)

As CI is 95%, so Z^2 is 4

p = estimated proportion of an attribute that is present in the population = 0.4

q = complement of p = $1 - p$ = 0.6

d = absolute precision = 0.05

$$n = \frac{4 \times 0.4 \times 0.6}{0.05 \times 0.05} = 384$$

If there is 10% nonresponse rate, then the final sample size will be

0.9 n = 384

Final n = 426.66 (approximately 427)

- Common error done by students in this step

n = 384

1.1 n = 422.4 (approximately 423)

Second approach is wrong as if you back calculate with second approach, then you will attain a sample size of 380.

Practical Example

Q 8. Suppose we require a 95% confidence interval for the mean of a continuous variable with a standard deviation of 15 to be no wider than 10 (i.e. $d = 5\%$).

Answer:

For mean

$$n = \frac{Z^2 \sigma^2}{d^2} = \frac{4 \times 15 \times 15}{5 \times 5} = 36$$

where, n = sample size

Z^2 = abscissa of normal curve (1 – desired confidence interval)

σ^2 = variance (square of standard deviation) of an attribute in population

d = absolute precision

Inference: In order to estimate the mean of a continuous variable (SD = 15) with 95% confidence interval no wider than 10, 36 participants would be required.

MEASURES OF ASSOCIATION

Theoretical Overview

1. **Absolute risk**
   a. Incidence of a disease in a population
   b. Indicates the magnitude of risk in a group of people with certain exposure
   c. **Does not indicate** whether exposure is associated with an increased risk of disease as it **does not involve comparison**
2. **Relative risk**

		Then follow to see whether			
		Disease develops	Disease does not develop	Total	Incidence rates of disease
First select	Exposed	a	b	$a + b$	$a/a + b$
	Not exposed	c	d	$c + d$	$c/c + d$
	$a/(a + b)$ = incidence in exposed		$c/(c + d)$ = incidence in nonexposed		

$$\text{Relative risk} = \frac{\text{Incidence of disease in exposed}}{\text{Incidence of disease in nonexposed}} = a/(a + b)$$

RR	Association	Relationship
1	No	$I\,(E) = I\,(NE)$
> 1	+	$I\,(E) > I\,(NE)$
<1	−	$I\,(E) <I\,(NE)$

3. **Attributable risk**
   Suggests:
   a. In exposed persons, how much of the total of disease is actually due to exposure.
   b. How much risk (or incidence) of disease can be prevented if exposure to the agent is eliminated
   c. Indicate the potential for prevention
   d. Important in clinical practice and public health
4. **Population attributable risk**
   It is incidence of disease in total population minus incidence of disease in nonexposed group.
   Incidence in total population = (Incidence in exposed group) (Percent of population exposed) + (Incidence in nonexposed group) (Percent of population nonexposed)

5. Proportion attributable risk
a. In proportion denominator is present
b. Incidence among exposed group serves as denominator
c. Numerator is attributable risk

Proportion population attributable risk
Proportion of disease in total population that can be attributed to exposure

6. Odds ratio (OR)
Odds = Probability that the event will occur/probability that the event will not occur

$$= P/1 - P$$

A. Unmatched odds ratio $= \dfrac{\text{Odds of being exposed among diseased}}{\text{Odds of being exposed among nondiseased}}$

$$OR = \frac{\text{Probability of exposure among diseased/probability of no exposure among diseased}}{\text{Probability of exposure among nondiseased/probability of no exposure among nondiseased}}$$

$$= \frac{(a/a + c)/(c/a + c)}{(b/b + d)/(d/b + d)} = ad/bc$$

Category	Cases	Controls
Exposed	a	b
Not exposed	c	d

B. Matched odds ratio:
- If exposure is dichotomous (a person is either exposed or not exposed), only the following 4 types of case control pairs are possible:
  - Concordant pairs
    1. Pairs in which both case and the control were exposed
    2. Pairs in which neither the case nor the control was exposed
  - Discordant pairs
    3. Pairs in which the case was exposed but the control was not
    4. Pairs in which the control was exposed and the case was not

Case	Control	
	Exposed	**Not exposed**
Exposed	a	b
Not exposed	c	d

Practical Overview 9

Common Steps in Calculation of Measures of Association:
Step 1: Read the question carefully to see which measure of association is asked to be calculated. Also try to frame the study design in mind.
Step 2: Make the 2 by 2 table as per the study design and label the cells.
Step 3: Assign values provided in the question to the cells.
Step 4: Use the formulae to derive the required results.

Practical Example

Q 9. A study is undertaken to determine if prenatal exposure to marijuana is associated with LBW in infants. Mothers of 50 infants weighing >2.5 kg and <2.5 kg each are questioned about their marijuana use during pregnancy. Study finds that 20 mothers of LBW infants and 2 mothers of normal birth weight infants used the drug during pregnancy. What is the OR?

Answer:

	Cases	Controls
Exposed	20	2
Nonexposed	30	48
Total	50	50

$$OR = \frac{20 \times 48}{2 \times 30} = 16$$

Interpretation: This means that an infant of LBW was 16 times as likely as an infant of normal birth weight to have had a mother who used marijuana during pregnancy.

Q 10. A study was done in New Delhi and Shimla to see effect of pollution on development of COPD at age of 50 years. Children born in the year 2016 were made into the birth cohort of 2016 and birth cohorts were compared of Delhi and Shilmla in the year 2066. There were initially 1000 children each in the 2 groups. 50 in Delhi had COPD and 5 in Shimla had COPD in 2066. Assuming that none were smokers during their lifetime and all stayed in their respective places without any migration or travel. Calculate the RR for COPD taking pollution as the exposure.

Answer:

		Then follow to see whether			
		Disease develops	Disease does not develop	Totals	Incidence rates of disease
First select	Exposed	50	950	1000	$a/a + b$ (50/1000)
	Not exposed	5	995	1000	$c/c + d$ (5/1000)
	$a/(a + c)$ = incidence of exposed (50/55)			$c/(b + d)$ = incidence of nonexposed (950/1945)	

$$\text{Relative risk} = \frac{\text{Incidence of disease among exposed}}{\text{Incidence of disease among nonexposed}} = \frac{a/(a+b)}{c/(c+d)}$$

$$= \frac{50/1000}{5/1000} = 10$$

KAPPA STATISTIC

Theoretical Overview

Kappa statistic is how much better the level of agreement is between two observers than that which results just from chance.

Steps	Components	Components (details)	Steps
1	Numerator	How much better is the observed agreement than the agreement expected by chance alone?	(% agreement observed) – (% agreement expected by chance alone)
2	Denominator	What is the maximum the observers could have improved upon the agreement expected by chance alone?	100% – (% agreement expected by chance alone)
3	Kappa statistic	Of the maximum improvement in agreement expected beyond chance alone that could have occurred, what proportion has in fact occurred?	

$$\text{Kappa statistic} = \frac{(\text{\% agreement observed}) - (\text{\% agreement expected by chance alone})}{100\% - (\text{\% agreement expected by chance alone})}$$

Interpretation

Value of kappa	Strength of agreement
<0.20	Poor
0.21–0.40	Fair
0.41–0.60	Moderate
0.61–0.80	Good
0.81–1.00	Very Good

Practical Overview 10

Step 1: Calculate the percentages of each row and column out of the grand total of all the four cells

Grading by observer 2	Pancreatic cancer	Grading by observer 1		
		Yes	No	Total
	Yes	A	B	A + B
	No	C	D	C + D
	Total	A + C	B + D	A + B + C + D

Step 2: Calculate percentage observed agreement = $\dfrac{(A + D)}{(A + B + C + D)} \times 100$

Step 3: Calculation of % percentage expected by chance alone

Kappa statistic = $\dfrac{(\% \text{ agreement observed}) - (\% \text{ agreement expected by chance alone})}{100\% - (\% \text{ agreement expected by chance alone})}$

Practical Example

Q 11. 100 patients suffering from pancreatic carcinoma underwent CECT abdomen. Two radiologists reviewed the reports. Calculate the kappa.

Grading by radiologist 2	Pancreatic cancer	Grading by radiologist 1		
		Yes	No	Total
	Yes	40	5	45
	No	15	40	55
	Total	55	45	100

Answer:

Step 1: Calculate the percentages of each row and column out of the grand total of all the four cells.

Grading by radiologist 2	Pancreatic cancer	Grading by radiologist 1		
		Yes	No	Total
	Yes	40	5	45 (45%)
	No	15	40	55 (55%)
	Total	55 (55%)	45 (45%)	100

Step 2: Calculate percentage observed agreement = $\dfrac{(A + D)}{(A + B + C + D)} \times 100$

$$= \dfrac{40 + 40}{100} \times 100 = 80\%$$

Step 3: Calculation of percent agreement expected by chance alone

Radiologist 1 has labelled 55% of all CECT abdomen as positive and 45% as negative, whereas Radiologist 2 has labelled 45% as positive and 55% as negative.

Suppose Radiologist 1 would have read the CECT as Radiologist 2 would have read, we would expect that radiologist 1 would read disease present as 55% of all CECT labelled positive by radiologist 2 and also 55% of all CECT labelled negative by radiologist 2.

Therefore, for radiologist 1 we expect that 55% of 45 (24.75) and 45% of 55 (24.75) as positive and negative respectively.

$$\text{Agreement expected by chance alone} = \frac{24.75 + 24.75}{100} \times 100 = 49.5$$

$$\text{Kappa statistic} = \frac{(\% \text{ agreement observed}) - (\% \text{ agreement expected by chance alone})}{100\% - (\% \text{ agreement expected by chance alone})}$$

$$= \frac{80 - 49.5}{100 - 49.5} = \frac{30.5}{50.5} = 0.6$$

SURVIVAL ANALYSIS

Purpose: For the analysis of cohort data, when the interest is not in calculating the rate at which event occurs, rather it is time to occurrence of event and survival.

Uses
1. To look at natural history of disease
2. To evaluate new interventions by comparing survival in two groups

Examples: For calculating
1. Time to death after treatment of lung cancer.
2. Time to development of signs of disease after exposure.

Important Terms

Event: Death, conception, or recovery from a disease or second CHD event after first CHD event

Survival time: Time from a predetermined start point, (e.g. entry into a study, date of diagnosis, or date of birth) until the occurrence of event of interest.

Censoring: It is required for the observations in which total survival time Cannot be ascertained. This can happen in situations like participants lost to the follow-up, died during the follow-up time for some other cause, not experiencing the event during the follow-up duration.

Methods for survival analysis: Life table method and Kaplan-Meier curve.

Life table methods: Split the follow-up duration into intervals, and then calculate survival probability within each interval. Survival curve plotted with this method is a smooth one.

Steps for life table method

1. Plot a table in the pattern as shown (divide the **total follow up** in **intervals,** and at the end of each pre-specified intervals duration estimate the number at risk at the start of each interval, number of participants died and number of participants censored)
2. For each interval
   a. Calculate the probability of death
      Probability of death = number of deaths/(number at risk – 0.5 × number censored)
   b. Calculate the survival probability
      Survival probability = 1 – probability of death
   c. Cumulative survival at the end of each interval
      = Survival probability for 2nd year × survival probability for 1st year
      = $(1 - P_2)(1 - P_1)$
3. Follow the steps for number of years specified in question or years of interest.

Interval	Time band	Number at risk	Number of death	Number censored	Probability of death	Probability of survival	Cumulative survival
1	0, 1 year	a	b	c	$P_1 = b/(a - 0.5 \times c)$	$1 - P_1$	$1 - P_1$
2	1, 2 year	d	e	f	$P_2 = d/(e - 0.5 \times f)$	$1 - P_2$	$(1 - P_1) \times (1 - P_2)$

Example

Q 12. A cohort study enrolled 38 patients with coronary heart disease to see the occurrence of fatal episode of CHD and survival after first episode of CHD. These 38 patients have been followed up to see the survival. The following table is showing the number of participants at the beginning of each year, number of events, and number censored during the one-year duration. Calculate the cumulative survival at the end of 5 years through the life table method.

Interval	Time band	Number at risk	Number of death	Number censored	Probability of death	Probability of survival	Cumulative survival
1	0,1	38	1	0	A	B	C
2	1,2	37	1	0	D	E	F
3	2,3	36	0	3	G	H	I
4	3,4	33	1	0	J	K	L
5	4,5	32	1	0	M	N	O

Solution:

Step 1: For the life table method, the entire follow-up duration is divided into one year intervals, and number at risk, number died and number censored for each interval is plotted in table (it is already given in the table)

Step 2: For each interval

For interval 1

Probability of death in the interval 1(*A*)

= number of deaths/(number at risk − 0.5 × number censored)

= 1/38 − 0.5 × 0 = 0.026316

Probability of survival in the interval 1 (*B*)

= 1 − probability of death

= 1 − 0.026316 = 0.973684

Cumulative survival for surviving 1st year (*C*) = 0.973684

For interval 2

Probability of death in the interval 2 (*D*) = 1/37 − 0.5 × 0 = 0.027027

Probability of survival in the interval 2 (*E*) = 1 − 0.027027 = 0.972973

Cumulative survival for surviving 2 years (*F*), i.e. probability of surviving 2nd year × probability of surviving 1st year = Cell *E* × Cell *C* = 0.972973 × 0.973684 = 0.947368

For interval 3

Probability of death in the interval 3 (*G*) = 0/36 − 0.5 × 3 = 0

Probability of survival in the interval 3 (*H*) = 1 − 0 = 1

Cumulative survival for surviving 3 years (*I*), i.e. probability of surviving 3rd year × probability of surviving first 2 years = Cell *H* × Cell *F* = 1 × 0.947368 = 0.947368

For interval 4

Probability of death in the interval 4 (*J*) = 1/33 − 0.5 × 0 = 0.030303

Probability of survival in the interval 4 (*K*) = 1 − 0.030303 = 0.969697

Cumulative survival for surviving 4 years (*L*), i.e. probability of surviving 4th year × probability of surviving first 3 years = Cell *K* × Cell *I* = 0.969697 × 0.947368 = 0.9186599

For interval 5

Probability of death in the interval 5 (*M*) = 1/32 − 0.5 × 0 = 0.03125

Probability of survival in the interval 5 (*N*) = 1 − 0.03125 = 0.96875

Cumulative survival for surviving 5 years (O), i.e. probability of surviving 5th year × probability of surviving first 4 years = Cell *N* × Cell *L* = 0.96875 × 0.9186599 = 0.88995178

Interval	Time band	Number at risk	Number of death	Number censored	Probability of death	Probability of survival	Cumulative survival
1	0,1	38	1	0	0.026316*A*	0.973684*B*	0.973684*C*
2	1,2	37	1	0	0.027027*D*	0.972973*E*	0.947368*F*
3	2,3	36	0	3	0*G*	1*H*	0.947368*I*
4	3,4	33	1	0	0.030303 *J*	0.969697 *K*	0.9186599 *L*
5	4,5	32	1	0	0.03125 *M*	0.96875 *N*	0.88995178 *O*

Thus, cumulative survival (using the life table method) at the end of 5 years is 0.88995178

Kaplan-Meier method: In this method, cumulative survival probability is estimated after each individual's death or after every event. For calculating survival by this method, essential prerequisite is knowledge of exact date of death and censoring.

The difference from the life table method: Probability of death and survival is not calculated at a pre-specified interval, rather it is calculated at the point of occurrence of event.

Steps for Kaplan-Meier Analysis

1. For the Kaplan-Meier analysis, first plot the table in the format as given in the following table

S. No.	Follow-up duration (in months)	Number at risk	Number of death	Number censored	Probability of death	Probability of survival	Cumulative survival
1.	5	40	1	0	P_1	$1 - P_1$	$1 - P_1$
2.	12	39	0	1	P_2	$1 - P_2$	$(1 - P_1) \times (1 - P_2)$

The above table is showing two events, first event in the form of death and second censored observation at 12 months. At 5 months, 40 participants are at risk, one has died, and no censored observation. At 12 months, no death and one censored observation. Thus, follow-up data is divided into two intervals—the 1st interval is from the time of start to 5 months, and the 2nd interval is from 5 months till 12 months.

2. Now calculate the following probabilities at 5 months and at 12 months duration
   a. Calculate the probability of death
      Probability of death = number of deaths/(number at risk − 0.5 × number censored)
   b. Calculate the survival probability
      Survival probability = 1 − probability of death
   c. Cumulative survival at 5 months = $1 - P_1$
      Cumulative survival at 12 months = $(1 - P_2) \times (1 - P_1)$

3. Follow the steps for the follow up duration of the study at the time of occurrence of event.

Example

Q 13. A cohort study enrolled 38 patients with coronary heart disease to see the occurrence of fatal episode of CHD and survival after 1st episode of CHD. These 38 patients have been followed up to see the survival. The following table is showing the number of participants at risk, number of events, and number censored at the time of occurrence of event. Calculate the cumulative survival at the end of 5 years using Kaplan-Meier method?

S. No.	Follow-up duration (in months)	Number at risk	Number of death	Number censored	Probability of death	Probability of survival	Cumulative survival
1.	5	38	1	0	A	B	C
2.	12	37	1	0	D	E	F
3.	30	36	0	3	G	H	I
4.	42	33	1	0	J	K	L
5.	54	32	1	0	M	N	O

Step 1: For Kaplan-Meier analysis, plot the table at the point of occurrence of each event and censored observations (as given in the Table). In this, total follow-up duration is divided into five intervals. First interval is from the start time till the occurrence of first event at 5 months; second interval from 5 months to 12 months; third interval is from 12 months to 30 months; fourth interval from 30 months to 42 months; fifth interval from 42 months to 54 months.

Step 2: For each interval

For interval 1

Probability of death at 5 months (A)

= number of deaths/(number at risk − 0.5 × number censored)

= $1/(38 − 0.5 × 0) = 0.026316$

Probability of survival for the duration of 5 months (B)

= 1 − Probability of death

= $1 − 0.026316 = 0.973684$

Cumulative survival for surviving 1st five months (C) = 0.973684

For interval 2

Probability of death in the interval 2 (D) = $1/(37 − 0.5 × 0) = 0.027027$

Probability of survival in the interval 2 (E) = $1 − 0.027027 = 0.972973$

Cumulative survival for surviving till 12 months (F), i.e. probability of surviving 2nd interval × probability of surviving 1st interval = Cell E × Cell C = 0.972973 × 0.973684 = 0.947368

For interval 3

Probability of death in the interval 3 (G) = $0/(36 − 0.5 × 3) = 0$

Probability of survival in the interval 3 (H) = $1 − 0 = 1$

Cumulative survival for surviving till 30 months (I), i.e. probability of surviving 3rd interval × probability of surviving till 2nd interval = Cell H × Cell F = 1 × 0.947368 = 0.947368

For interval 4

Probability of death in the interval 4 (J) = $1/(33 − 0.5 × 0) = 0.030303$

Probability of survival in the interval 4 (K) = $1 − 0.029412 = 0.969697$

Cumulative survival for surviving till 42 months (*L*), i.e. Probability of surviving 4th interval × probability of surviving till 3rd interval = Cell *K* × Cell *I* = 0.96967 × 0.947368 = 0.9186599

For interval 5

Probability of death in the interval 5 (*M*) = 1/(32 – 0.5 × 0) = 0.03125

Probability of survival in the interval 5 (*N*) = 1 – 0.03125 = 0.96875

Cumulative survival for surviving till 54 months (*O*), i.e. probability of surviving 5th interval × Probability of surviving till 4th interval = Cell *N* × Cell *L* = 0.96875 × 0.9186599 = 0.88995178

Thus, cumulative survival (using Kaplan-Meier method) at the end of 54 months is 0.891641.

Important

Using the life table method, the cumulative survival curve is calculated at predefined intervals, and graph is plotted at specific intervals. Thus, the cumulative survival curve follows a continuous decline in the survival probability, there is no sharp decline.

While in Kaplan-Meier method, survival probability suddenly drops at the time of the event. There is no continuous decline, rather a staircase pattern.

SENSITIVITY, SPECIFICITY AND PREDICTIVE VALUES

Theoretical Overview

A. Definitions:
1. **Sensitivity/Usefulness:** Ability of the test to identify correctly those **who have** the disease/TP (true positives)
2. **Specificity:** Ability of the test to identify correctly those **who do not have** the disease/TN (true negatives)
3. **PPV/positive predictive value:** If the test results are positive in this patient, **what is the probability that this patient has the disease,** or in other words, what proportion of patients who test positive actually have the disease in the question.
4. **NPV/negative predictive value:** If the test results are negative in this patient, **what is the probability that this patient does not have the disease.**

		Disease present by gold standard test	
		Yes	**No**
Test results	Positive	a [True positive (TP)]	b [False positive (FP)]
	Negative	c [False negative (FN)]	d [True negative (TN)]

B. Some key concepts:
1. Sensitivity more:
   a. TP more, FN less
   b. Specificity is less
2. Specificity more:
   a. TN more, FP less
   b. Sensitivity is less

3. Sensitivity is inversely proportional to specificity
4. As prevalence increases, PPV increases, NPV decreases, sensitivity and specificity are not affected
5. As specificity and sensitivity increase, PPV increases but more increase occurs when specificity increases as compared to sensitivity
6. PPV is also called post-test probability of a disease/precision rate
   a. Pre-test probability is equivalent to prevalence
   b. Most of the gain in predictive value occurs with increase in prevalence at the lowest rates of disease prevalence
   c. PV is affected maximum by prevalence as compared to sensitivity and specificity
   d. Public health significance: Screening programme is most productive and efficient if it is used for a high risk target population

Practical Overview 11

1. Sensitivity = *TP/(TP + FN)*
2. Specificity = *TN/(TN + FP)*
3. PPV = *TP/(TP + FP)*
4. NPV = *TN/(TN + FN)*

Steps of calculating specificity, sensitivity, PPV, NPV:
1. Read the question carefully
2. Make a 2 × 2 table
   a. Gold standard by convention is written on the top
   b. Test result is written on the left-hand side
3. Label the boxes as *TP, FN, FP, TN*
4. Assign values given in the question
5. Use formulae given above to calculate the values

Practical Example

Q 14. In a test of 150 people for HIV, western blot found that 50 people are suffering from HIV and 100 were not suffering from HIV. Out of this 50, 30 had positive results with ICT kit and only 70 were found to be negative as per the kit from the 100 labelled as negative from the western blot. What is the sensitivity, specificity, PPV and NPV?

1. Step one is to read the question carefully
2. **Make a 2 × 2 table:**
   a. **Gold standard by convention is written on the top**
   b. **Test result is written on the left-hand side**

		Gold standard test		
		Positive	**Negative**	**Total**
Screening test	Positive			
	Negative			
	Total			

3. **Label the boxes as** *TP, FN, FP, TN*

		Gold standard test		Total
		Positive	**Negative**	**Total**
Screening test	Positive	*TP*	*FP*	
	Negative	*FN*	*TN*	
	Total			

4. **Assign values given in the question**

		Gold standard test		Total
		Positive	**Negative**	**Total**
Screening test	Positive	30 (*TP*)	30 (*FP*)	60
	Negative	20 (*FN*)	70 (*TN*)	90
	Total	50	100	150

5. **Use formulae given above to calculate the values**
   a. Sensitivity = *TP/TP + FN* = 30/50
   b. Specificity = *TN/TN + FP* = 70/100
   c. PPV = *TP/TP + FP* = 30/60
   d. NPV = *TN/TN + FN* = 70/90

Theoretical overview	
Screening tests in series	**Screening tests in parallel**
• One after the other (2nd screening test is applied only on those individuals tested positive on the 1st)	• Simultaneously all the tests are applied
• Sensitivity decreases	• Sensitivity increases
• Specificity increases	• Specificity decreases
• PPV increases	• PPV decreases
• NPV decreases	• NPV increases
• Combined sensitivity = Sn (*A*) × Sn (*B*)	• Combined sensitivity = Sn (*A*) + Sn (*B*) − [Sn (*A*) × Sn (*B*)]
• Combined specificity = Sp (*A*) + Sp (*B*) − [Sp (*A*) × Sp (*B*)]	• Combined specificity = Sp (*A*) × Sp (*B*)

LIKELIHOOD RATIOS

1. Includes both sensitivity and specificity
2. LR$^+$
   a. How much odds of disease increase when test is positive

   b. $\dfrac{\text{Sensitivity}}{(1 - \text{specificity})}$

3. LR$^-$
   a. How much odds of disease decrease when test is negative

   b. $\dfrac{(1 - \text{sensitivity})}{\text{Specificity}}$

4. Post-test odds:
   a. Chances that patient has the disease
   b. Odds (post) = Odds (pre) × likelihood ratios

Presentation of Data

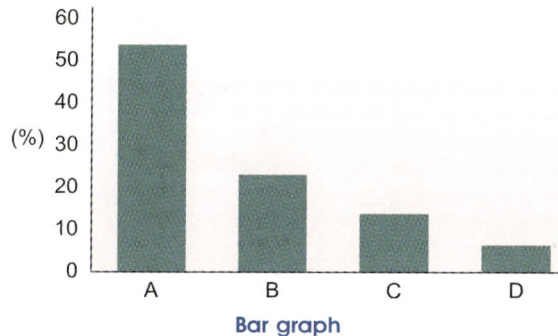

Bar graph

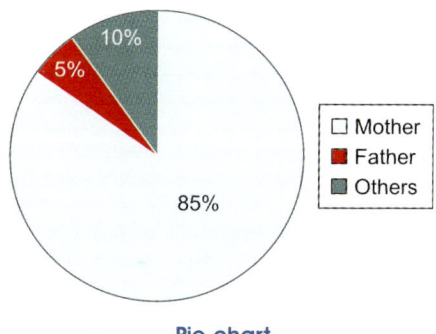

Pie chart

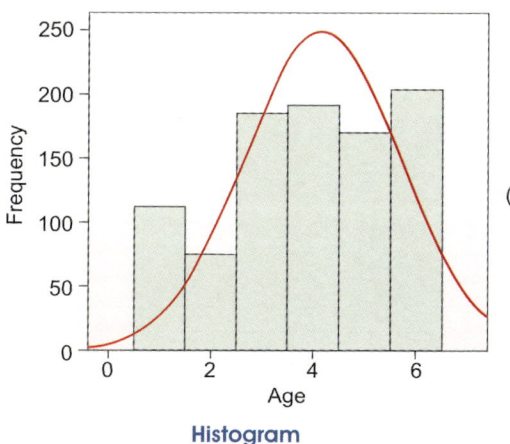

Histogram

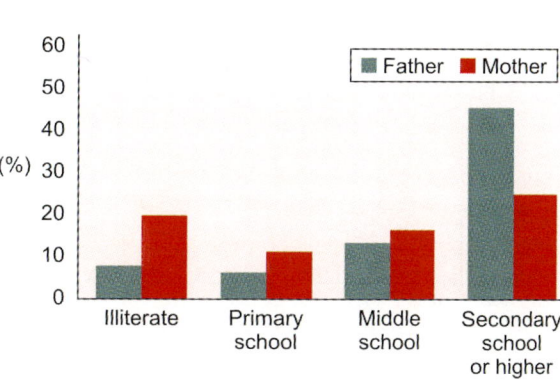

Compound bar graph

Stem and Leaf Diagram

Frequency	Stem and Leaf
51.00	1. OOOOOOOOOOOOOOOOOOOOOOOOOOOOOOOOOOOOOOOOOOOOOOOOOOO
30.00	2. OOOOOOOOOOOOOOOOOOOOOOOOOOOOOO
89.00	3. OOOOOOOOOOOOOOOOOOOOOOOOOOOOOOOOOOOOOOOOOOOOOOOOOOOOOOOOOOOOOOOOOOOOOOOOOOOOOOOOOOOOOOOOOOO
84.00	4. OOOOOOOOOOOOOOOOOOOOOOOOOOOOOOOOOOOOOOOOOOOOOOOOOOOOOOOOOOOOOOOOOOOOOOOOOOOOOOOOOOOOOO
76.00	5. OOOOOOOOOOOOOOOOOOOOOOOOOOOOOOOOOOOOOOOOOOOOOOOOOOOOOOOOOOOOOOOOOOOOOOOOOOOOOO
78.00	6. OOOOOOOOOOOOOOOOOOOOOOOOOOOOOOOOOOOOOOOOOOOOOOOOOOOOOOOOOOOOOOOOOOOOOOOOOOOOOOOO

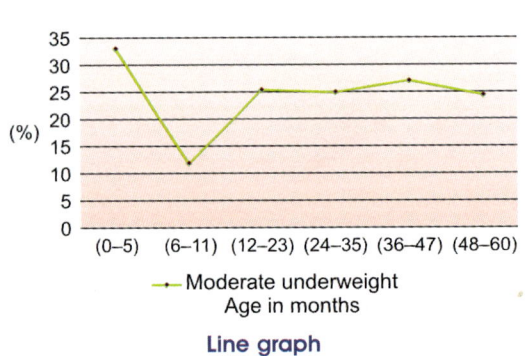

Line graph

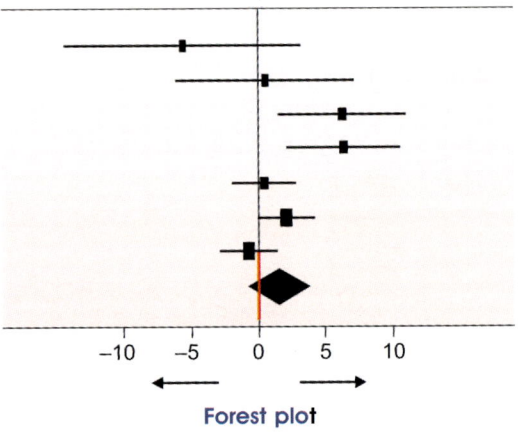

Forest plot

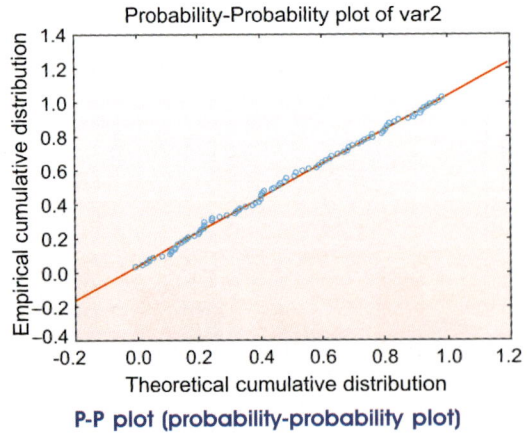

P-P plot (probability-probability plot)

Source: https://en.wikipedia.org

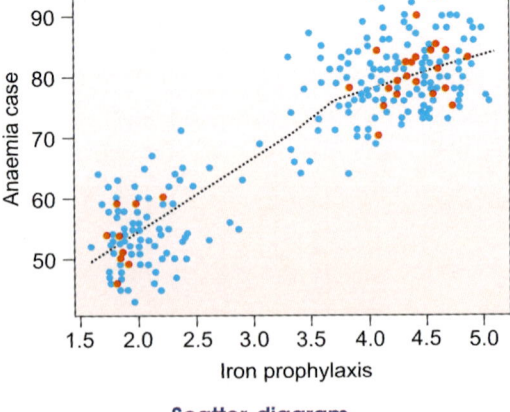

Scatter diagram

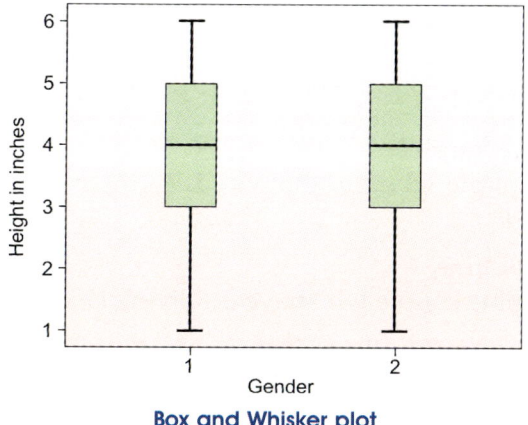

Box and Whisker plot

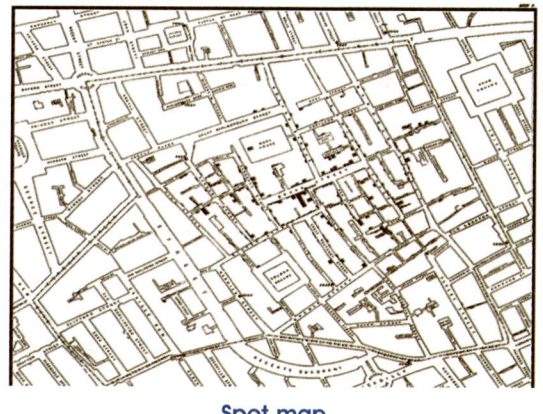

Kaplan-Meier curve

Spot map

Source: https://en.wikipedia.org

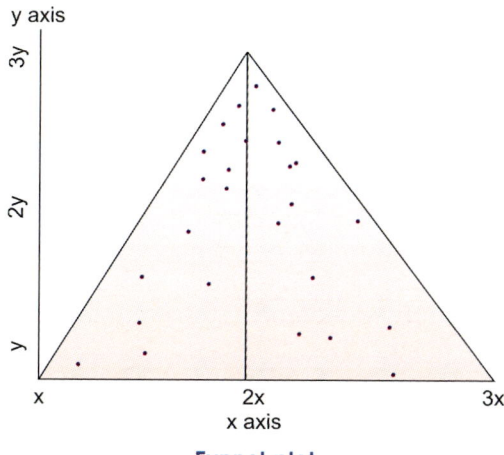

Funnel plot

Source: https://en.wikipedia.org

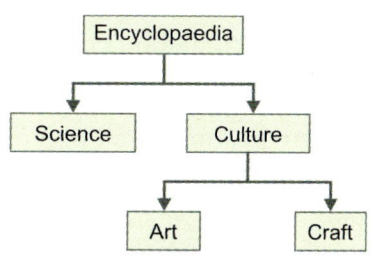

Tree diagram

Source: https://en.wikipedia.org

Others

FAMILY WELFARE

Q 1. What is an eligible couple?

A currently married couple wherein the wife is in the reproductive age, i.e. 15 to 49 years (15 to 45 years).

Q 2. What is a target couple?

Target couple is an eligible couple who have 2–3 living children.

Q 3. What is unmet need for family planning?

It is defined as the percent of women of reproductive age, married or in a union, those who want to stop or delay childbearing but are not using any method of contraception.

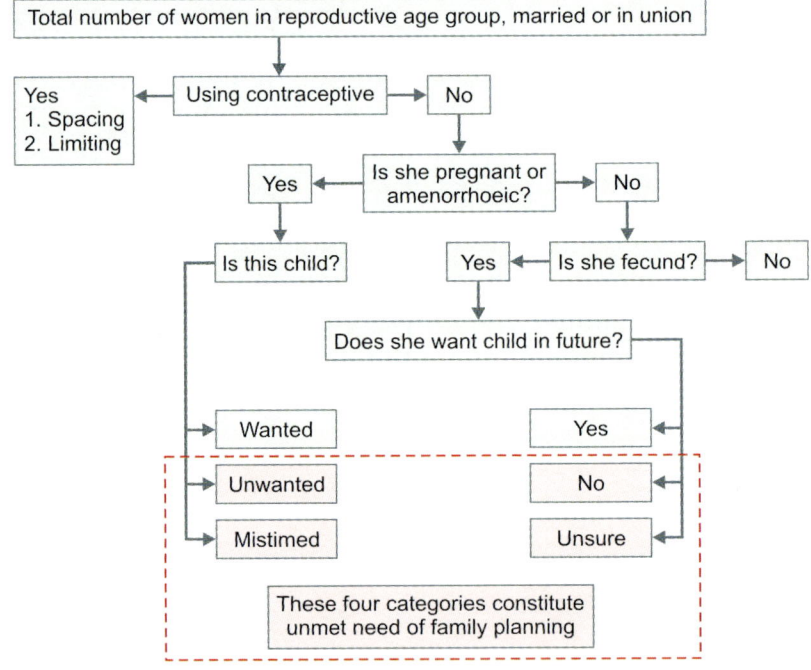

Example:

A village has a population of 800 of women of reproductive age, either married or in a union. Nonusers of contraception were 600. The total number of women who are not pregnant and menorrhoeic were 500. Hundred women do not want a child in future and 120 were unsure. Of all pregnancy, five were unwanted and 110 were mistimed. What is unmet need for family Planning of this village?

Solution:

Total number of women in reproductive age, either married or in a union = 800
Percent of women not pregnant and menorrhoeic who do not want child in future [A]
= (100/800) × 100 = 12.5%

Percent of women not pregnant and menorrhoeic who unsure whether she wants child in future [B] = (120/800) × 100 = 15%

Percent of unwanted pregnancy [C] = (5/800) × 100 = 0.6%

Percent of mistimed pregnancy [D] = (110/800) × 100 = 13.7%

Total unmet need [A + B + C + D] = 12.5% + 15% + 0.6% + 13.7% = 41.8%

Percent of women using contraception = (200/800) × 100 = 25%

Total demand for family planning = 41.8% + 25% = 66.8%

Q 4. What is contraceptive prevalence rate?
Contraceptive prevalence is the percentage of women who are currently using, or whose sexual partner is currently using, at least one method of contraception. It is usually reported for married or in-union women aged 15 to 49.

Contraceptive prevalence rate = [Number of women (aged 15–49) using a contraceptive method/total number of women (aged 15–49)] × 100

Example:
A village has a total population of 5000, 1800 women are in reproductive age. Users of contraception were 300. 800 women were either married or in a union. What is contraceptive prevalence rate?

Solution:
Total number of women aged 15–49 using a contraceptive method = 300

Total number of women 15–49 age group = 1800

Contraceptive prevalence rate = (300/1800) × 100 = 16.7%

Contraceptive prevalence rate of currently married or in union = (300/800) × 100 = 37.5%

Q 5. What is couple protection rate?
The estimated protection to women in the age group of 15–49 years, from pregnancy or childbirth, provided by family planning services during a one year period, based upon the contraceptives use during that period.

Q 6. What is Pearl index?
It is an index to measure the effectiveness of a contraceptive method. The number of unintentional pregnancies related to 100 women years measures it.

Pearl index = (Number of on contraceptive pregnancies/number of 28-day usable cycle) × 1300

For example, if 100 women use contraceptive for 1 year each and if three pregnancies occur during this one year in this group, the Pearl index will be 3.0.

Q 7. What are the measures of fertility?
  a. **Crude birth rate (CBR):** Annual number of live births per 1000 mid-year population
  b. **General fertility rate (GFR):** Annual number of live births per 1000 women of child bearing age (15–49 years old, or 15–44 years old) mid-year population

c. **General marital fertility rate (GMFR):** Annual number of live births per 1000 married women of childbearing age (15–49 years old, or 15–44 years old) mid-year population

d. **Age-specific fertility rates (ASFR):** Annual number of live births per 1000 women in particular age groups (usually age 15–19 years, 20–24 years, etc.)

e. **Gross reproduction rate (GRR):** Number of daughters who would be born to a woman completing her reproductive life at current ASFRs

f. **Net reproduction rate (NRR):** Expected number of daughters, per newborn prospective mother, who may or may not survive to and through the ages of childbearing

g. **Total fertility rate (TFR):** Number of live births per woman completing her reproductive life, if her childbearing at each age reflected current ASFRs

Q 8. What is vital statistics?

Vital statistics are conventionally numerical records of marriage, birth, sickness, and death by which the health and growth of the community can be studied.

Q 9. What are the measurements of mortality?

a. **Infant mortality rate** = (Number of deaths under 1 year of age in a year/number of live births in a year) × 1000

b. **Neonatal mortality rate** = (Death under 28 days of birth in a year/number of live births in the same year) × 1000

c. **Post-neonatal mortality rate** = (Total no. of deaths between 28 days and 1 year of age/number of live births in the year) × 1000

d. **Maternal mortality ratio** = (Number of death of females due to complications of pregnancy, childbirth or within 42 days of delivery from puerperal causes in a year/total number of live births in a year) × 1000

e. **Maternal mortality rate:** The number of maternal deaths to women in the ages 15–49 years per lakh of women in that age group.

f. **Lifetime risk:** The probability that one woman of reproductive age (15–49 years) will die due to childbirth or puerperium assuming that chance of death is uniformly distributed across the entire reproductive span.

Example:

The mid-year population of a city was 4,00,000. In the same year the number of live births was 12,000; number of deaths 6,400 and number of infant deaths 1500. Calculate the crude birth rate, crude death rate, and infant mortality rate.

Solution:

Crude birth rate (CBR) = (12,000/4,00,000) × 1000 = 30 per 1000 midyear population

Crude death rate (CDR) = (6,400/4,00,000) × 1000 = 16 per 1000 midyear population

Infant mortality rate (IMR) = (1500/12,000) × 1000 = 125 per 1000 live birth

IMMUNIZATION

Age	Vaccine
At birth	BCG; OPV 0; Hep B0
6 weeks	Penta 1/DPT 1; Hep B1; OPV 1; ROTA 1; IPV 1; PCV 10**
10 weeks	Penta 2/DPT 2; Hep B2; OPV 2; ROTA 2
14 weeks	Penta 3/DPT 3; Hep B3; OPV 3; ROTA 3; IPV2; PCV 10**
In place of DPT and Hep B some states also give pentavalent (DPT + Hep B + HIB)	
9 months	Measles 1; JE 1*; PCV 10**, MR vaccine
16–24 months	Measles 2; JE 2*; DPT booster; OPV booster
5 years	DPT booster
10–16 years	TT 2 doses (age of 10 years: TT_1; age of 16 years: TT_2)

At 9 months 1 dose of vitamin A (1 lakh IU/1 ml) and every 6 months 2 lakh IU till 60 months
  * Only in the endemic districts of the country
 ** Just started in a few states
*** In some states in place of measles, MR vaccine is given

Q 1. How to calculate vaccine requirement in doses?

1. Write the total population of village.
2. Write annual target of beneficiaries (pregnant women and infants)
   a. For infants, actual headcount has to be taken.
   b. For PW the headcount provides a point estimate for only 6 months (as pregnancies in the the first trimester may be undetected). Hence, multiply the headcount by 2 to arrive at an estimate for 12 months.
3. Divide the annual target of pregnant women and infants by 12 to get the monthly target.
4. For example, if the monthly target for a village is 1 infant and 1 pregnant woman, then the beneficiaries for each vaccine 1 and vitamin A for such a village is calculated as follows:

Vaccine	*Injection*
a. 1 TT = Monthly target of pregnant women × 2 doses	(2)
b. 1 BCG = Monthly target of infants × 1 dose	(1)
c. 1 Pentavalent = Monthly target of infants × 3 doses	(3)
d. 1 DPT booster = Monthly target of infants × 2 doses	(2)
e. 1 OPV = Monthly target of infants × 4 doses [including booster]	
f. 1 IPV = Monthly target of infants × 2 doses	(2)
g. 1 Hep B = Monthly target of infants × 3 doses	(3)
h. 1 Measles = Monthly target of infants × 2 doses	(2)
i. 1 JE = Monthly target of infants × 1 dose	(1)
j. 1 Vitamin A = Monthly target of infants × 9 doses	

Therefore, about 16 injections are required for a target of each infant per month.

Based on the specific needs, add the calculations of beneficiaries for the following doses:

OPV-0, Hep B-Birth, TT-10, TT-16

Example:

A village of population 1000, wherein headcount was undertaken in July 2015, and 40 children of age group 0–1 years and 20 pregnant women were identified. What would be the annual and monthly target of infants and pregnant women for the immunization services? Also, estimate the BCG, DPT, OPV, measles and TT vaccine requirement in doses for the above situation.

Solution:
1. The total population of A = 1000
2. Annual target of beneficiaries
   a. Annual target for infants = 40
   b. Annual target for pregnant women = $20 \times 2 = 40$
3. The monthly target of beneficiaries
   a. Monthly target for infants = $40 = 3.3 \approx 3$
   b. Monthly target for pregnant women = $40 = 3.3 \approx 3$
4. For 1 infant and 1 pregnant woman, the beneficiaries for each vaccine 1 and vitamin A for such a village is calculated as shown above:

Therefore, 3 infants and 3 pregnant women, a total of about $16 \times 3 = 48$ injections are required for a target of each infant and pregnant woman per month.

Q 2. How to calculate the monthly vaccine requirement in vials?
1. To calculate the requirement of vaccines in vials, the doses of vaccines packaged per vial are to be known.
2. Thereafter, wastage of 25% is to be considered.
3. This amount has to be added to the initial requirement and is multiplied with a wastage factor of 1.33.
4. For BCG/DPT/TT/Pentavalent/IPV, one vial has 10 doses. Therefore, calculation will be:

   TT/BCG/DPT/Hep B = (Beneficiaries per month × 1.33)/10
5. For OPV one vial has 20 doses. Therefore, calculation will be:

   OPV = (Beneficiaries per month × 1.33)/20
6. For measles one vial has 5 doses. Therefore calculation will be:

   Measles = (Beneficiaries per month × 1.33)/5
7. For vitamin A, wastage taken is 10% and so a wastage factor is 1.11

   Vitamin A = [(monthly target of infants × 1 ml) + (monthly target of infants × 2 ml × 8)] × 1.11

Example:

A village of population 1000, wherein headcount was undertaken in July 2015, and 40 children of age group 0–1 years and 20 pregnant women were identified. What would be the annual and monthly target of infants and pregnant women for the immunization services? Also estimate the BCG, pentavalent, IPV, DPT, measles and TT vaccine requirement in vials for the above situation.

Solution:

1. The total population of village = 1000
2. Annual target of beneficiaries
   a. Annual target for infants = 40
   b. Annual target for pregnant women = 20 × 2 = 40
3. The monthly target of beneficiaries
   a. Monthly target for infants = 3.3 ≈ 3
   b. Monthly target for pregnant women = 3.3 ≈ 3
4. Calculating the monthly vaccine requirement in vials:
   a. For BCG/DPT/TT/pentavalent/IPV vaccine each = 3 × 1.33 = 0.79 ≈ 1 each
   b. For measles vaccine = 3 × 1.33 = 0.79 ≈ 1

Q 3. How to calculate the requirement of syringes per month for immunization?
The proper calculation of syringes is required during the immunization sessions.

1. For syringes = 10% wastage rate or 1.11 WMF (wastage multiplication factor)
2. The BCG vaccination requires 0.1 ml auto disabled (ADS) syringe per beneficiary:
   0.1 ml ADS = Beneficiaries for BCG × 1.1
3. The TT + DPT + Hep B + IPV + Measles vaccination requires 0.5 ml auto-disabled syringe (ADS) per beneficiary
   0.5 ml ADS = Beneficiaries for (TT + DPT + Hep B + Measles + IPV) × 1.1
4. Reconstitution syringes:
   0.5 ml ADS = (BCG + Measles vials) × 1.1

Example:
A village of population 1000, wherein headcount was undertaken in July 2015, and 40 children of age group 0–1 year and 20 pregnant women were identified. What would be the annual and monthly target of infants and pregnant women for the immunization services? Also, estimate the BCG, DPT, Hep B, measles and TT vaccine requirement for the syringe for the above situation.

Solution:

1. The total population of village = 1000
2. Annual target of beneficiaries
   a. Annual target for infants = 40
   b. Annual target for pregnant women = 20 × 2 = 40
3. The monthly target of beneficiaries
   a. Monthly target for infants = 3.3 ≈ 3
   b. Monthly target for pregnant women = 3.3 ≈ 3
4. Calculating the monthly syringe requirement:
   a. 0.1 ml ADS = [(1 BCG)] 3 × 1.1 = 3.3 ≈ 4
   b. 0.5 ml ADS = [(2 TT + 5 DPT + 3 Hep B + 2 measles + 2 IPV)] × 3 × 1.1 = 46.2 ≈ 47
   c. 0.5 ml ADS = (1 BCG + 1 measles vials) × 1.1 = 2.2 ≈ 3

Q 4. How to calculate fully immunized coverage, left out and drop out rate in a village?

The immunization coverage is often studied in children from 12 to 23 months in a village.

Fully immunized is defined as the percentage of children (12–23 months age) receiving one dose of BCG, 3 doses of pentavalent/OPV/Hep B each and 1 measles vaccine.

Left out rate is defined as the percentage of children 12–23 months age not receiving any vaccination.

Drop-out rate is defined as the percentage of children who received the first dose but did not receive the next dose in immunization. For example, BCG to measles drop out rate is BCG coverage minus measles coverage divided by BCG coverage.

Example:

A village of population 1000, wherein headcount was undertaken in July 2015, and 15 children of age group 12–23 months were identified. Of the total, three did not receive any vaccination and other 2 did not receive measles vaccine. What would be the full coverage, left out rate and drop out rate of BCG to measles for the immunization services in this village?

Solution:

1. The total 12–23 months children = 15
2. Number of children received no vaccine = 5
3. Number of children did receive measles = 2
4. Full coverage is receiving one dose of BCG, 3 doses of pentavalent/OPV/Hep B each and 1 measles vaccine.
   a. Full coverage = [{15 – (5 + 2)}/15] × 100 = 53.3%
5. Left out rate not receiving any vaccination = (5/15) × 100 = 33.3%
6. Drop-out rate is BCG coverage minus measles coverage divided by BCG coverage.
   a. BCG coverage = [(15 – 5)/15] × 100 = 66.7%
   b. Measles coverage = [{15 – (5 + 2)}/15] × 100 = 53.3%
   c. Drop out BCG measles rate = [(66.7–53.3)/66.7] × 100 = 20.1%

NUTRITION

Dietary Calculations for Adult

In case of adult people, dietary calculations are done by counting their daily requirement of calories and proteins.

   (a)   In case of protein, generally we take a standard of 1 gm/kg.
   (b)   In case of calories, there is different calorie requirement in different categories.

	Level of activity	Calories (kcal/day)
a. Man	(a) Sedentary	2320
	(b) Moderate	2730
	(c) Heavy	3490
b. Woman	(a) Sedentary	1900
	(b) Moderate	2230
	(c) Heavy	2850

Pregnant women need extra 350 kcal/day during her pregnancy period.
During lactation (a) 0–6 months—extra 600 kcal/day
(b) 6–12 months—extra 520 kcal/day.

Methods of dietary assessment:
a. Food record
b. 24-hour dietary recall
c. Food frequency questionnaire
d. Brief instruments
e. Diet history

Distribution of total calories according to nutrient source

Foodstuff	Percentage of total calories
Carbohydrate	55–65
Protein	15–20
Fats	20–25

Dietary Calculations for Obese

For the obese person, we use Mifflin-St Jeor equation to calculate resting metabolic rate. For obese people, we take example of a person whose BMI >30.

Men

RMR = (9.99 × weight in kilograms) + (6.25 × height in centimetres) – (4.92 × age) + 5

Women

RMR = (9.99 × weight in kilograms) + (6.25 × height in centimeters) – (4.92 × age) – 161
Then, for total energy expenditure:

Total energy expenditure = RMR × activity factor × injury Factor.

For example: If any person with BMI >30 is 95 kg in weight and 1.6 m in height and his age is 20 years, then

RMR = (9.99 × 95) + (6.25 × 160) – (4.92 × 20) + 5 = 1855.65

Dietary Calculations for under Five Years Child

For energy calculation of an under five child, we use the rule of thumb, which is based upon their weight.

According to this rule:

For first 10 kg of weight = 100 kcal/kg
Next 10 kg weight = 50 kcal/kg
For rest of weight = 20 kcal/kg

Example:
1. Energy requirements for a 9 kg child
   = 100 × 9 = 900 kcal/day
2. Energy requirements for an 18 kg child
   = 10 × 100 + 50 × 8 = 1400 kcal/day
3. Energy requirements for a 32 kg child
   = 10 × 100 + 10 × 50 + 12 × 20 = 1740 kcal/day

Dietary Calculations for Malnourished Child

In such cases at first, we have to calculate how much child is malnourished. For this, we use WHO weight for age growth chart. [Annexure 1, 4, 7, 10]

With the help of these charts, we can calculate how much child is underweight. Then we calculate how much extra energy he needs and then the amount is increased gradually.

Example:

According to WHO weight for age growth chart, a boy child "Anil" of 5 years of age should have weight approx. 18 kg.

So using the rule of thumb the required energy will be = 10 × 100 + 8 × 50 = 1400 kcal/day.

But for a malnourished child weight will be less than normal.

Suppose it is 14 kg for a boy "Bharat" of 5 years, then by using rule of thumb the required energy will be = 10 × 100 + 4 × 50 = 1200 kcal/day.

However, there is need of extra calorie for this malnourished boy "Bharat" to gain weight. Therefore, calories will be calculated based on the median weight of the child as shown in WHO weight for age growth charts.

Therefore, in the above example the boy "Bharat" will require 1400 kcal/day, which has additional 200 kcal/day for weight gain.

We increase the calories demand gradually in malnourished children.

Dietary Calculations for Preterm Baby

In case of preterm delivery, baby generally has low birth weight. Therefore, we cannot calculate his energy requirements according to the general formula.
1. At first, we count the months of preterm delivery.
2. Then we subtract them from WHO weight for age growth chart, age bar.
3. Then we count the weight from estimated age.

If the baby of "Suman" is delivered at 34th week of pregnancy. Therefore, we subtract rest of 6 weeks, i.e. 1.5 months from the age bar from WHO weight for age growth chart. Then we calculate the actual weight of the baby and calculate the energy requirements.

Example: Suppose a boy "Chandan" is delivered at 32 weeks of gestation on 2nd December, 2014. We measured the weight of the child on 3rd, December, 2016 to assess the underweight status and calculate the daily requirement of calories.

In the above example, the boy "Chandan" is 2 years of age and weight is 9 kg. On plotting the age and weight on WHO weight for age growth chart without considering gestational age the child will be malnourished.

Though the fact the boy "Chandan" was preterm, therefore we adjusted the age by deducting 2 months from 2 years, i.e. 24 months. Therefore, for interpreting the child's weight on WHO weight for age growth chart, the age to be considered is 22 months instead of 24 months.

Therefore, this child requires calorie with respect to median weight at 22 months for boy, which is 12 kg. Using the rule of the thumb the calorie is 1100 kcal/day.

Dietary Calculations for Elderly

In this case, the dietary calculation is slightly different. After 40 years resting metabolism decreases gradually.

Categories	Sub categories	Required calories (kcal/day)	41–50 years Decrease by 5% (kcal/day)	51–60 years Further decrease by 5% (kcal/day)	61–70 years Further by 10% (kcal/day)	So on each decades further by 10% (kcal/day)
Man	Sedentary	2320	2320 – 5% of 2320 = 2320 – 116 = 2204	2204 – 5% of 2204 = 2204 – 110 = 2094	2094 – 10% of 2094 = 2094 – 210 = 1884	1884 – 10% of 1884 = 1884 – 188 = 1696
	Moderate	2730	2594	2464	2218	1996
	Heavy	3490	3316	3150	2835	2551
Woman	Sedentary	1900	1805	1715	1543	1389
	Moderate	2230	2118	2012	1811	1630
	Heavy	2850	2708	2573	2316	2084

Balanced Diet for Elderly Person for a Day

Foodstuffs	Quantity (raw) grams	
	Males	Females
Cereals	350	225
Pulses	50	40
Vegetables	200	150
Green leafy vegetables	50	50
Roots and tubers	100	100
Fruits	200	200
Milk and milk products	300	300
Sugar	20	20
Fats and oils	25	20

Dietary Guidelines for Diabetes

3 Major meals and 3 minor meals

Recommended calorie intake for diabetics (kcal/kg body wt/day)		
Category	Sedentary activity	Moderate activity
Overweight/Obese	20	25
Ideal weight	30	35
Underweight	40	40

Body Mass Index (BMI)

It is calculated as weight in kilograms (kg) divided by height in metres squared (m²), rounded to one decimal place.

Category	Indian Council of Medical Research released updated guidelines (in 2012) based on the World Health Organization Asia Pacific Guidelines[Asian]	World Health Organization criteria for [Europids]
	BMI in kg/m²	
Underweight	<18.5	<18.5
Normal	18.5 – 22.9	18.5 – 24.9
Generalized obesity		
Overweight	23.0 – 24.9	25 – 29.9
Obesity	≥25	≥30
Abdominal obesity		
Waist circumference (cm)	≥90 cm for men, ≥80 cm for women	≥102 cm for men, ≥88 cm for women
Waist–hip ratio	-	>0.95 in men, >0.80 for women

DASH Diet for Hypertension

Daily nutrient goals used in DASH studies (for a 2100 calorie eating plan)	
Total fats	27% of calories
Saturated fats	6% of calories
Protein	18% of calories
Carbohydrate	55% of calories
Cholesterol	150 mg
Sodium	2,300 mg
Potassium	4,700 mg
Magnesium	500 mg
Fiber	30 gm

Public Health Laboratory

Venkatashiva Reddy B, Munesh Kumar Gupta

NUTRITION

MILK QUALITY

Composition of Different Natural Milk per 100 ml

Nutrient	Buffalo	Cow	Human
Fat (g)	6.5	4.1	3.4
Protein (g)	4.3	3.2	1.1
Lactose (g)	5.1	4.4	7.4
Calcium (mg)	210	120	28
Iron (mg)	0.3	0.2	0.04 to 0.15
Vitamin C (mg)	1	2	3
Minerals (g)	0.8	0.8	0.1
Water (g)	81	87	88
Energy	117	67	65

Composition of Different Packed Milk per 100 ml

Nutrient	Full cream milk	Toned milk	Double toned milk	Skimmed milk
Fat (g)	6.0	3.0	1.5	Trace
Protein (g)	4.8	4.4	4.4	4.8
Carbohydrate (g)	3.2	3.2	3.2	2.4
Energy	90.8	57.4	44.0	30

MILK BORNE DISEASES

- Diarrhoeal diseases
- Typhoid and para-typhoid fevers
- Tuberculosis
- Brucellosis
- Streptococcal poisoning
- Staphylococcal poisoning

pH of Milk

Principle: Average pH of milk is 6.6 due to lactic acid.
Instrument: pH meter

Chloride Content of Milk

Principle: Indicate diseases state of animal
Reagent: Potassium chromate and silver nitrate
Interpretation: Brick red colour in milk indicates a positive test

Fat Content of Milk [Gerber Method]

Principle: Dissolution of protein and release of fat
Reagent: Sulfuric acid and isoamyl alcohol
Procedure: Centrifugation
Interpretation: Fat rising into the calibrated tube and percentage recorded.

Vansapati in Milk

Reagent: Hydrochloric acid and sugar
Interpretation: Red discolouration in milk indicates a positive test

Detergent in Milk

Reagent: Eosin and buffer
Procedure: Centrifugation
Interpretation: Red or pink colour in milk indicates a positive test

Urea in Milk

I. Reagent: p-Dimethyl amino benzaldehyde
   Interpretation: Yellow colour in milk indicate a positive test
II. Reagent: Soyabean or arhar powder
   Interpretation: A change in colour of litmus paper from red to blue indicates the presence of urea in milk.

Glucose in Milk

Procedure: Take a teaspoonful of milk in a test tube. Dip a strip of diastix in it for 30 seconds.

Interpretation: A change in colouration from blue to green indicates a positive test

Sugar in Milk

Reagent: Hydrochloric acid and resorcinol

Procedure: Take 3 ml of the milk in a test tube. Add 2 ml of hydrochloric acid or muriatic acid in it. Heat the test tube after adding 50 mg of resorcinol.

Interpretation: A red colouration in milk indicates a positive test

Cereal Starch in Milk

Reagent: Aqueous solution of iodine
Procedure: Take 3 ml of the milk in a test tube. Add 1 drop of 1% aqueous solution of iodine
Interpretation: A deep blue colouration in milk indicates a positive test.

Dalda in Milk

Reagent: Hydrochloric acid
Procedure: Take 3 ml of milk in a test tube. Add 10 drops of hydrochloric acid. Mix up one teaspoonful of sugar.
   Interpretation: A red colouration in milk indicates a positive test

Viable Bacterial Count in Milk

Procedure: Pour plate method
Interpretation: Bacterial count more than 50000 cfu/ml in pasteurized milk indicates a positive test

Coliforms in Milk

Principle: Production of acid changes the colour of culture medium
Media: MacConkey's broth
Procedure: Inoculation
Interpretation: Purple to yellow colour change of media indicates a positive test

Milk Quality

Principle: Increasing number of bacterial flora will reduce the colour of dye
Reagent: Methylene blue
Procedure: Centrifugation
Interpretation: The rapid reduction of dye is directly proportional to the number of bacteria in milk

FOOD QUALITY TESTING

Physical and Rheological Parameters

Types of food	Test	Property
Carbohydrates, e.g. flour	Sieve test	Refraction
Proteins, e.g. cereal, pulse	Visual observation	Insect infestation and admixture
Oils and fats	Lovibond tintometer	Colour and Lovibond scale

Test for Adulteration

Adulteration in Oils and Fats

1. **Food item:** Mustard oil

   Adulterant: *Argemone mexicana*

   Toxin: Sanguinarine

   Reagent: Nitric acid

   Procedure: Take some quantity of oil in a test tube. Add equal quantity of nitric acid and shake carefully:

   Interpretation: Red to reddish brown color in lower (acid) layer indicates a positive test.

2. **Food item:** Ghee

   Adulterant: Coal tar dye

   Reagent: Nitric acid

   Procedure: Add 5 ml of sulphuric acid and hydrochloric acid to one teaspoon full of melted sample in a test tube and shake well.

   Interpretation: Pink colour in case of sulfuric acid and crimson colour in case of hydrochloric acid indicates a positive test.

   Public health problem: Cancer

3. **Food item:** Butter

   Adulterant: Vanaspati

   Reagent: Nitric acid

   Procedure: Take a teaspoon full of a melted sample of butter with the equal quantity of concentrated hydrochloric acid in a test tube and add to it a pinch of sugar. Shake for one minute and let it rest for five minutes.

   Interpretation: A crimson red colour indicates a positive test.

   Public health problem: Heart diseases

4. **Food item:** Mustard oil

   Adulterant: Cotton seed oil

   Reagent: Amyl alcohol and carbon disulphide

   Procedure: Take about 3 ml of the mustard oil in a test tube. Add 2 ml of amyl alcohol in it and 1 ml of carbon disulphide and a little amount of sulphur. Heat it for 3 minutes.

   Interpretation: A red colouration indicates a positive test.

5. **Food item:** Mustard oil

   Adulterant: Mineral oil

   Reagent: Alcoholic potash

   Procedure: Take about 3 ml of the mustard oil in a test tube. Add 20 drops of alcoholic potash. For 3 minutes, heat the test tube. Shake the test tube after adding 10 drops of distilled water.

   Interpretation: The turbidity appearance indicates a positive test.

6. **Food item:** Edible oil

   Adulterant: Rancidity

   Reagent: Hydrochloric acid and phloroglucinol

   Procedure: Take 3 ml of the edible oil in a test tube. Add 3 ml of hydrochloric acid, in it. Shake well. Add 3 ml of 0.1% phloroglucinol solution in it. Shake again for 2 minutes and keep it aside. Examine after 30 minutes.

   Interpretation: A pink or red colouration in acid layer indicates a positive test.

7. **Food Item:** Ghee

   Adulterant: Dalda

   Reagent: Hydrochloric acid

   Procedure: Take 3 ml of ghee in a test tube. Add 10 drops of hydrochloric acid, and ¼th of teaspoon of sugar. Shake well. Examine after 5 minutes.

   Interpretation: The red colouration indicates a positive test

Adulteration with Colours in Food

1. **Food item:** Turmeric powder

   Adulterant: Metanil yellow colour

   Reagent: Muratic acid or hydrochloric acid

   Procedure: Take ¼th of teaspoon of turmeric powder in a test tube. Add 3 ml of alcohol in it. Shake the tube thoroughly to mix up the contents. Add 10 drops of muratic acid or hydrochloric acid in the test tube.

   Interpretation: A pink colouration indicates a positive test.

2. **Food item:** Red chilli powder

   Adulterant: Rhodamine B colour

   Reagent: Carbon tetrachloride and hydrochloric acid

   Procedure: Take ¼th teaspoon of the red chilli powder in a test tube. Add 3 ml of distilled water in it, and 10 drops of carbon tetrachloride. Shake it well.

   Interpretation: The red colour will disappear on shaking, and if the red colour reappears with hydrochloric acid, it indicates a positive test.

3. **Food item:** Green vegetable

   Adulterant: Malachite green colour

   Reagent: Liquid paraffin

   Procedure: Take a cotton piece soaked in liquid paraffin, and rub the outer surface of the green vegetable.

   Interpretation: If the cotton turns green indicates a positive test.

4. **Food item:** Edible oil

   Adulterant: Prohibited colour

   Reagent: Hydrochloric acid

   Procedure: Take 20 drops of the edible oil in each of 4 test tubes. Make 3 different solutions, mixing up 1 part of distilled water, 3 parts of distilled water and 4 parts of distilled water. Add 2 ml of each solution in each of the test tubes and add 2 ml of hydrochloric acid in the 4th test tube. Shake it well.

   Interpretation: Rosy colouration in any tube indicates a positive test.

5. **Food item:** Jaggery

   Adulterant: Metanil Yellow Colour

   Reagent: Alcohol and hydrochloric acid

   Procedure: Take ¼th of a teaspoon of the jaggery in a test tube. Add 3 ml of alcohol and shake well. Pour 10 drops of hydrochloric acid in it.

   Interpretation: A pink colouration indicates a positive test.

Adulteration in Cereals and Legumes

1. **Food item:** Rice

   Adulterant: Urea

   Reagent: Arhar or soya bean

   Procedure: Take 30 numbers of rice in a test tube. Add 5 ml of distilled water in it. Shake well. After 5 minutes, filter the water-contents, and add ½ teaspoon of powder of arhar or soya bean in it. Leave it for 5 minutes, and then dip a red litmus paper.

   Interpretation: A blue colouration of litmus paper indicates a positive test.

2. **Food item:** Maida/rice

   Adulterant: Boric acid

   Reagent: Hydrochloric acid

   Procedure: Take a small amount of sample in a test tube. Add some water and shake. Add a few drops of hydrochloric acid and dip a turmeric paper strip.

   Interpretation: A red colouration of turmeric paper strip indicates a positive test.

3. **Food item:** Wheat flour

   Adulterant: Excess bran

   Procedure: Sprinkle wheat flour on water surface

   Interpretation: Bran will float on the surface indicating a positive test.

4. **Food item:** Wheat flour

   Adulterant: Chalk powder

   Reagent: Hydrochloric acid

   Procedure: Take a small amount of sample in a test tube and shake sample with diluted hydrochloric acid

   Interpretation: The occurrence of effervescence indicates a positive test.

5. **Food item:** Gram powder

   Adulterant: Khesari powder

   Reagent: Muratic acid

   Procedure: Take ½ teaspoon of the gram powder in a test tube and add 3 ml of distilled water in it. Then pour 3 ml of muratic acid in the test tube. Keep the test tube in water. Check the test tube after 15 minutes.

   Interpretation: A violet colouration indicates a positive test

Adulteration in Other Food Items

1. **Food item:** Coffee powder

   Adulterant: Cereal starch

   Reagent: Potassium permanganate solution, muriatic acid, and iodine.

Procedure: Take ¼th of a teaspoon of coffee powder in a test tube and add 3 ml of distilled water in it. Heat it. Add about 33 ml of potassium permanganate solution and muriatic acid to decolorize the mixture. Add a drop of 1% aqueous solution of iodine.

Interpretation: A blue colouration indicates a positive test

2. **Food item:** Coffee powder
   Adulterant: Scorched persimmon stones
   Reagent: Sodium carbonate.
   Procedure: Take 1 teaspoon of the coffee powder and spread it on a moisturized blotting paper. Pour 3 ml of 2% aqueous solution of sodium carbonate.
   Interpretation: A red colouration indicates a positive test.

WATER

WATER QUALITY TESTING

			Drinking water standards				
S. No.	Parameter	Unit	Recommended value				
			BIS (IS 10500—2012)		ICMR		WHO 2013
			Requirement (acceptable limit)	Maximum permissible limits in the absence of alternate source	Desirable limit	Maxium permissible limits in the absence of alternate source	Maximum
1.	pH		6.5 to 8.5	6.5 to 8.5	7 to 8.5	6.5 to 9.2	6.5 to 8.5
2.	Total dissolved solids	mg/L	500	2000	500	1500–3000	<600
3.	Colour		5 Hazen Unit	15 Hazen Unit	–	–	<15 TCU
4.	Turbidity	NTU	1	5	–	–	<5
5.	Total hardness as $CaCO_3$	mg/L	200	600	600	300	<100–300
6.	Calcium	mg/L	–	–	75	200	–
7.	Magnesium	mg/L	–	–	50	–	–
8.	Chloride	mg/L	250	1000	200	1000	–
9.	Sulphate	mg/L	200	400	200	400	–
10.	Nitrate	mg/L	45	45	20	100	<50
11.	Nitrite	mg/L	–	–	–	–	<3
12.	Iron	mg/L	0.3	0.3	0.1	1	

(Contd.)

			Drinking water standards				
S. No.	Parameter	Unit	Recommended value				
			BIS (IS 10500—2012)		ICMR		WHO 2013
			Requirement (acceptable limit)	Maximum permissible limits in the absence of alternate source	Desirable limit	Maximum permissible limits in the absence of alternate source	Maximum
13.	Fluoride	mg/L	1.0	1.5	1	1.5	<1.5
14.	Arsenic	mg/L	0.01	0.05	–	0.05	0.01
15.	Manganese	mg/L	–	–	0.1	0.5	–
16.	Zinc	mg/L	5	15	0.1	5	–
17.	Copper	mg/L	0.05	1.5	0.05	1.5	–
18.	Chromium	mg/L	0.05	0.05	–	–	–
19.	Lead	mg/L	0.01	0.01	–	0.5	–
20.	Mercury	mg/L	0.001	0.001	–	0.001	–
21.	Cadmium	mg/L	0.003	0.003	–	0.01	0.003
22.	Cyanide	mg/L	0.05	0.05	–	0.05	–
23.	Sodium	mg/L	–	–	–	–	50
24.	Residual free chlorine	mg/L	0.2	1	–	–	–
25.	Boron	mg/L	–	–	–	–	2.4
26.	Selenium	mg/L	0.01	0.01	–	–	–
27.	Total coliform	MPN/ 100 ml	Nil	Nil	–	–	–
28.	Gross alpha radiological activity	Bq/L	–	–	–	–	<0.5
29.	Gross beta radiological activity	Bq/L	–	–	–	–	<1 Bq/L

SAFE WATER/WHOLESOME WATER

1. Aesthetically acceptable
2. Chemically safe
3. Organic substances absent
4. Free from bacteria
5. Radioactive elements absent

Physical Water Quality Assessment

Parameters

1. **Dissolved oxygen**

Method: The Winkler method with Azide modification

Principle: Oxygen oxidizes the divalent manganous to its higher valency which precipitates as a brown hydrated oxide after addition of NaOH and KI. Upon acidification, manganese reverts to divalent state and liberates iodine from KI equivalent to dissolved oxygen. The liberated iodine is titrated against sodium thiosulfate.

Procedure: Collect sample in BOD bottle. Add 2 ml $MnSO_4$, 2 ml alkali iodide-azide and close stopper. Mix well. Add 2 ml concentrated sulfuric acid and mix well. Take 200 ml sample in a conical flask and titrate against sodium thiosulfate (0.025 N).

Quantity: Dissolved oxygen in mg/L = [(0.2 × 1000) × ml of thiosulfate]/200

2. **Biochemical oxygen demand**

Methodology: Bioassay test

Principle: The biochemical oxygen demand test is based upon determination of dissolved oxygen.

Procedure: Aerate the required volume of diluted water by bubbling compressed air for 1–2 days to attain dissolved oxygen saturation. Add 1 ml each per litre of dilution water, phosphate buffer, magnesium sulphate, calcium chloride, ferric chloride and mix well. Determine dissolved oxygen.

D_0 = Dissolved oxygen in sample on 0th day

D_1 = Dissolved oxygen in sample on 5th day

C_0 = Dissolved oxygen in blank on 0th day

C_1 = Dissolved oxygen in blank on 5th day

Quantity: BOD in mg/L $(D_0 - D_1) - (C_0 - C_1)$ mg × decimal fraction of sample used

3. **Colour**

Method: Visual comparison method or spectrophotometric method

Principle: Unit for colour measurement is based on platinum cobalt scale

Procedure: Visual comparison with known concentration of coloured solutions prepared by diluting stock platinum cobalt solution

4. **Total dissolved solids**

Method: Evaporation method

Principle: At 180° + 20°C temperature all mechanically occluded water is lost

5. **Turbidity**

Method: Nephelometers

Principle: Comparison of the intensity of light scattered by the sample under defined conditions with the intensity of light scattered by a standard reference suspension under the same conditions.

Chemical Water Quality Assessment

Parameters

1. **pH**

Method: pH meter

Principle: pH of hydrogen ion exponent is 6.5–8.5

2. **Chloride**

   Method: Argentometric method

   Principle: Chloride is titrated with standard silver nitrate, using potassium chromate as an indicator.

3. **Nitrate**

   Method: Ultraviolet spectrophotometric method

   Principle: Add 1 ml of 1 N hydrochloric acid per 50 ml of sample and read absorbance or transmittance at 220 nm and 275 nm

4. **Fluoride**

   Method: Colorimetric SPADNS method

   Principle: Under acidic conditions fluorides (HF) react with zirconium SPADNS solution and colour of SPADNS reagent gets bleached.

5. **Sulfate**

   Method: Spectorphotometric method

   Principle: Sulfate ions are precipitated as $BaSO_4$ in acidic media. The absorption of light is measured by spectrophotometer at 420 nm.

6. **Ammonia**

   Method: Nesslerization method

   Principle: The proper selection of light path and wavelength permits the photometric determination of ammonia.

7. **Phosphates**

   Method: Vanadomolybdophosphoric acid method

   Principle: In a dilute orthophosphate solution, ammonium molybdate reacts under acid conditions to form a heteropoly acid. In the presence of vanadium, yellow vanadomolybdophosphoric acid is formed. The intensity of yellow colour is proportional to phosphate concentration.

8. **Iron**

   Method: Colorimetric method

   Principle: Iron is detected at wavelength 510 nm

9. **Manganese**

   Method: Colorimetric method

   Principle: Manganese is detected at wavelength 525 nm.

10. **Hardness**

    Methods: Calcium can be estimated by EDTA titrimetric methods and magnesium can be estimated by Gravimetric method

    Total hardness in mg $CaCO_3$/L = 2.497 [Ca mg/L] + 4.118 [Mg mg/L]

11. **Chlorine**

    Method: Orthotoluidine test

    Principle: Orthotoluidine in 10% hydrochloric acid when added to water containing chlorine turns yellow

12. **Arsenic**

    Method: Arsenic detection field kit

    Principle: Based on mercuric bromide stain method

ENVIRONMENT INSTRUMENTS

Chloroscope

Use: To detect free, residual and total chlorine content in water.

Principle: The yellow colour is matched with standard colours by rotating the disc of chloroscope through the viewing window.

Procedure: To 0.1 ml orthotoluidine solution, add 10 ml of chlorinated sample water in a test tube. Observe colour change after 5 minutes.

Disadvantage: Impurities like iron, manganese, and nitrate likely to give false yellow colour.

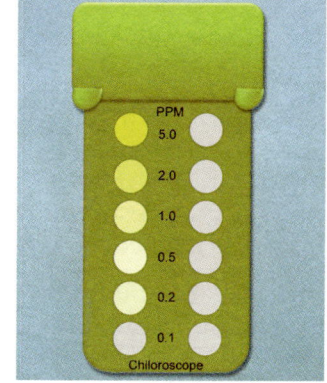

H₂S Strip Test Kit

Use: Bacteriological examination of drinking water.

Principle: H_2S reacts with iron forming iron sulfide that is black in colour.

Procedure: Unseal the H_2S test kit bottle. Fill the bottle up to 20 ml mark with sample water. Keep the bottle at room temperature for 24 hours.

Interpretation: Change in water colour to black indicates water is unsafe for drinking.

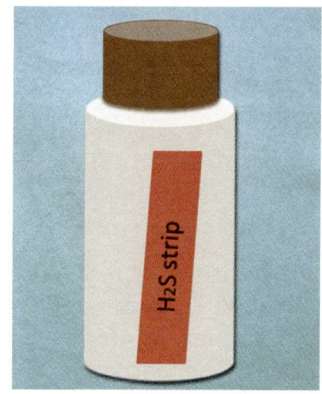

Maximum and Minimum Thermometers

Use: To record the maximum and minimum temperature reached over a period of time.

Design: Maximum minimum thermometers are typically U-shaped parallel tubes of glass. One side registers the minimum temperature, while the other registers the maximum temperature. The bend at bottom of thermometer contains liquid mercury that moves up and down based on contractions of the oil or alcohol located in two bulbs at the top of thermometer.

Principle: The contractions of alcohol or oil are the result of thermal changes in the environment causing it to expand or contract.

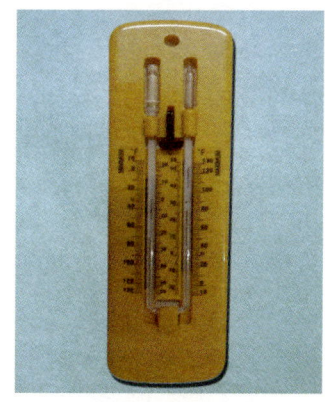

Hygrometer

Use: To measure relative humidity

Design: This instrument consists of two similar thermometers, which are mounted side by side on a stand, namely wet bulb thermometer and dry bulb thermometer. The bulb of the wet bulb thermometer is covered with a gauze or wick and is kept moist.

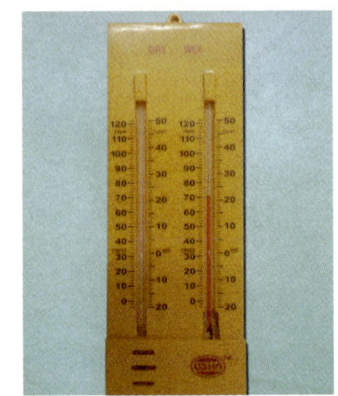

Principle: The dry bulb measures air temperature. The wet bulb temperature is usually lower than the dry bulb temperature. After obtaining readings of dry and wet bulbs, the corresponding relative humidity can be found from specially constructed psychometric charts.

Interpretation: If both readings are the same, it indicates that the atmosphere is 100 percent saturated with moisture.

Sling Psychrometer

Use: To measure the relative humidity

Design: The sling or whirling psychometer consists of two mercury thermometers mounted side by side on a suitable wooden frame.

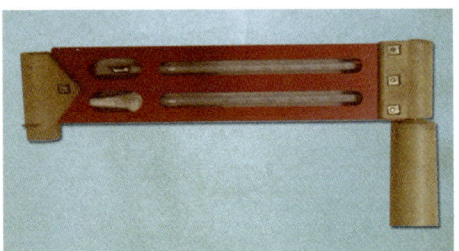

Principle: By rotating, the bulbs are exposed to air at a definite velocity, which is required to obtain accurate readings.

Procedure: Wet bulb is first moistened with distilled water and the instrument is whirled or rotated standing with the back to sun for about 15 seconds at the rate of 4 revolutions per second, to obtain the desirable speed of 5 m/sec. The reading of wet bulb is then noted. The instrument is again whirled for about 10 seconds and the wet bulb reading is noted. This is repeated several times until two successive readings of the wet bulb are identical. The reading of dry bulb is then noted. By using suitable charts the relative humidity of the air may be obtained from the readings of psychometer.

Hydrometer

Use: In alcohol hydrometer shows the degree to which the yeast is converting sugar into ethanol.

Principle: Measure the ratio of a sample liquid density to the density of water.

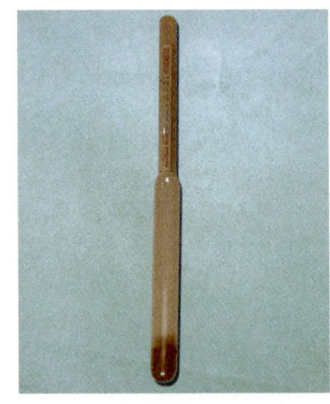

Procedure: Retrieve sample and insert hydrometer. Obtain the original specific gravity reading. Calculate the temperature using specific gravity temperature correction chart. Repeat to obtain final gravity reading when the fermentation process is complete or nearly complete.

Lactometer

Use: To measure specific gravity of milk

Principle: Specific gravity of milk is 1.025 to 1.035 at 25–35°C. After 12 hours of milking, it rises to 0.0013.

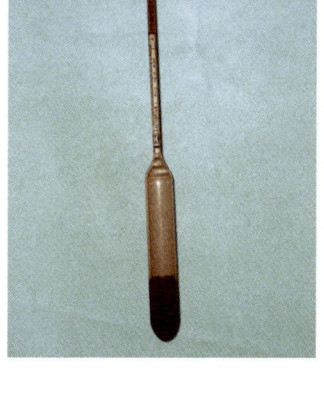

Design: Lactometer is a cylindrical vessel made by blowing a glass tube. One side of glass tube looks like a bulb filled with mercury and the other side is a thin tube with scales.

Procedure: Dip lactometer in milk, point up to which it sinks in pure milk is marked, put lactometer in water, the point up to which it sinks in water is marked.

Interpretation: It sinks less in milk than in water as we know milk is denser than water. If it sinks up to the mark 'M' that means milk is pure or if not that means milk is impure. If the milk is mixed in water, then it would sink higher than marked 'M'. If it stands at mark 3 that means milk is 75% pure and respectively 2 for 50% purity and 1 means 25% purity.

Iodine Testing Kit

Use: To measure the amount of iodine in salt.

Principle: Colour of salt changes depending on the amount of iodine in presence of reagent.

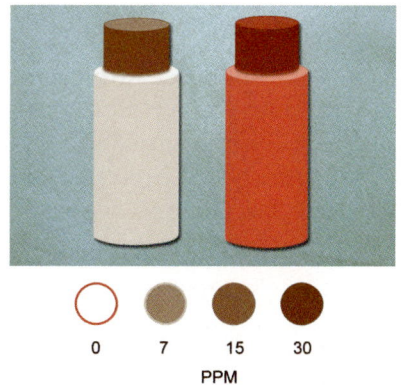

Content:

1. 1 ampoule of 10 ml test solution

2. 1 red ampoule of recheck solution

3. Colour chart with circular spots

Procedure:

1. Take 1 spoonful of salt

2. Add a few drops of white solution on salt

3. Colour of salt changes depending on amount of iodine

4. Use colour to compare iodine content

5. If the colour does not change add red solution, to remove alkalinity

6. Again add a few drops of white solution on salt, colour of salt changes depending on the amount of iodine

Tinotometer

Use: Colorimetric water analysis

Principle: Comparator for colour grading and colorimeteric chemical analysis with the use of light.

Content:

1. Comparator box
2. Disc
3. Glass tubes
4. Brush
5. Light source
6. Other

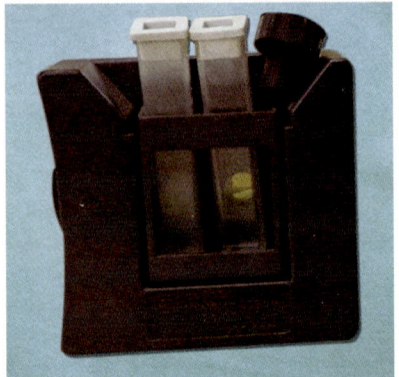

Procedure: A water sample is taken in a glass tube. The glass tube is inserted in the comparator and compared with a series of coloured glass discs to record the nearest possible match.

Horrock's Apparatus

Use: To find out dose of bleaching powder required for disinfection of water.

Content: 6 white cups (200 ml capacity each), 1 black cup with circular mark, metal spoons (each holds 2 g of bleaching powder), stirring rods, 1 special pipette, 2 droppers, starch and iodide indicator solution.

Procedure

1. Take spoonful of bleaching powder in the black cup and make a thin paste by adding some water up to the circular mark by vigorous stirring.
2. Fill 6 white cups with water to be tested.
3. With special pipette, add one drop of stock solution to the 1st cup, two drops to the 2nd cup and so on.
4. Stir water in cups using separate rods.

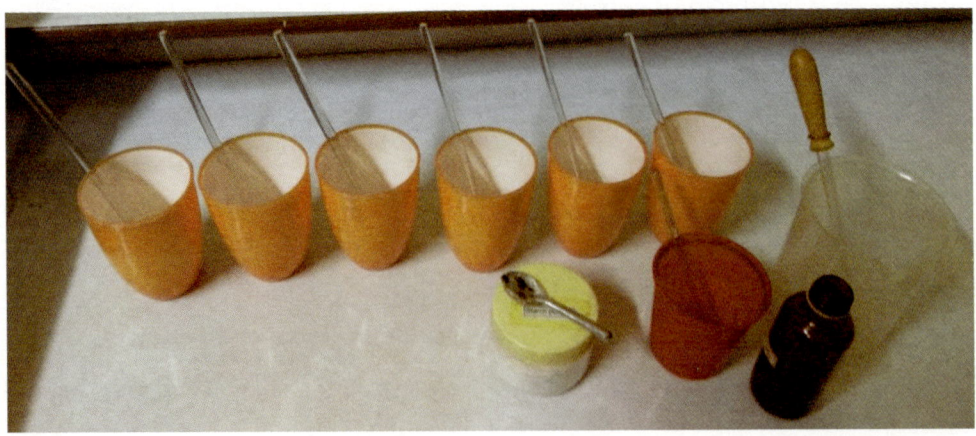

5. Wait for half an hour for action of chlorine.
6. Add 3 drops of starch iodide indicator to each of white cups. Development of blue colour indicates the free residual chlorine.
7. Note the first cup, which shows blue colour. For example, let the third cup shows the blue colour, then 3 spoonful (6 g) of bleaching powder is needed to disinfect 455 litres of water.

PUBLIC HEALTH MICROBIOLOGY

STAINING TECHNIQUES AND INTERPRETATION

Gram Stain

Principle: Gram-positive cell wall has high content of teichoic acid and peptidoglycan, whereas gram-negative cell wall has lipopolysaccharide. Lipid component of gram-negative cell wall is dissolved by alcohol (decolouriser). Primary stain (crystal violet) comes out from gram-negative cell wall due to formation of pores, whereas gram-positive cell wall retains the primary stain. Thus, gram-positive cell wall takes the colour of primary stain (violet) and gram-negative takes the colour of secondary stain (red).

Procedure
1. A new slide is used to make smear which is labelled with laboratory serial number
2. A drop of normal saline is placed on a slide in which microbial colony is mixed with the help of loop. This mix colony is spread over slide to make a uniform thin smear covering 2 × 3 cm. Smear is allowed to air dry which is further heat fixed by passing the slide 3–4 times over the flame of a Bunsen burner. Do not overheat.
3. Place the slide on staining rack and pour 1% crystal violet covering the smear. Slide is kept for 1 minute, rinse smears with water.
4. Gram's iodine (iodine + potassium iodide) is added over smear which makes complex with crystal violet. Slide is kept for one minute.
5. Smear is decolourised with 70% alcohol by adding drop by drop. Process is done till there is no further flowing of violet colour from slide (most crucial step).
6. Smear is covered with safranine. Smear is kept for 30 seconds. Only decolourised smear takes the colour of safranine (secondary stain), wash off the stain with clean water.
7. Wipe the back of the slide clean, and place it in a draining rack for the smear to air-dry (do not blot dry).
8. Examine the smear microscopically, using the 100X oil immersion objective.
9. Gram-positive organism takes the violet colour of primary stain, whereas gram-negative organism takes the colour of pink-red (colour of secondary stain)

Ziehl-Neelsen Stain

Principle: Mycobacterial cell wall contains a high content of mycolic acid (long chain fatty acids) which is impermeable to common dye. Permeability is increased by phenol (carbol fuschin = basic fuschin + phenol) and intermittent heating. Mycobacterial cell wall is resistant to decolourisation by 25% sulfuric acid and takes the colour of primary stain (pink). Rest organisms are easily decolourised and takes the colour of secondary stain (blue/green).

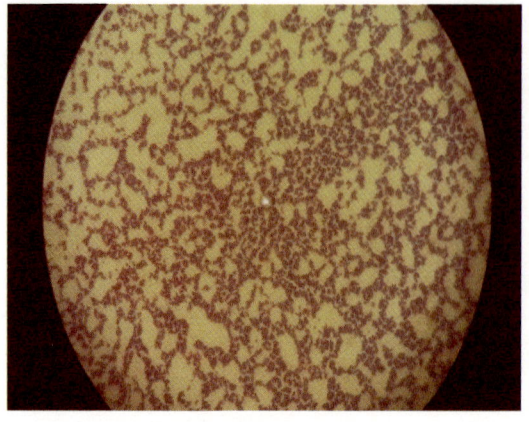

Gram-positive cocci

Gram-positive organism: *Staphylococcus aureus, Streptococcus pyogenes, Corynebacterium diphtheriae*

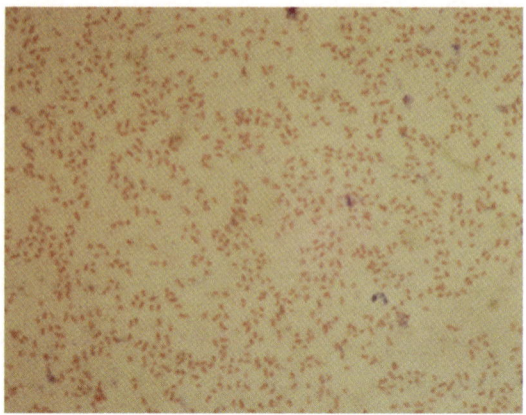

Gram-negative bacilli

Gram-negative organism: *Escherichia coli, Salmonella typhi, Shigella dysenteriae, Vibrio cholerae*

Procedure

1. A new slide is used to make smear which is labelled with laboratory serial number.
2. Yellowish purulent material from sputum sample is picked up with the help of a broomstick. Material is spread to make uniform thin smear covering 2 × 3 cm. The smear is allowed to air dry which is further heat fixed by passing the slide 3–4 times over the flame of a Bunsen burner. Do not overheat. Do not touch the smear.
3. Place the slide on a staining rack and pour 1% carbol fuschin covering the entire slide. Intermittent heating is done by passing a flame under the rack until fumes appear (without boiling). Do not overheat and allow it to stand for 8–10 minutes. Rinse smears with water.
4. Decolourise the smear with 25% sulfuric acid till there is complete absence of colour (slide become as colourless in case of clinical samples) (most crucial step)
5. Wash well with clean water.
6. Cover the smear with 1% methylene blue or malachite green stain for 1–2 minutes. (slide takes the colour of secondary stain—methylene blue/malachite green)
7. Wash off the stain with clean water.
8. Wipe the back of the slide clean, and place it in a draining rack for the smear to air-dry (do not blot dry).
9. Examine the smear microscopically, using the 100X oil immersion objective. (minimum examine 2 × 1 cm area of smear)

Albert Stain

Albert stain is used to demonstrate the metachromatic granules/volutin granules of *Corynebacterium diphtheriae* in clinical samples.

Principal: In Albert staining, two solutions are used. Solution I contains toluidine blue O and malachite green, malachite green—basic dye have affinity for acidic tissue

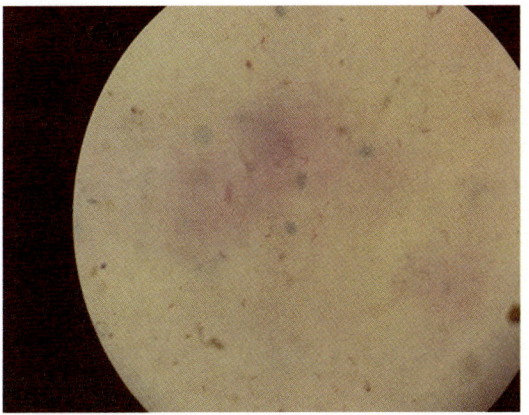

Mycobacterium tuberculosis (25% H$_2$SO$_4$)

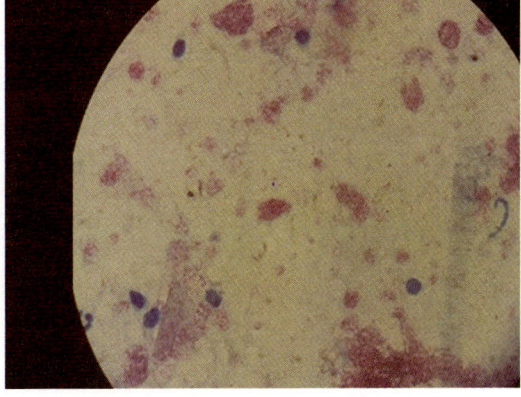

Mycobacterium leprae (5% H$_2$SO$_4$)

component such as cytoplasm. Toluidine blue O stains volutin granules, whereas malachite green stains cytoplasm as green. Solution II contains Albert iodine. After addition of Albert iodine, granules appear blue as metachromatic property is not observed.

Procedure
1. Smear is prepared on clean glass slides with patients details
2. Smear is dried and heat fixed by passing 3–4 times over bunsen burner flame
3. Solution I is poured over smear and kept for 8–10 minutes
4. Excess stain is drained off. Slide is not washed with water
5. Solution II is poured over slide for 2 minutes
6. Slide is washed with water. It is air dried and examined under oil immersion (100X)

Result: *Corynebacterium diphtheriae* reveal as green and volutin granules appear blue.

Wright's Stain (Wright-Giemsa)

Wright's stain is Romanowsky's stain having both eosin and methylene blue. Eosin stains the cytoplasm pink, whereas methylene blue stains the nucleus. It is a histological stain that facilitates the differentiation of blood cell types.

Procedure
1. Peripheral blood smear is first fixed in methanol/ethyl alcohol for 3–5 minutes
2. Smear is air dried
3. 1.0 ml of the Wright stain solution is poured upon the smear for 1–3 minutes.
4. 2.0 ml of distilled water or Wright stain phosphate buffer pH 6.8 is poured
5. Slide is kept on staining rack for 15–20 minutes
6. Slide is rinsed with water or Wright stain phosphate buffer pH 6.8 until a faint pinkish red appears on the edges.
7. Dry thoroughly using paper to blot dry.
8. Smear is air dried and examined under 100X oil immersion lens.

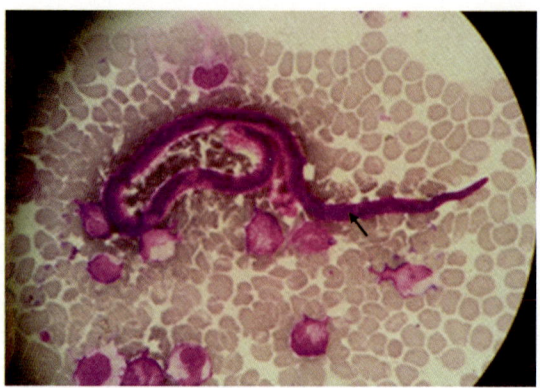

Microfilariae

STAINS FOR MALARIA

Leishmann Stain

Principle: It has acidic and basic components which get attached to basic component and acidic component of the organism. With aging and exposure to acid/alkali, a number of oxidation products as methylene azure, methylene blue eosinate are formed which give contrast colour staining. Eosin stains the RBCs pink, methylene blue stains the cytoplasm of malarial parasite blue and azure with eosin stains nuclear chromatin red.

Procedure
1. Place the slide on a staining rack—ensuring that the smear is uppermost.
2. Cover the smear completely (i.e. flood the slide) with Leishman stain from a dropping bottle, and leave it to act for 1–2 min. This fixes the smear.
3. Add to the slide a volume of buffered distilled water, which is approximately twice that of the stain already present. By gently rocking the staining rack evenly, mix the buffered distilled water and stain.
4. Allow the mixture to act for 10–15 min. Ensure that there is sufficient diluted stain on the slide to prevent its drying out during this period. If not, add more stain and buffered distilled water.
5. Wash off the mixture from the slide with buffered distilled water and allow it to remain on the slide, for approximately 1 min. until the smear has a pinkish tinge.
6. Pour off the water, dry the smear by standing the slide upright on a piece of filter paper, leaning against the staining dish or some other objects, e.g. a bottle.

Example: All stages of *Plasmodium vivax* (trophozoite, schizont, gametocytes) are seen in peripheral blood film, whereas in *Plasmodim falciparum*, only early trophozoite and gametocyte stages are seen.

JSB Stain (Jaswant Singh and Bhattacharjee)

Principle: It is the standard method used by the laboratories under the National Malaria Eradication Programme in India. This stain is superior to the Field's stain because the parasites stain clearer and both thick and thin smears can be stained. However, preparations fade quite rapidly. Therefore, this stain is not recommended when permanent slides are desired. The malaria parasites are stained similar to staining with Giemsa (the red chromatin dots with light blue cytoplasm).

Smear preparation

a. *Thick smear:* Clean slides are taken which are marked with patient's details. Figure is punctured with a needle. The first blood drop is wiped off and the second drop is placed at one point which is spread to make a dot. Thickness of a smear should be such through which newspaper can be read. Thick smear is air dried but never fixed.

b. *Thin smear:* A drop of blood after wiping the first drop is placed over a cleaned slide which is spread over with the help on another slide by keeping it at 45° angle. For a better smear, tailing should be made on thin smear. Thin smear is air dried but it is methanol fixed.

Procedure: Two solutions are made for JSB staining.

a. *Solution I* containing 0.5 gm of methylene blue, 0.5 gm of potassium dichromate, 3 ml of sulfuric acid (1% by volume 3), 10 ml of potassium hydroxide (1%), and 500 ml of water

b. *Solution II* containing 1 gm of eosin in 500 ml of tap water

For thick films

1. Thick blood smear is immersed in solution I for 10 seconds
2. Slide is washed for 2 seconds in a jar containing acidulated tap water (pH 6.2–6.6) by the addition of 5% acetic acid or citric acid
3. Smear is stained with solution II for 1 second
4. Wash in the same jar (repetition of 2nd step)
5. Slide is immersed again in solution I for 10 seconds
6. Again wash in acidulated tap water till the smear gives pink background
7. Smear is dried and examined under microscope

For thin films

1. Thin blood smear is fixed in methanol for 1–2 seconds and it is dried
2. Dried smear is immersed in solution I for 30 seconds
3. Slide is washed for 2 seconds in a jar containing acidulated tap water (pH 6.2–6.6) by the addition of 5% acetic acid or citric acid
4. Smear is stained with solution II for 1 second
5. Wash in the same jar for 4 seconds (repetition of 3rd step)
6. Slide is immersed again in solution I for 30 seconds
7. Again wash in acidulated tap water till the smear gives pink background
8. Smear is dried and examined under microscope

Field Stain

Principle: Polychromated methylene blue and eosin stains specifically to basophilic and acidophilic cellular elements to demonstrate blood cells and hemoparasites.

Procedure:

1. Place a drop of blood on a microscope slide and spread to make an area of approximately 1 cm². (The film should be spread thin enough so that it appears transparent.)

2. Air dry the film. Do not fix in methanol.
3. Stain the slide into Field's stain A for 3 seconds, wash the slide in water for 3 seconds; agitate gently.
4. Stain the slide into Field's stain B for 3 seconds and wash gently in tap water for a few seconds to remove excess stain, drain the slide and air dry the slide.

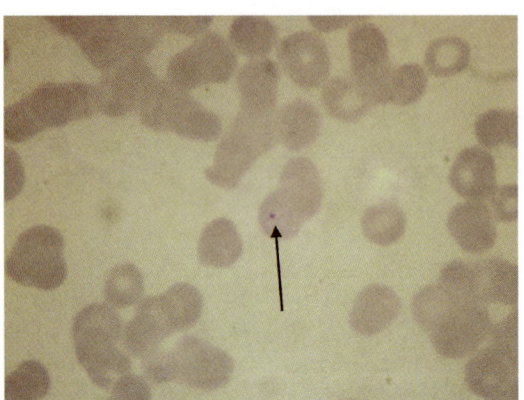

Plasmodium vivax trophozoite stage

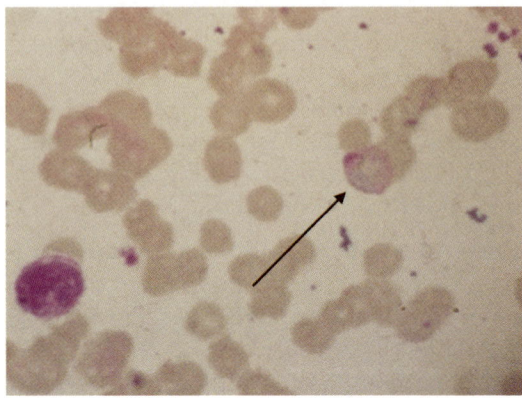

Female gametocyte of *Plasmodium vivax*

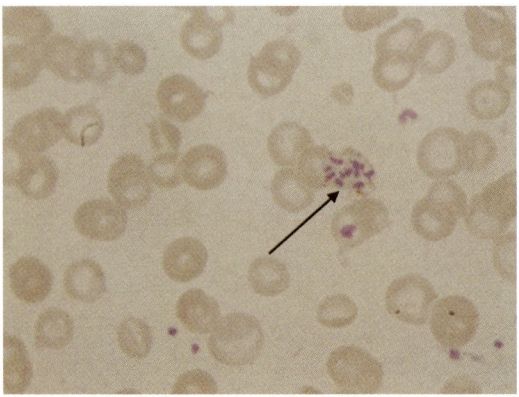

Plasmodium vivax schizont stage

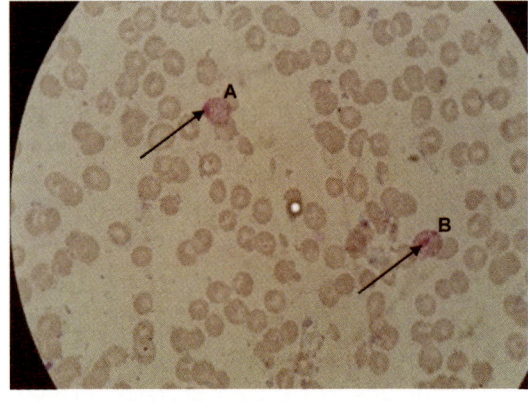

Female gametocyte (A) and male gametocyte (B) of *Plasmodium vivax*

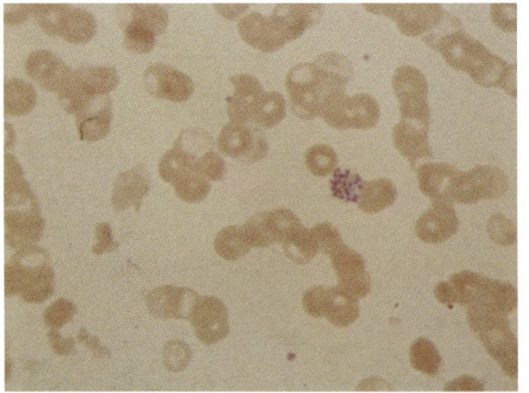

Plasmodium vivax mature schizont

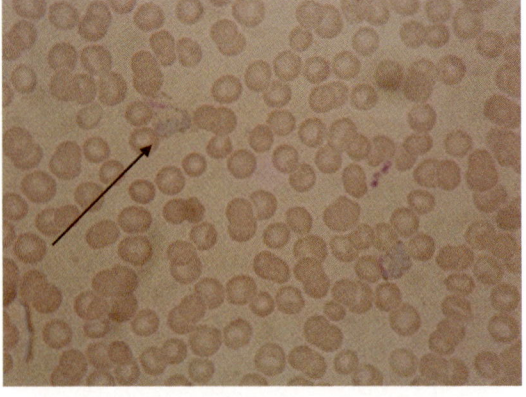

Amooeboid stage of *Plasmodium vivax*

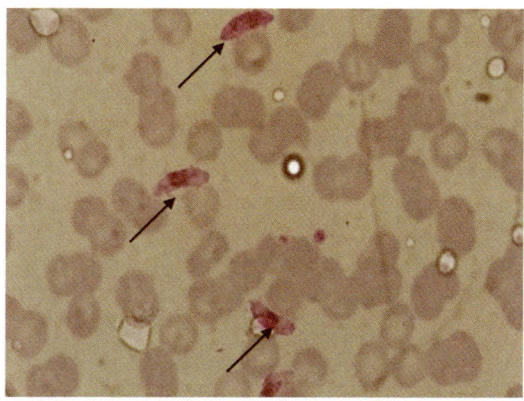

Gametocyte of *Plasmodium falciparum*

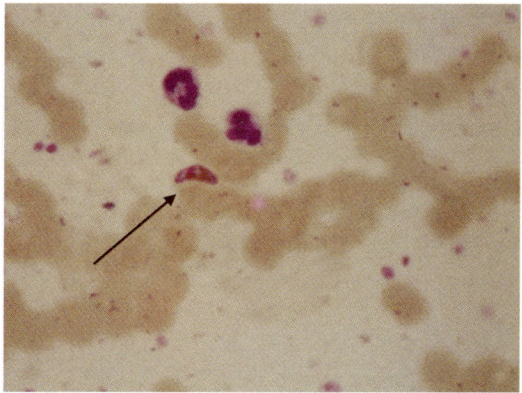

Gametocyte of *Plasmodium falciparum*

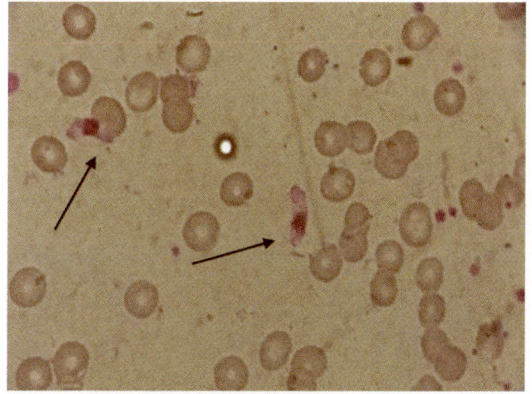

Gametocyte of *Plasmodium falciparum* (attached to RBCs)

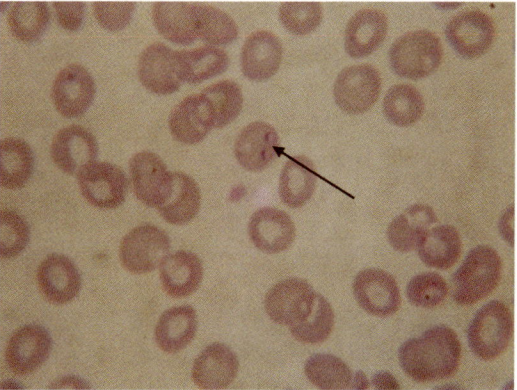

Plasmodium falciparum trophozoite stage

Microbial Colonies

Organism: *Staphylococcus aureus*—most common cause of suppurative lesion

Colony characteristics: On blood agar, 1–2 mm size, smooth, round, opaque colony having entire margin.

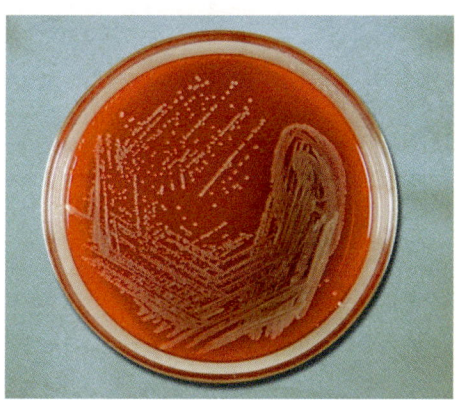

Organism: *Streptococcus pyogenes*—most common cause of bacterial pharyngitis

Consequences: Rheumatic fever, rheumatic heart disease, post-streptococcal glomerulonephritis

Colony characteristics: On blood agar, pinpoint small smooth, round, opaque only having entire margin showing beta hemolysis.

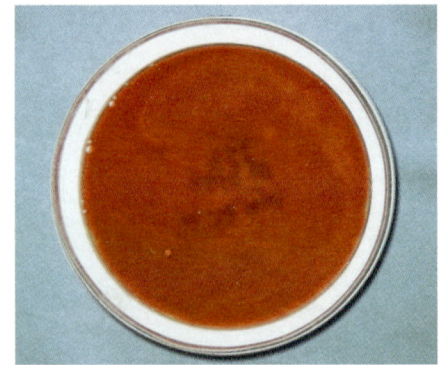

Organism: *Pseudomonas aeruginosa*—common cause of hospital acquired infection

Colony characteristics: On nutrient agar, 2–3 mm size, green coloured, smooth transversly streched colony having entire margin.

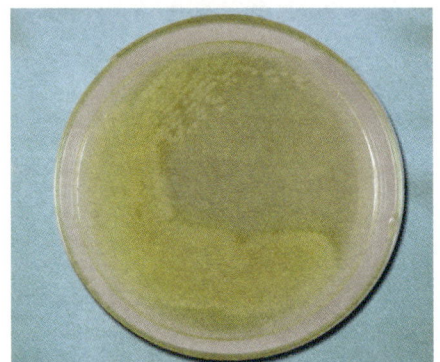

Organism: *Salmonella typhi*—causative agent of enteric fever

Colony characteristics: On MacConkey agar, 2–3 mm size, smooth, round, translucent non-lactose fermenter colony (same colour of media) having entire margin.

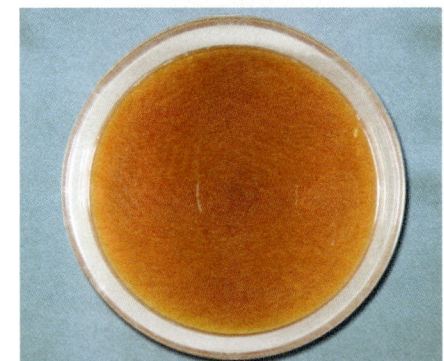

Biochemical test:

From right to left: TSI (red/yellow + H_2S), SIM (motile, indole negative), glucose (pink colour—fermented), lactose (no colour change—nonfermented), sucrose (no colour change—nonfermented), mannitol (pink colour—fermented), urease (negative), citrate (negative)

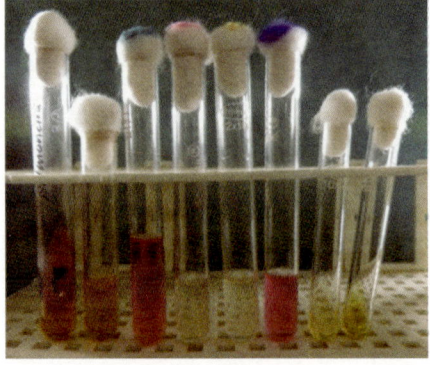

Organism: Shiggella—most common cause of dysenteriae

Colony characteristics: On MacConkey agar, 1 mm size, smooth, round, translucent nonlactose fermenter colony (same colour of media) having entire margin.

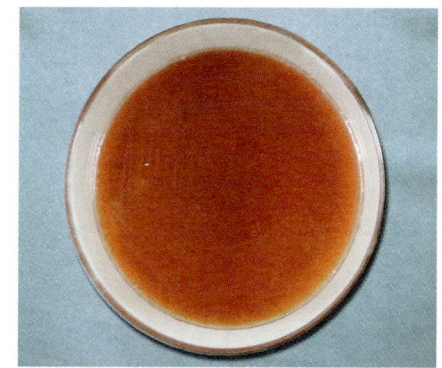

Biochemical test

From right to left: TSI (red/yellow), SIM (non-motile, indole negative, no H_2S), Glucose (pink colour—fermented), lactose (no colour change—nonfermented), sucrose (no colour change—nonfermented), mannitol (no colour change—nonfermented), urease (negative), citrate (negative)

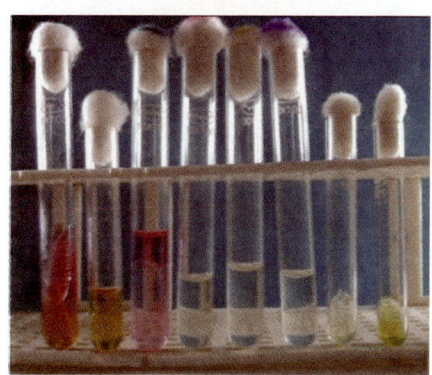

Organism: *Vibrio cholerae*—most common cause of cholera

Colony characteristics: On MacConkey agar, 2–3 mm size, smooth, round, translucent non-lactose fermenter colony (same colour of media) having entire margin.

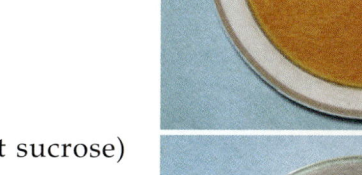

On TCBS (thiosulfate citrate bile salt sucrose) agar, it gives yellow colony.

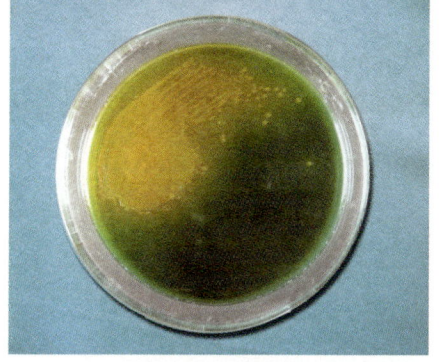

Biochemical test:

From right to left: TSI (yellow/yellow), SIM (motile, no H_2S), Glucose (pink colour—fermented), lactose (no colour change—non-fermented), sucrose (pink colour—fermented), mannitol (pink colour—fermented), urease (negative), citrate (utiliser—colour changed to blue).

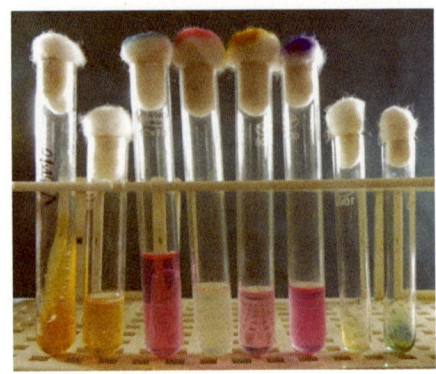

Hanging Drop Preparation

- Done to detect motility of micro-organism
- Can be performed from clinical sample especially in case of cholera
- For microbial identification

Procedure to detect *Vibrio cholerae* in field:

1. A clean concavity slide is taken which is marked with laboratory serial number/patients information
2. A very small amount of stool sample from a patient suspected of cholera is taken and placed on clean coverslip.
3. On all four sides, wax is applied to prevent drying
4. Concavity slide is fixed on such a way that stool sample hangs in concavity of the slide
5. Slide is inverted and examined for the presence of darting motility
6. If darting motility is observed, then anti-O antisera for *Vibrio cholerae* (without preservative) is added
7. In presence of antiserum, no motility is observed.

If no motility after addition of antisera → *Vibrio cholerae*

If motility persists even after addition of antisera → other causative agent of diarrhoea, cholerae

Procedure to determine the motility of micro-organism

1. A clean concavity slide is taken which is marked with laboratory serial number/patients information
2. A small drop of peptone water in whom microbial pathogens have been inoculated already for 2 hours at 37°C, is placed on clean coverslip.
3. On all four sides, wax is applied to prevent drying
4. Concavity slide is fixed on such a way that stool sample hangs in concavity of the slide

5. Slide is inverted and examined for the presence of motility at the margins of drop (400X)

If no motility is observed $\rightarrow$ Nonmotile microbial pathogen

If motility is observed $\quad \rightarrow$ Motile microbial pathogen

Example:
Nonmotile organism: Shigella
Motile organism: *Vibrio cholerae*
Darting motility: *Salmonella typhi*

Public Health Museum

Arti Gupta

FAMILY WELFARE

Spot: Male condom

Type: Barrier method

Trade name: Nirodh, Durex

Composition: Rubber latex

Mechanism of action: Prevents sperm from meeting the ovum

Advantages
- Easy availability
- Safe and inexpensive
- Protects from STD

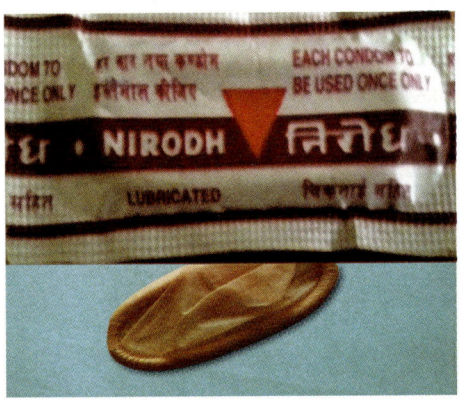

Disadvantage: Slip or tear during intercourse

Failure rate: 14–20%

Spot: Female condom

Type: Vaginal barrier method

Trade name: Velvet, confidom

Composition: Polyurethane

Mechanism of action: Prevents passage of semen into vagina

Advantage: Protects from STD

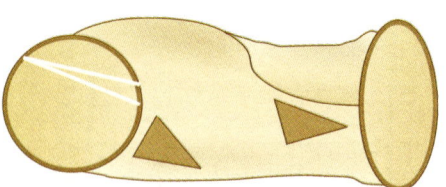

Disadvantages
- Cost
- Low acceptability

Failure rate: 5–21%

Spot: Diaphragm

Type: Vaginal barrier method

Trade name: Dutch cap

Composition: Rubber

Mechanism of action: Prevents passage of semen into cervix

Advantage: Protects from STD
Disadvantages
• Need of physician
• Toxic shock syndrome
Failure rate: 6–18%

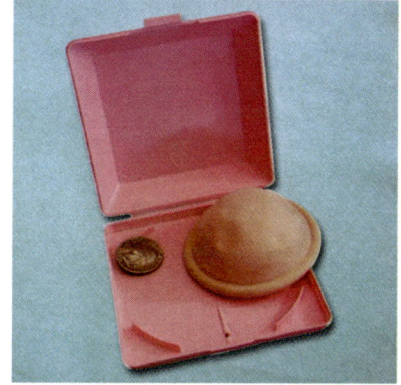

Source: [https://en.wikipedia.org/wiki/
Diaphragm_(birth_control)#/media/
File:Contraceptive_diaphragm.jpg]

Spot: Vaginal contraceptive gel

Type: Vaginal barrier method

Trade name: Gynol, today

Composition: Nonoxynol 9

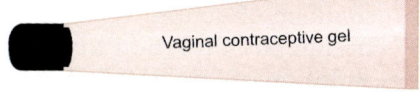

Mechanism of action: Prevents passage of semen into cervix, spermicidal

Failure rate: 18–26%

Spot: Lippies loop

Type: First generation intra-uterine devices (IUD)

Composition: Plastic (polyethylene) impregnated with barium sulfate

Mechanism of action: Sterile inflammatory response: Spermicidal.

Advantage: Long acting

Disadvantages: Pain, bleeding

Failure rate: 3–5%

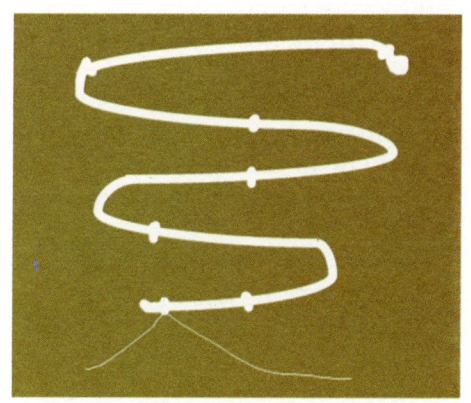

Spot: Copper T

Type: Second generation intra-uterine devices

Example: CuT-380A, Nova T, Multiload

Composition: Copper wire or sleeves are put on the plastic (polyethylene) frame

Mechanism of action

- Sterile inflammatory response spermicidal.
- Release free copper impact endometrium
- Alter cervical and endometrial secretions

Advantage: Long acting

Disadvantages: Pain, bleeding

Failure rate: 0.8%

Ideal candidate: Multiparous woman

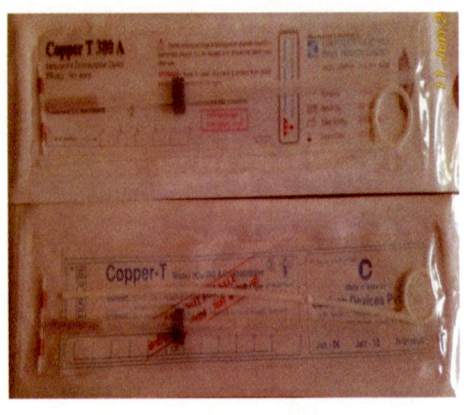

Spot: LNG-20 Mirena

Type: Third generation IUD

Composition: T shape and vertical arm containing 52 mg of levonorgestrel

Mechanism of action:
- Foreign body reaction to endometrium
- Inhibition of implantation
- Sperm—capacitation and survival

Advantage: Long acting

Disadvantages: Pain, bleeding

Failure rate: <0.8%

Ideal candidate- Multiparous woman

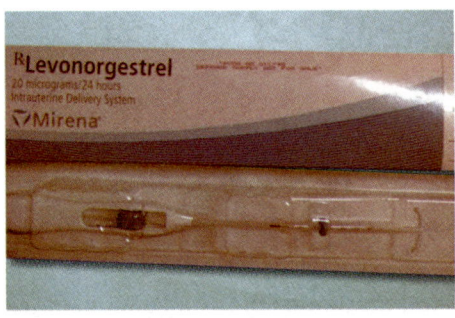

PC- Dr Divya Narayana, Family Welfare Officer, Command hospital, Air force, Bangalore, India.[PC*]

Spot: Mala N

Available in Government Supply

Type: Second generation combined oral contraceptive pill

Composition: Mala-N (30 g EE + 0.30 mg norgestrel per pill)

Mechanism of action: Inhibit ovulation

Advantages

- Early reversibility of fertility
- Decreases menstrual blood loss.

Disadvantages

- Patient compliance is required.
- No protection against STD
- Side-effects like nausea, vomiting, breast tenderness, headache, weight gain.

Ideal candidate: Nulliparous woman

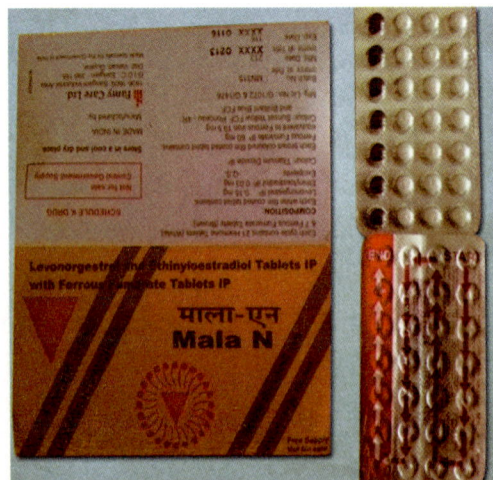

Spot: Mala D

Type: Second generation combined oral contraceptive pill

Composition: 30 g EE + 0.15 mg levonorgestrel per pill

Mechanism of action: Inhibit ovulation

Advantages

* Early reversibility of fertility
* Decreases menstrual blood loss

Disadvantages

* Patient compliance is required.
* No protection against STD
* Side effects like nausea, vomiting, breast tenderness, headache, and weight gain.

Ideal candidate: Nulliparous woman

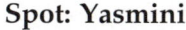

Spot: Yasmini

Type: Fourth generation oral contraceptive pill

Composition: Drospirenone

Mechanism of action: Inhibit ovulation

Advantages: Less side effect compared to second and third generations combined oral contraceptive pill

Ideal candidate: Nulliparous woman

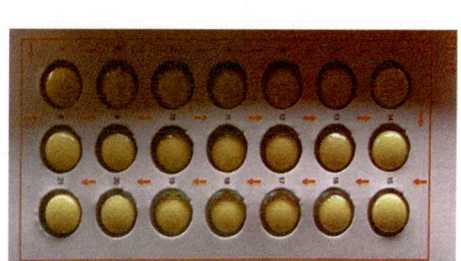

Spot: Emergency contraception

Type: Oral contraceptive pill

Other example: i-pill

Composition: 1.5 mg of levonorgestrel

Mechanism of action: Blocks the actions of the hormones LH and FSH

Advantages

* High efficacy
* No estrogen side-effects

Disadvantages: Fatigue, headache, dizziness, breast tenderness

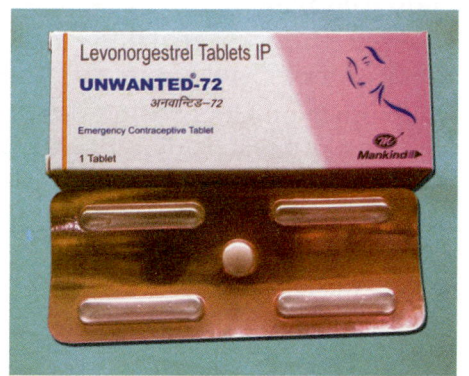

Spot: Injectable contraceptive

Type: Hormonal

Composition: DMPA (depot medroxy progesterone acetate) 150 mg, NET-EN (norethisterone enantate) 200 mg

Mechanism of action: Inhibit ovulation thickens cervical mucus, alters the endometrial receptivity for implantation

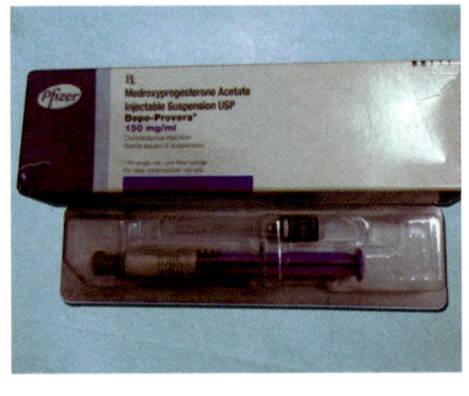

Advantages

- Effective, reversible 2 to 3 monthly
- No daily pill-taking is required
- No estrogen side-effects
- Quantity and quality of breast milk is not affected

Disadvantages

- Changes in menstrual pattern
- Breast tenderness, weight gain, acne

Spot: Norplant

Type: Progestin-only method of contraception

Composition: 6 capsules each 36 mg LNG.

Mechanism of action: Inhibit ovulation thickens cervical mucus, alters the endometrial receptivity for implantation

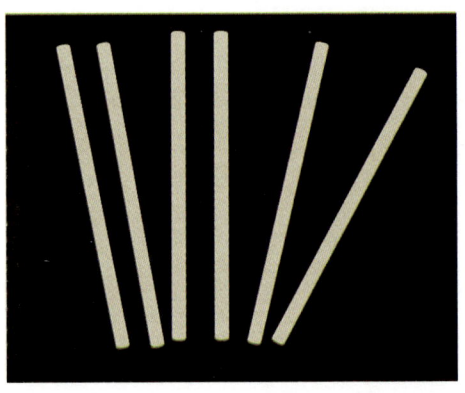

Advantages: Very effective, long acting, reversible no daily pill-taking is required

Disadvantages: Weight gain, breast tenderness, disruption of menstrual cycles, requires surgical procedure

Spot: Abortion pills

Composition: Mifepristone is a synthetic steroid. Misoprostol is a prostaglandin

Mechanism of action: Mifepristone works by blocking progesterone, misoprostol causes contractions of the womb

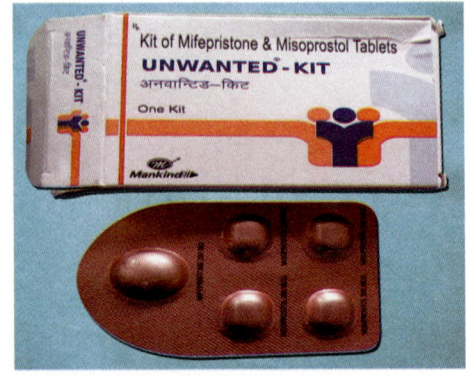

Advantages

- Easy availability
- Less invasive

Disadvantages: Headache, gastritis

Failure rate: 0.5–1%

Spot: Centchroman

Type: Nonhormonal, nonsteroidal oral contraceptive

Composition: Ormeloxifene

Mechanism of action: Anti-estrogenic, asynchrony between ovulation and the development of the endometrium

Advantages

- Effective for dysfunctional uterine bleeding
- Advanced breast cancer.

Disadvantage: Delayed menstruation

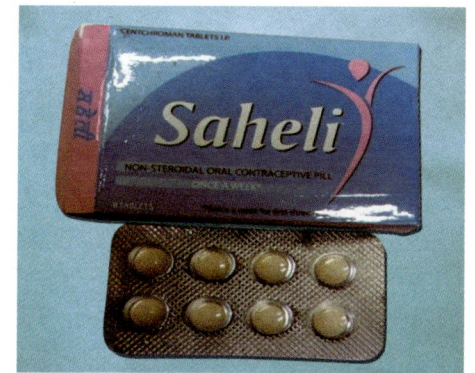

Spot: Vaginal ring

Type: Polymeric hormone delivery devices

Composition: Drospirenone

Mechanism of action: Stops sperm from meeting an egg, therefore, inhibiting fertilization and stops ovulation

Disadvantage: Require to be changed every month

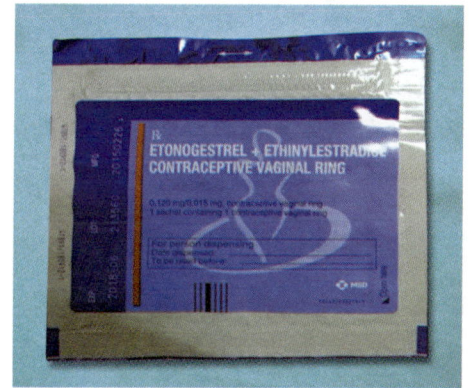

Spot: Ginette35

Type: Antiandrogen and oral contraceptive

Composition: Cyproterone acetate 2 mg, ethinylestradiol 0.035 mg

Mechanism of action: Inhibit ovulation

Advantages: Less side effect compared to second and third generations combined oral contraceptive pill, effective for acne and hirsutism

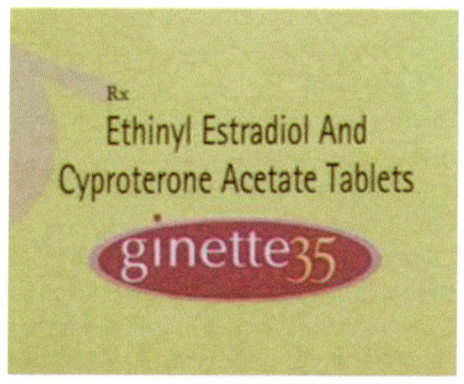

IMMUNIZATION

Spot: BCG (Bacillus Calmette-Guérin) vaccine
Type: Live bacterial vaccine
Strain: Danish 1331
Dose: 0.1 ml (0.05 ml for less than 1 month)
Site: Left upper arm (insertion of deltoid)
Route: Intra-dermal using 26G needle
Diluent: 1 ml sodium chloride (normal saline)
Age of administration: Give at birth or as early as possible in the first 12 months
One vial: 10 doses
Disease prevented: Tuberculosis
Precaution: Discard vaccine 4 hours after constitution
Side effect: Suppurative lymphadenitis
Contraindication: Immunodeficient child

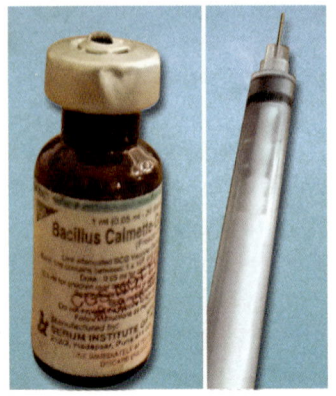

Spot: OPV (Oral Polio Vaccine)
Type: Live attenuated vaccine
Strain: Bivalent
Dose: 2 drops
Route: By mouth (oral administration)
Age of administration: At birth—zero dose
1½ months (6 weeks)—1st dose
2½ months (10 weeks)—2nd dose
3½ months (14 weeks)—3rd dose
1½ year—Booster dose
One vial: 20 doses
Disease prevented: Poliomyelitis
Precaution: Stored between + 2° and + 8°C
Side effect: Paralytic polio
Contraindication: Immunodeficient child

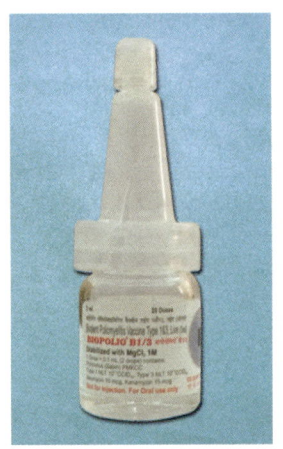

Spot: IPV (Injectable Polio Vaccine)
Type: Killed vaccine
Strain: Trivalent
Dose: 0.5 ml
Route: Intramuscular
Site: Anterolateral side of mid thigh—right
Age of administration: 14 weeks
One vial: 10 doses
Disease prevented: Poliomyelitis
Precaution: Discard vaccine after 6 hours
Contraindication: History of an allergic reaction, allergy to streptomycin, neomycin, or polymyxin B

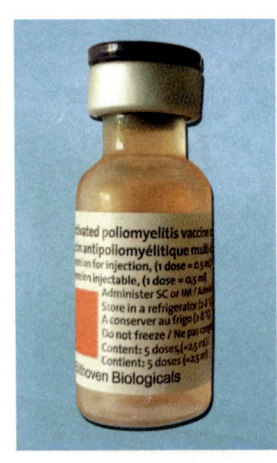

Spot: Pentavalent vaccine
Type: Killed vaccine
Dose: 0.5 ml
Site: Anterolateral side of mid thigh—left
Route: Intramuscular
Age of administration: 1½ months (6 weeks)—1st dose
2½ months (10 weeks)—2nd dose
3½ months (14 weeks)—3rd dose
One vial: 10 doses
Disease prevented: Diphtheria, tetanus, pertussis, hepatitis B, *Haemophilus influenzae* type B
Side effect: Fever
Precaution: Never use frozen vaccine

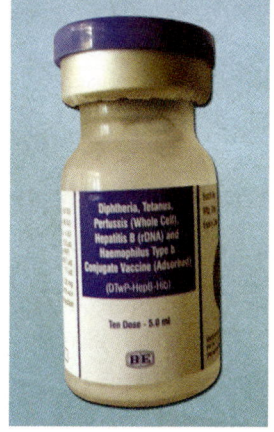

Spot: DPT vaccine
Type: Killed vaccine
Dose: 0.5 ml
Site: Anterolateral side of mid thigh—left
Route: Intramuscular
Age of administration: 1½ months (6 weeks)—1st dose
2½ months (10 weeks)—2nd dose
3½ months (14 weeks)—3rd dose
1½ year—1st booster dose
5–6 years—2nd booster dose (left upper arm)
One vial: 10 doses
Disease prevented: Diphtheria-pertussis-tetanus
Side effects: Fever, rarely seizures
Precaution: Never give DPT in buttocks

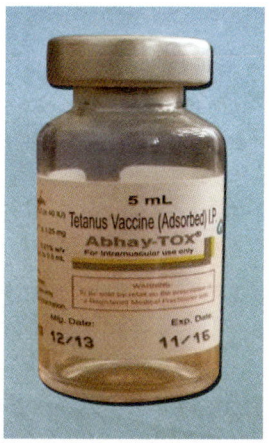

Spot: Hepatitis B vaccine
Type: Killed vaccine
Dose: 0.5 ml
Site: Anterolateral side of mid-thigh—left
Route: Intramuscular
Age of administration: Within 24 hours of birth—birth dose if not pentavental vaccine:
1½ months (6 weeks)—1st dose
2½ months (10 weeks)—2nd dose
3½ months (14 weeks)—3rd dose
One vial: 10 doses
Precaution: Never use frozen vaccine

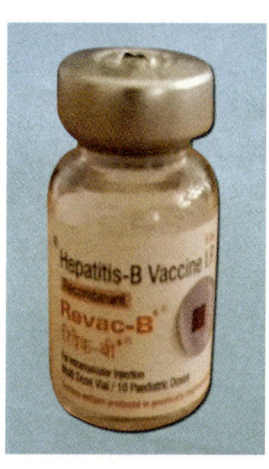

Spot: Measles vaccine

Type: Live vaccine

Strain: Edmonston—Zagreb

Dose: 0.5 ml

Site: Right upper arm

Route: Subcutaneous

Diluent: 2.5 ml double distilled water

Age of administration: First dose—9 completed months

If a child does not receive measles before the 12th month, give a dose as soon as possible before 5 years of age.

Second dose: 16–24 months

One vial: 5 doses

Disease prevented: Measles

Precaution: Discard vaccine 4 hours

Contraindication: Immunodeficient child

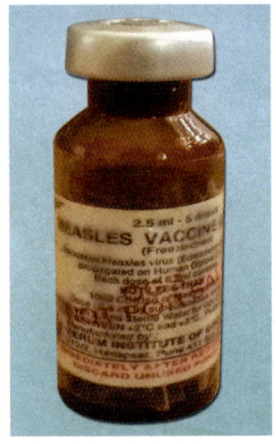

Spot: Tetanus vaccine

Type: Killed vaccine

Dose: 0.5 ml

Site: Upper arm, deltoid muscle

Route: Intramuscular

Age of administration

- 10 years and 16 years
- First dose early in pregnancy and 2nd at least 4 weeks later

One vial: 10 doses

Disease prevented: Tetanus

Precaution: Never use frozen vaccine give TT booster only if already received at least two TT injections within last 3 years

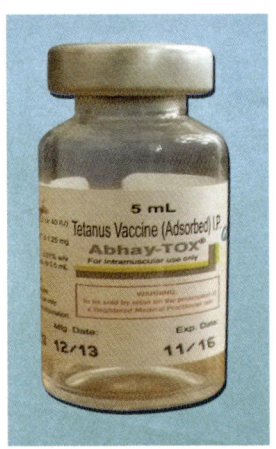

Spot: Rotavirus vaccine

Dose: 5 drops per dose

Route: Oral

Age of administration

1½ months (6 weeks)—1st dose

2½ months (10 weeks)—2nd dose

3½ months (14 weeks)—3rd dose

Disease prevented: Diarrhoea due to rotavirus

Presently in selected states

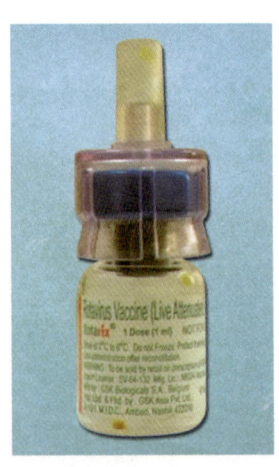

Spot: Measles rubella vaccine

Type: Live vaccine

Dose: 0.5 ml

Route: Subcutaneous injection

Diluent: 2.5 ml double distilled water

Age of administration: 9 months to less than 15 years

One vial: 5 doses

Disease prevented: Measles, rubella

Precaution: Discard vaccine 4 hours after constitution

Contraindication: Immunodeficient child

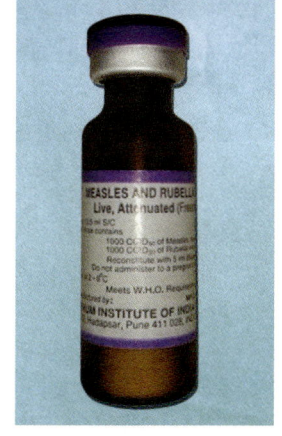

Spot: Vaccine vial monitor (VVM)

Use: For checking heat damage

Interpretation: Vaccine can be used if it is within expiry date and the colour of inner square of VVM is lighter than the colour of outer circle.

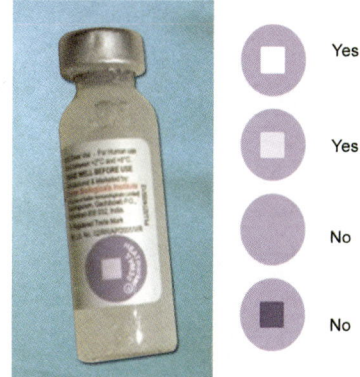

Spot: Alcohol thermometer

Use: To monitor the temperature of cold chain at PHC

Principle: Thermocouple

Monitoring frequency: Twice daily (morning and evening)

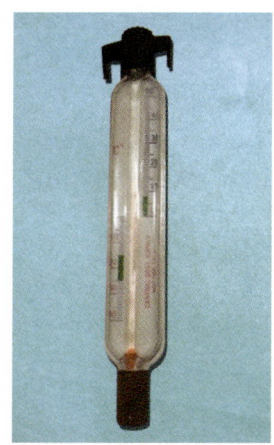

Spot: Vitamin A

Dose: 1st dose—1 ml, 2nd to 9th dose—2 ml

Route: Oral

Age of administration:

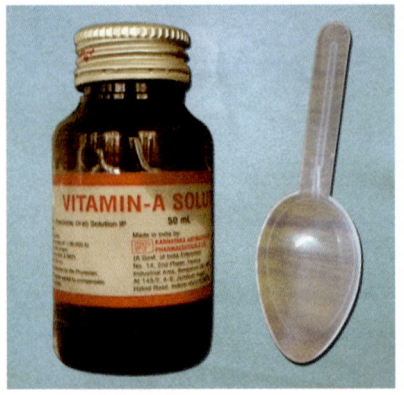

- First dose at 9 months with measles
- Second dose at 16 months with DPT/OPV booster, then one dose every 6 months up to the age of 5 years

Disease prevented: Vitamin A deficiency

Precaution: Use the bottle within 6–8 weeks once opened

Use only spoon provided with bottle observing marks for 1 ml and 2 ml

Spot: Deep freezer

Level: Large ILR at district; Small ILR at PHC

Capacity: Large 300 litres; Small 140 litres

Temperature: ± 20° to –40°C

Storage duration: 1 month

Use: Vaccine and diluents storage and temperature maintenance

Use to prepare icepacks

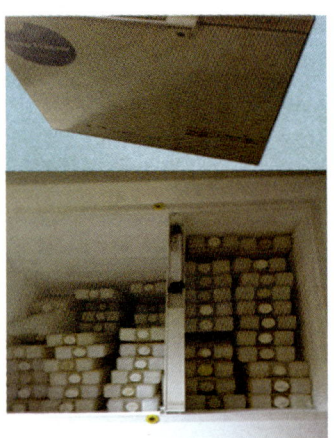

Spot: Ice-lined refrigerator

Level: Large ILR at district; small ILR at PHC

Capacity: Large 300/240 litres; Small 140 litres

Temperature: + 2° to + 8°C

Storage duration: 1 month

Use: Vaccine and diluents storage and temperature maintenance

Order of vaccines from top to bottom: Hep B—pentavalent, DPT, TT—JE—BCG—Measles—OPV

Follow early expiry first out (EEFO)

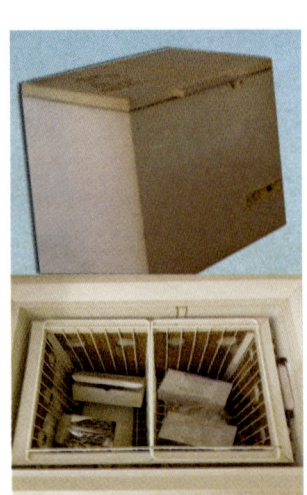

Spot: Vaccine carrier
Number of vaccine vials: 16–20 vials
Level: Subcentre
Temperature: + 2° to + 8°C
Storage duration: 48 to 72 hours
Fully frozen ice-packs: 4
Use: Vaccine transportation from PHC to immunization site
Red vaccine carrier: Used for reverse cold chain

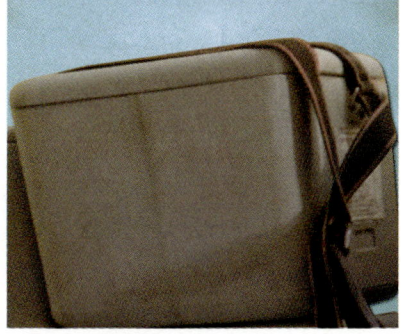

Spot: Day carrier
Number of vaccine vials: 6–8 vials
Level: Subcentre
Temperature: + 2° to + 8°C
Storage duration: 48 to 72 hours
Use: Vaccine transportation from PHC to immunization site
Fully frozen ice-packs: 2

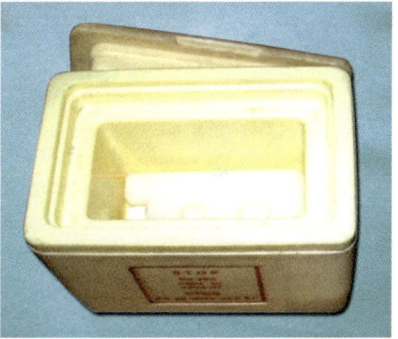

Spot: Ice-pack
Capacity: 320–340 ml
Horizontal mark: Water fill level
Level: Session site
Temperature: + 2° to + 8°C
Use: Temperature maintenance during vaccine transportation and immunization session
Storage duration: 1 to 3 hours

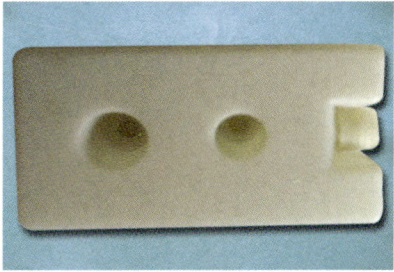

Spot: HUB cutter
Use: Used for cutting the nib from the syringe
Advantages: Prevent reuse of needle, prevent needle stick injury, prevent infections

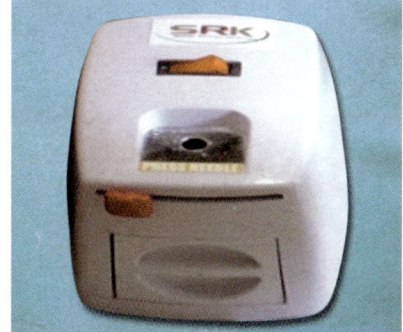

Image	Spot	Calorie (kcal) per 100 g edible portion	Protein (gm) per 100 g edible portion	Calorie (kcal) per household cooked measure	Protein (gm) per household cooked measure	Rich source/use	Limiting source
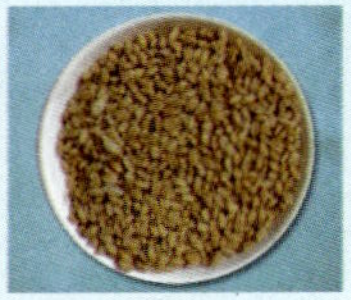	**Wheat**	341	12.1	85 per med. roti	3 per med. roti	Linolenic acid, vitamin B	Threonine and lysine amino acid
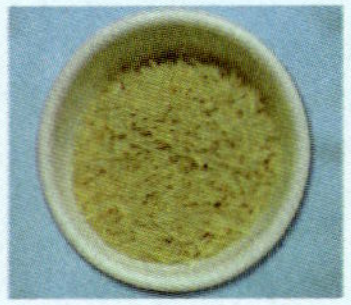	**Rice**	345	6.8	86 per ¾ katori	1.7 per ¾ katori	Lysine compared to other cereals, thiamine	Vitamins A, D, C, calcium, iron
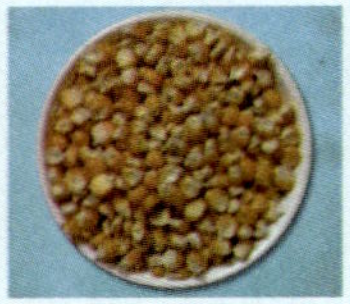	**Maize (corn, bhutta)**	342	11.1	≈85 per ¾ katori	≈3 per ¾ katori	Carotenoid pigment, High leucine can cause pellagra	Tryptophan and lysine
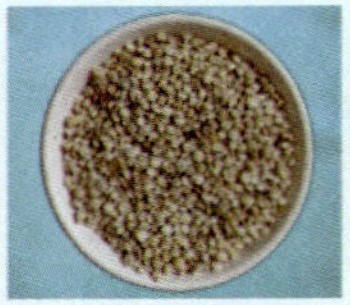	**Jowar (sorghum)**	340	9–14	≈85 per ¾ katori	≈3 per ¾ katori	High leucine can cause pellagra	Lysine and threonine
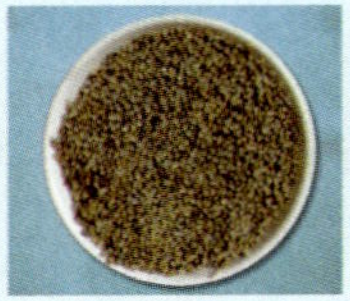	**Bajra (pearl millet)**	361	10–14	≈85 per ¾ katori	≈3 per ¾ katori	Vitamin B, calcium, iron	Lysine and threonine

Image	Spot	Calorie (kcal) per 100 g edible portion	Protein (gm) per 100 g edible portion	Calorie (kcal) per household cooked measure	Protein (gm) per household cooked measure	Rich source/use	Limiting source
	Ragi	328	7	111 calories per ¼ cup	≈2 per cup	Calcium, iron	–
	Bread	245	7.8	61 per slice	2 per slice	–	–
	Cornflakes	376	8	94 per ½ cup	2 per ½ cup	Carbohydrates	–
	Dalia/oats	346	11.8	87 per ½ cup	3 per ½ cup	Fibres	–
	Red gram (arhar dal)	335	22.3	86 per katori	6 per katori	Protein, vitamin B	Methionine and cysteine

(Contd.)

Image	Spot	Calorie (kcal) per 100 g edible portion	Protein (gm) per 100 g edible portion	Calorie (kcal) per household cooked measure	Protein (gm) per household cooked measure	Rich source/use	Limiting source
	Bengal gram (kala chana)	360	17.1	≈90 per katori	≈4 per katori	Protein, vitamin C, calcium	–
	Green gram (mung dal)	≈350	24	≈90 per katori	≈6 per katori	Protein	–
	Soya bean	432	43.2	108 per katori	11 per katori	Protein, iron, calcium	Methionine
	Cow pea (lobia)	≈350	≈20	≈90 per katori	≈5 per katori	Protein	–
	Kidney beans (rajmah)	337	25	≈85 per katori	≈6 per katori	Protein, calcium	–

(Contd.)

Image	Spot	Calorie (kcal) per 100 g edible portion	Protein (gm) per 100 g edible portion	Calorie (kcal) per household cooked measure	Protein (gm) per household cooked measure	Rich source/use	Limiting source
	Leafy (Spinach)	33.6	2	42 per katori	2.5 per katori	Iron	
	Seasonal Peas	≈51	≈2	≈51 per katori	≈2 per katori	Protein	—
	Cauliflower	≈25	≈2	≈25 per katori	≈2 per katori	Vitamins C and K	—
	Ladyfinger	≈33	≈1.9	≈33 per katori	≈2 per katori	—	—
	Brinjal	≈35	≈0.8	≈35 per katori	≈1 per katori	—	—

(*Contd.*)

Image	Spot	Calorie (kcal) per 100 g edible portion	Protein (gm) per 100 g edible portion	Calorie (kcal) per household cooked measure	Protein (gm) per household cooked measure	Rich source/use	Limiting source
	Roots and tuber: Potato, arbi	93	1	93 per katori	1 per katori	Carbohydrate	
	Egg	173	13.3	70 per pc (60 g)	6 per pc (60 g)	All 9 amino acids	Carbohydrate, vitamin C
	Chicken	109	26	109 per portion	26 per portion	Protein	–
	Fish	97	19.5	97 per two pc	16.6 per two pc	Unsaturated fatty acid, vitamins A and D	Less iron, carbohydrate
	Mutton	191	21.4	191	21.4	Protein, iron, zinc, vitamin B	Calcium

(Contd.)

Image	Spot	Calorie (kcal) per 100 g edible portion	Protein (gm) per 100 g edible portion	Calorie (kcal) per household cooked measure	Protein (gm) per household cooked measure	Rich source/use	Limiting source
	Oil/ghee	900	0	45 per tsp (per 5 gm)	0	Fat	Vegetable oils contain no vitamin A and D
	Almonds	655	20.8	163 per handful (25 gm)	5.2 per handful (25 gm)	Omega 3 fatty acid, vitamin B	–
	Full cream milk	90.8	3.2	215 per glass (250 ml)	8 per glass (250 ml)	Calcium	Vitamin C
	Curd	61.6	3.2	77 per katori (125 ml)	4 per katori (125 ml)	Calcium	Vitamin C
	Paneer	256	16	64 per pc (25 gm)	4 per pc (25 gm)	Protein	Vitamin C

(Contd.)

Image	Spot	Calorie (kcal) per 100 g edible portion	Protein (gm) per 100 g edible portion	Calorie (kcal) per household cooked measure	Protein (gm) per household cooked measure	Rich source/use	Limiting source
	Butter milk	15.6	0.8	39 per glass (250 ml)	2 per glass (250 ml)	Electrolytes	Vitamin C
	Sugar	400	0	20 per tsp (5 gm)	0	Pure sucrose	No other nutrients
	Groundnut	567	25.3	142 per handful (25 gm)	6.3 per handful (25 gm)	Proteins	
	Coconut fresh	444	4.5	444	4.5	Electrolytes	
	Banana	104	1.2	104 per pc (100 gm)	1.2 per pc (100 gm)	Potassium	

(Contd.)

Image	Spot	Calorie (kcal) per 100 g edible portion	Protein (gm) per 100 g edible portion	Calorie (kcal) per household cooked measure	Protein (gm) per household cooked measure	Rich source/use	Limiting source
	Apple	51	0.6	51	0.6	Iron	
	Mango	74	1	74	1	Carotenes	
	Jaggery	358	0	≈18 per tsp	0	Iron	
	Biscuit (1pc ≈5 gm)	509	8.4	25.5	0.42	Fat	

(Contd.)

Image	Spot	Calorie (kcal) per 100 g edible portion	Protein (gm) per 100 g edible portion	Calorie (kcal) per household cooked measure	Protein (gm) per household cooked measure	Rich source/use	Limiting source
	Sweet (1 pc = ≈50 gm)	–	–	175	5	Fat	
	Pastry	–	–	260	3	Fat	

DRUGS

Spot: Old anti-tubercular treatment: Category I
* For detail refer to chapter on tuberculosis

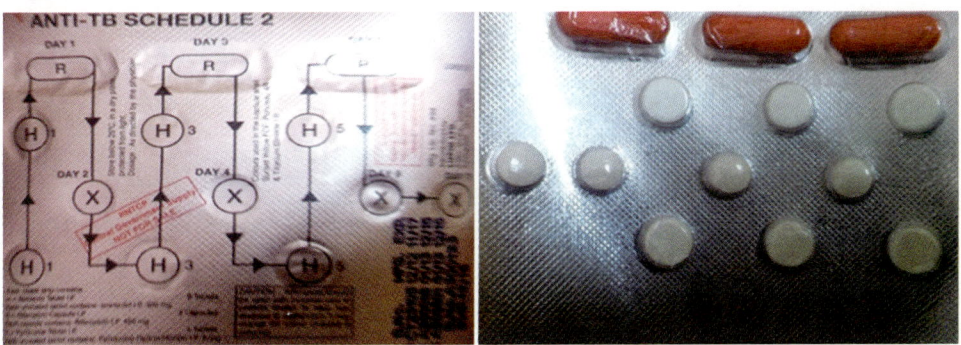

Spot: Old anti-tubercular treatment: Category II
*For detail refer to chapter on tuberculosis

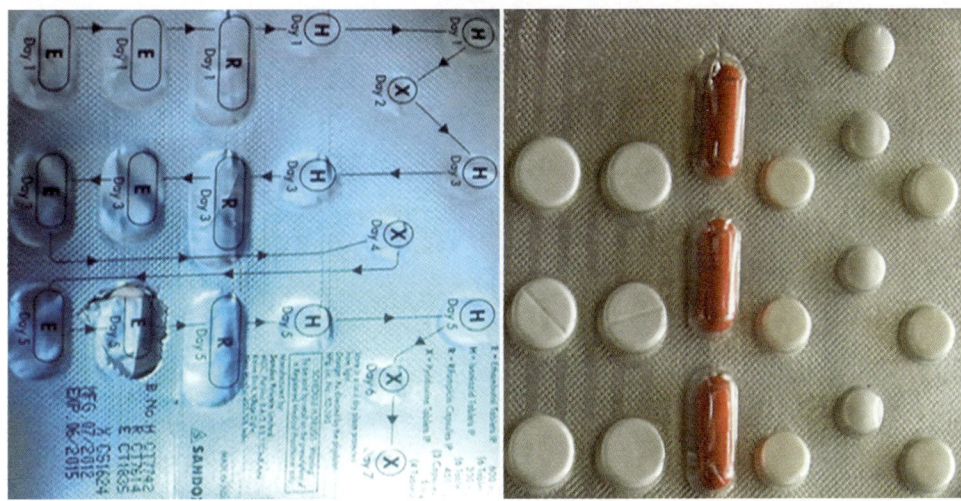

Spot: Anti-tubercular treatment for children
Orange—PC 13
Yellow—PC 14

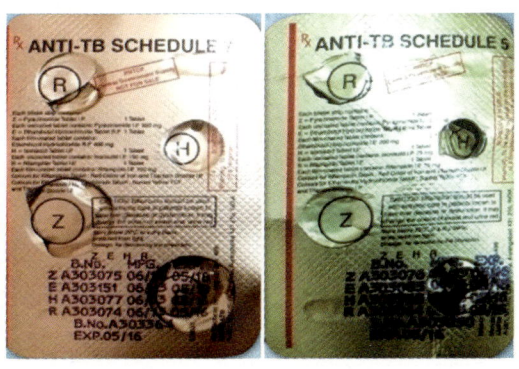

Spot: New anti-tubercular treatment schedule 9 for intensive phase

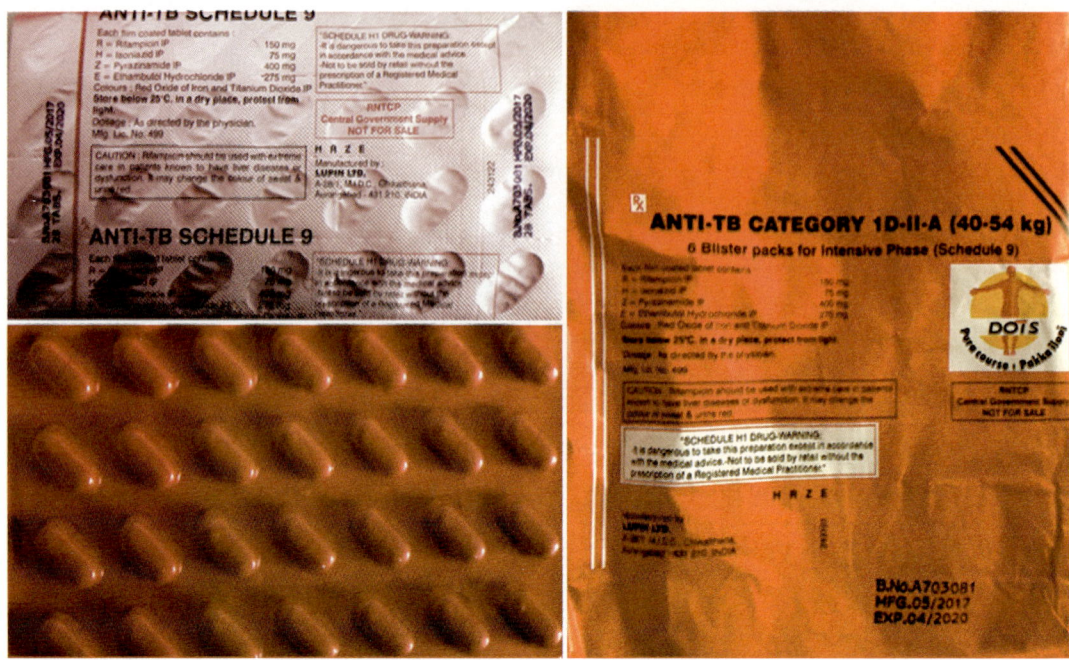

Spot: New anti-tubercular treatment schedule 10 for continuation phase

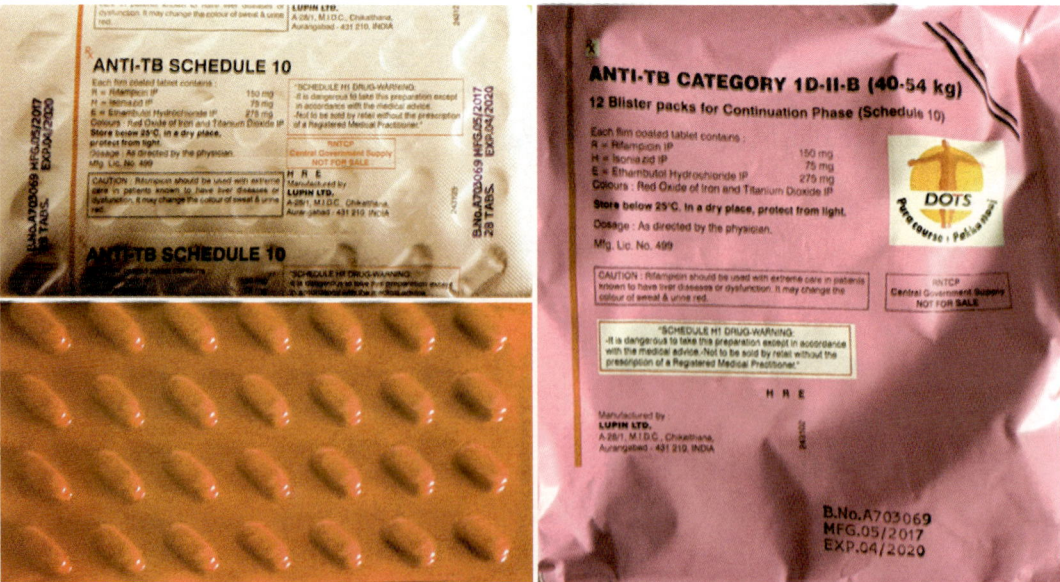

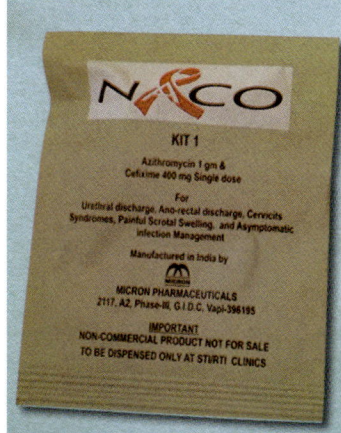
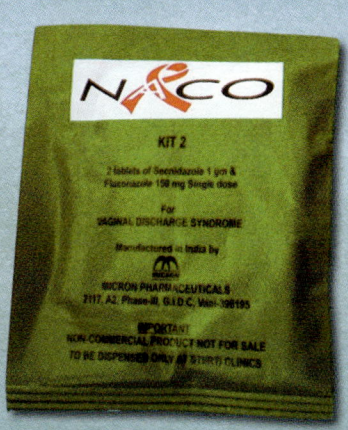
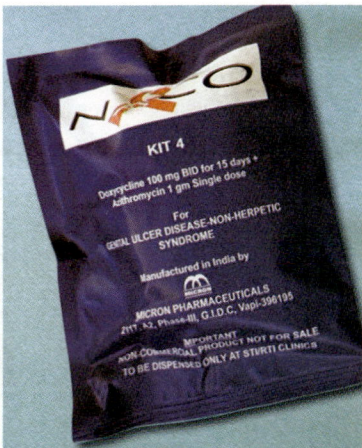

Spot: Pre-packed sexually transmitted and reproductive tract infection (STI/RTI) Kits

Kit 1 Grey for urethral discharge, anorectal discharge, cervicitis syndromes

Kit 2 Green for vaginal syndrome

Kit 3 White for syphilis

Kit 4 Blue for genital ulcer disease, e.g. chancroid

Kit 5 Red for herpetic genital ulcer disease

Kit 6 Yellow for lower abdominal pain

Kit 7 Black for inguinal bubo

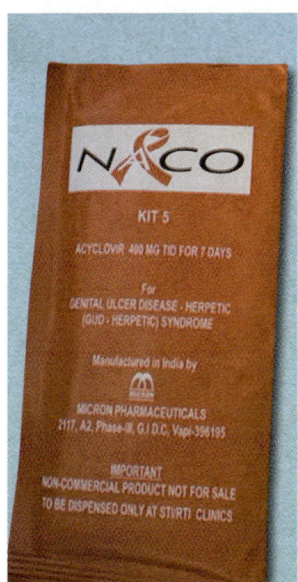
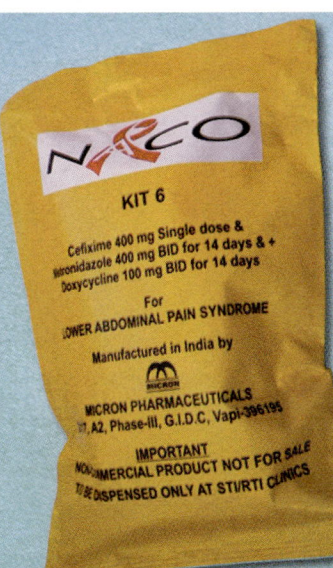
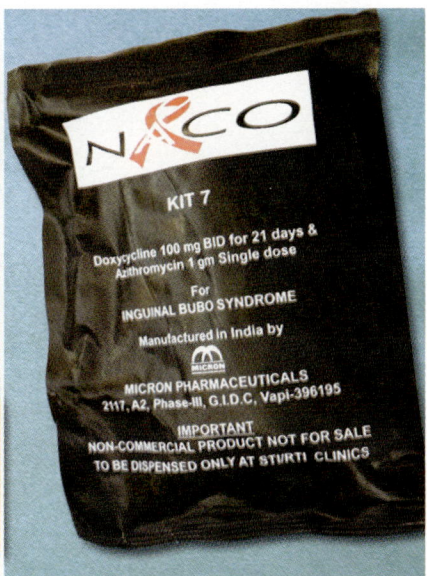

Spot: Artemisinin-based combination therapy
Use: Treatment of *P. falciparum* malaria
*For detail refer to chapter on fever

Spot: Chloroquine
Use: Treatment of *P. vivax* malaria
*For detail refer to chapter on fever

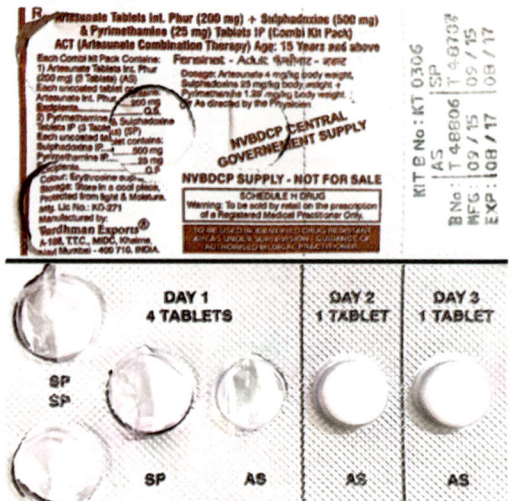

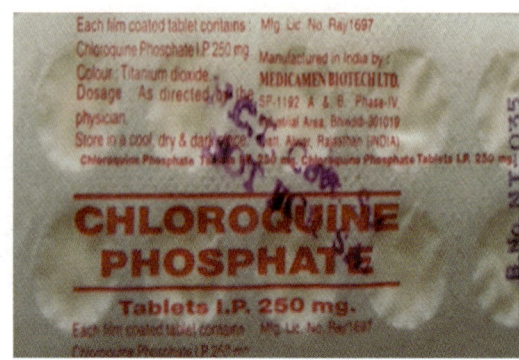

Spot: Antiretroviral therapy (ART) for HIV/AIDS for adult
*For detail refer to chapter on HIV

Spot: Antiretroviral therapy (ART) for HIV/AIDS for children
*For detail refer to chapter on HIV

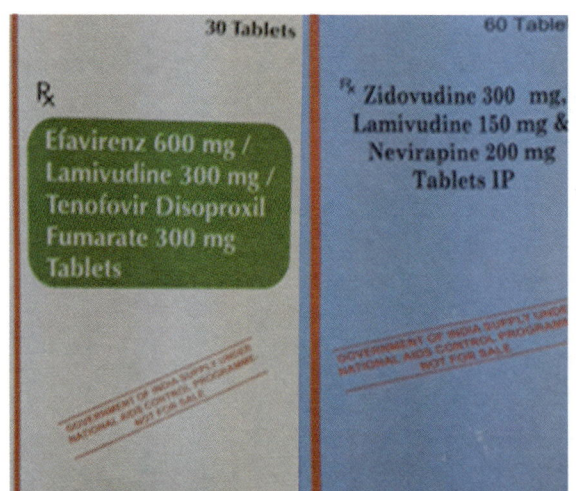

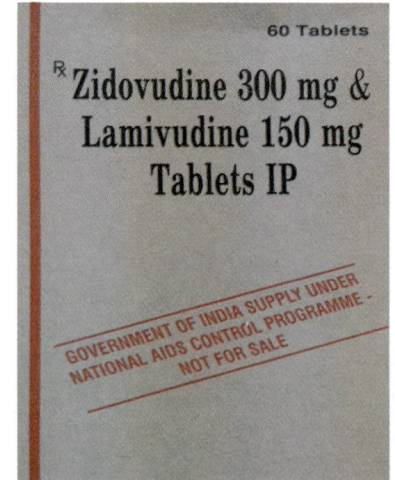

Spot: Oral rehydration spot (ORS)
*For detail refer to chapter on diarrhoea

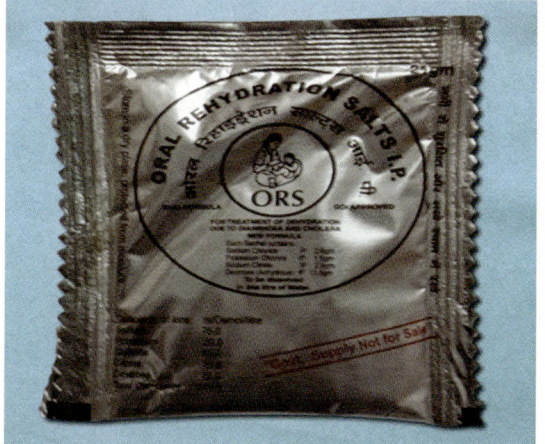

Spot: Zinc
*For detail refer to chapter on diarrhoea

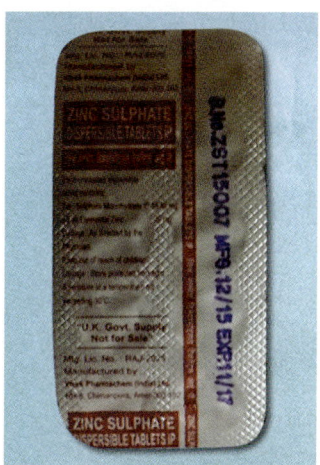

Spot: Iron folic acid (IFA) tablet
*For detail refer to chapter on anaemia

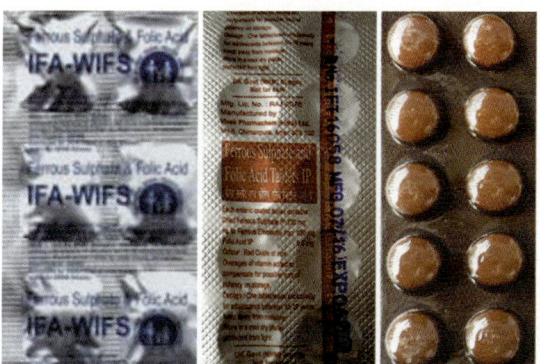

Spot: Albendazole tablet
*For detail refer to chapter on anaemia

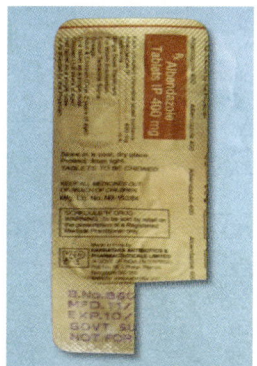

DISINFECTANTS/ANTISEPTICS

Spot: Phenol
Chemical composition: Carbolic acid
Use: Used for mopping floors and cleaning drains.

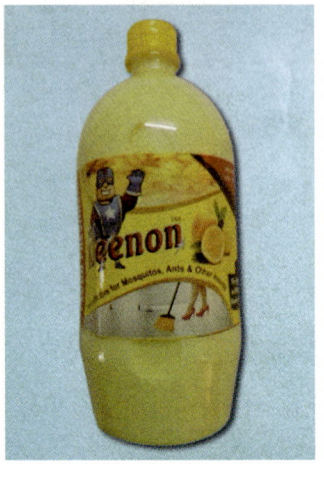

Spot: Potassium Permanganate
Use: Used to disinfect
- Foot before entering swimming pools
- Fruits and vegetables
- Aquariums

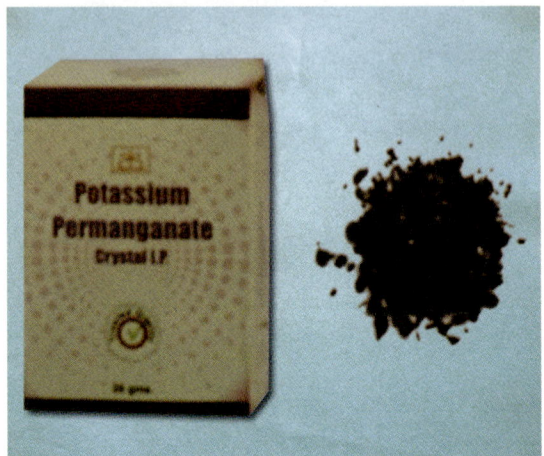

Spot: Antiseptic
Active component: Chloroxylenol
Use:
- Antiseptic against streptococci
- Disinfection instruments and others

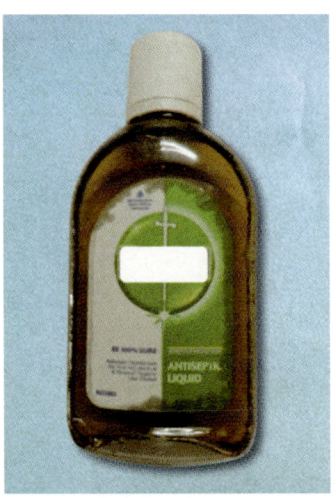

Spot: Antiseptic
Active component: Cetavlon and hibitane
Use:
- As antiseptic
- As disinfectant of plastic appliances like lippes loop
- Disinfectant for thermometers

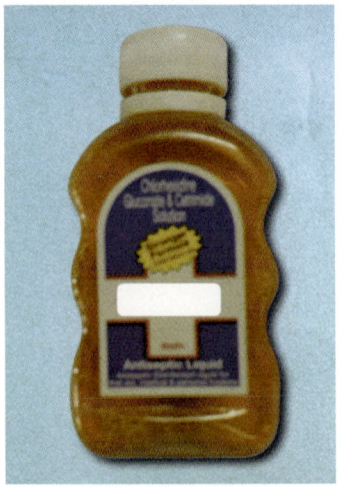

Spot: Hydrogen peroxide
Use: Used to disinfect surfaces in hospital settings, used as antiseptic to cleaning wounds and ulcers

Spot: Iodine
Active component: Complexes of iodine and solubilizers
Use:
• Bactericidal agents
• Antiseptics with sporocidal action

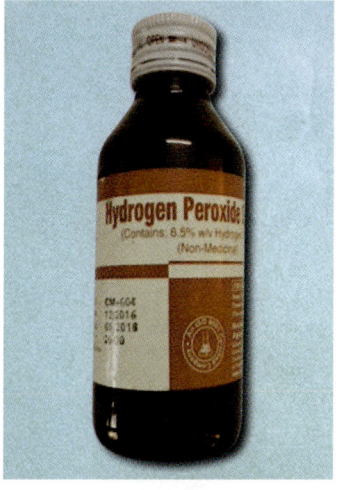

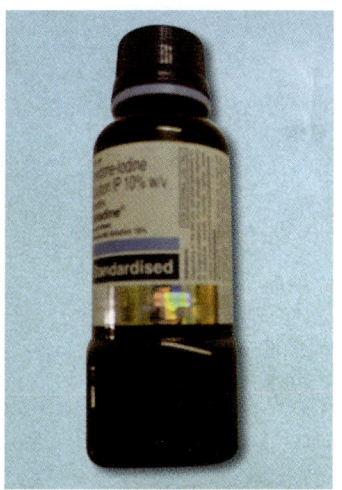

Miscellaneous

Spot: Bleaching powder
Active component: Calcium hypochlorite
Use:
• Disinfection of water, faeces and urine
• Cleaning floor
• Disinfecting instruments

Spot: Chlorine tablets
Use: One tablet of chlorine containing 0.5 g of chlorine is sufficient to disinfect about 20 litres of water in 1 hour

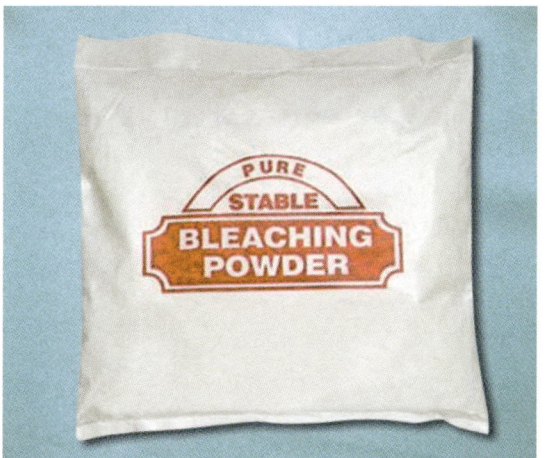

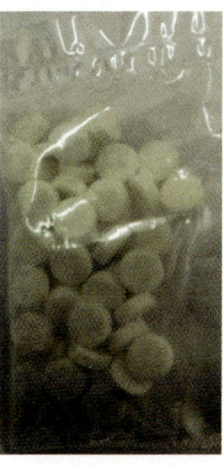

Spot: Anti-adult mosquito cream
Active component: DEET (N, N-diethyl-3-
methyl benzamide)

Spot: Rat poison
Active component: Bromadiolone

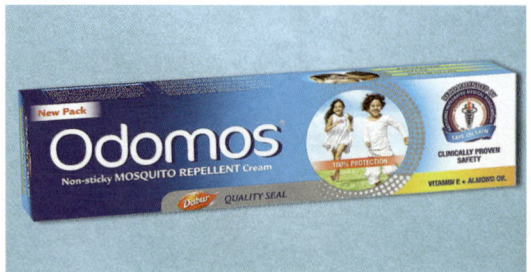

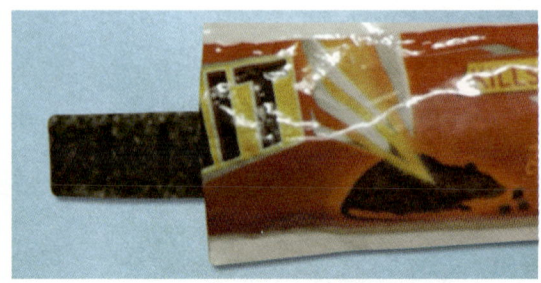

Spot: Anti-adult mosquito spray
Active component: Pyrethroid
compound

Spot: Anti-adult mosquito repellant
Active component: A pyrethroid
compound like malathion

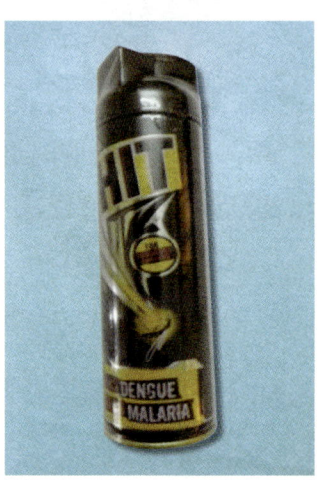

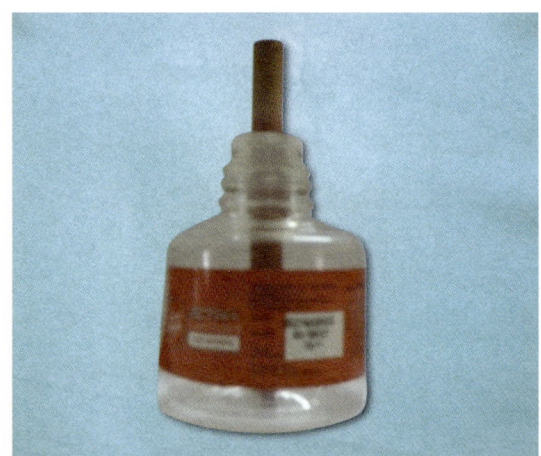

Spot: Spirit
Active component: Ethyl and isopropyl alcohols
Use:
- Antiseptics
- Disinfectants for skin
- Handwashing

Spot: Anti-cockroach
Active component: Imiprothrin cypermethrin

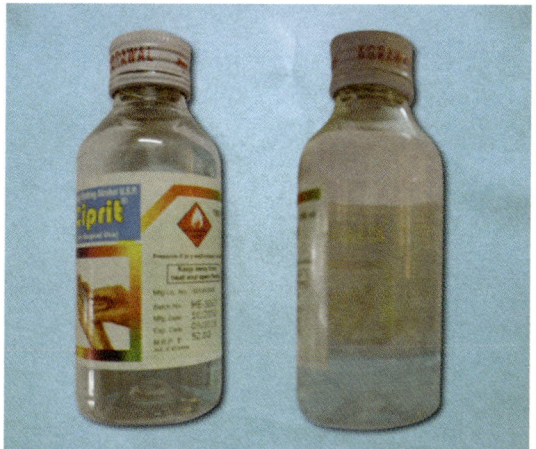

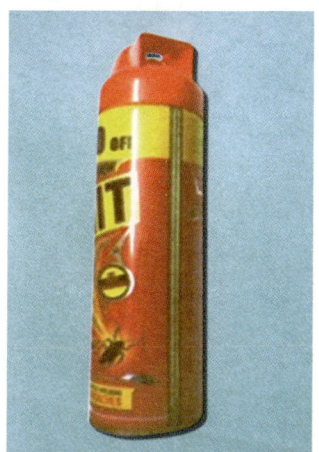

Spot: Anti-adult mosquito coil
Active component: Pyrethrum

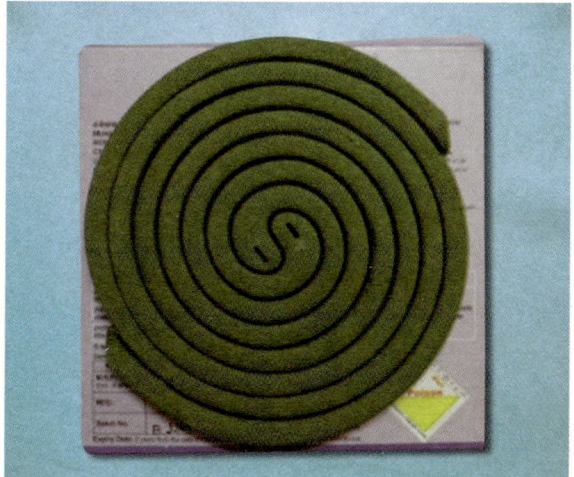

ENTOMOLOGY

Anopheles mosquito

Macroscopic		Microscopic

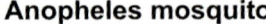

Female adult diseases transmitted

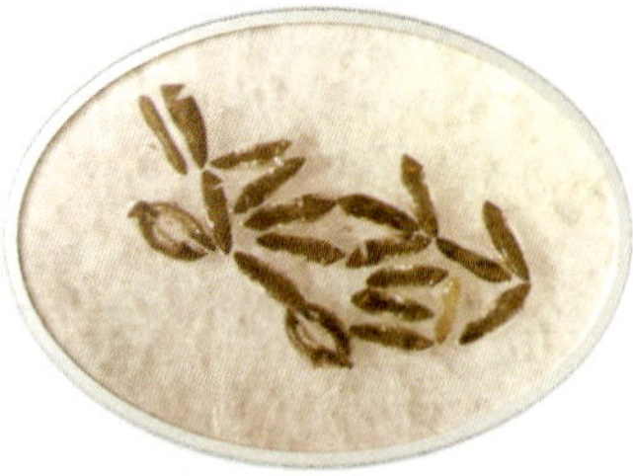

Egg

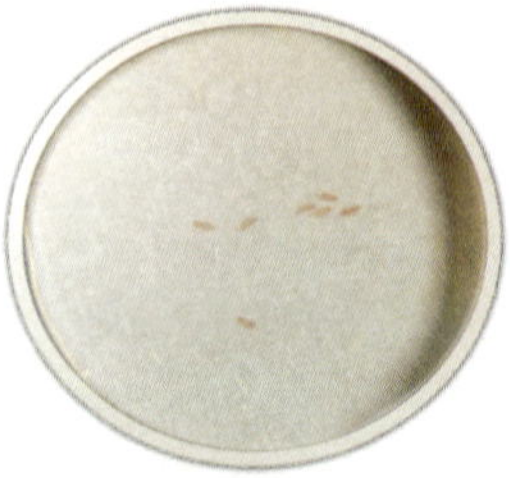

Eggs:
Laid singly, boat-shaped provided with lateral floats

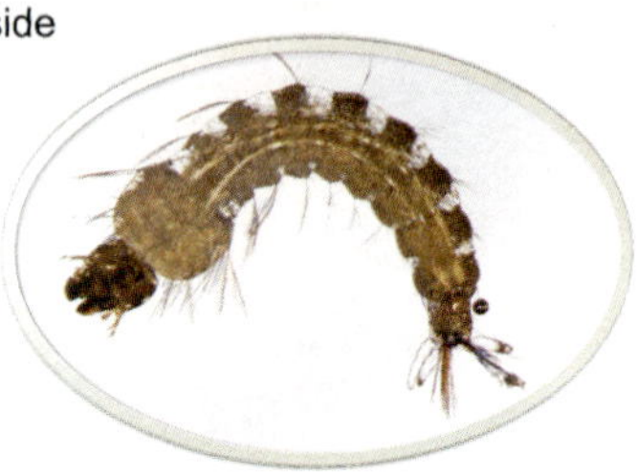

- Malaria
- Filaria (outside India)

Larva

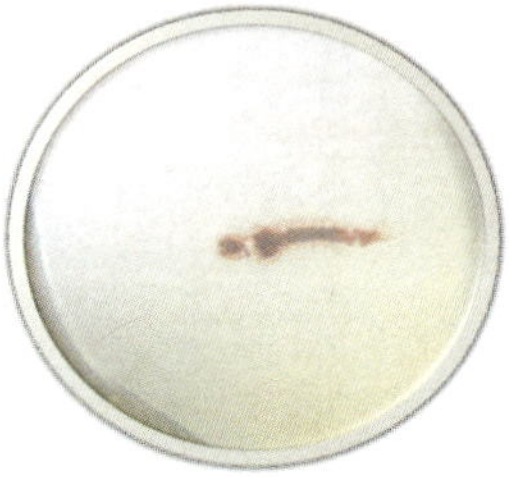

Larvae:
Rest parallel to water surface no siphon tube

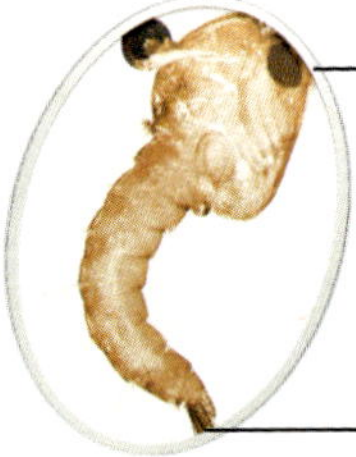

Pupa
Air trumpet

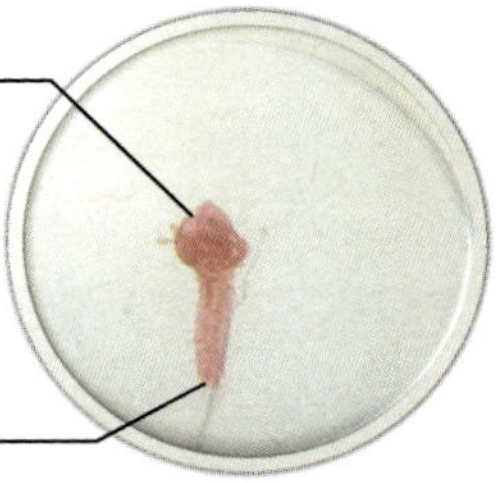

Pupa:
Siphon tube is broad and short

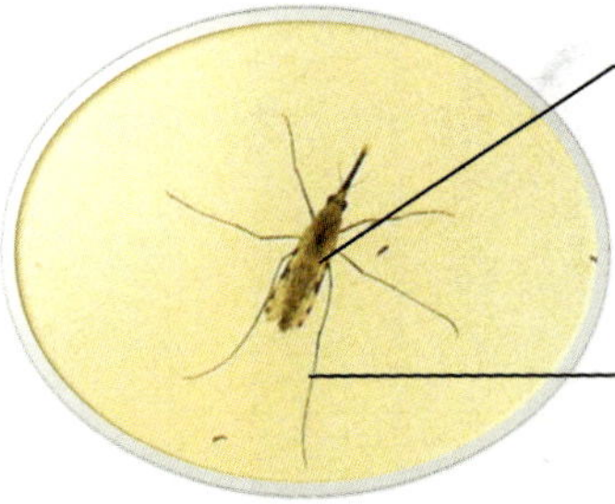

Siphon tube

Adult
Spotted wings

Legs

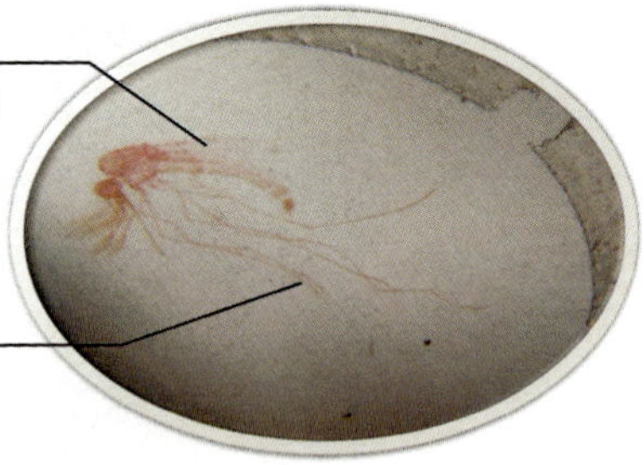

Source for the macroscopic images is https://pixnio.com.

Culex mosquito

Macroscopic	Microscopic

Female adult diseases transmitted

Egg

Eggs:
Laid in cluster raft like
no air floats

Larva

Siphon tube

• Bancroftian filariasis
• Japanese encephalitis
• West Nile fever
• Viral arthritis

Siphon tube

Larvae:
Siphon tube present also known as wriggler

Pupa
Air trumpet

Siphon tube

Siphon tube

Pupa:
Siphon tube is long

Adult
unspotted wings

Legs

Adult:
When at rest, rest parallel to surface, therefore posterior limbs are almost equal to anterior limbs
wings are unspotted.

Source for the macroscopic images is https://pixnio.com.

Others

Macroscopic   **Microscopic**

Diseases transmitted

Housefly

Housefly does not bite:

Modes of disease transmission
Mechanical
Vomit-drop
Defection

- Typhoid and paratyphoid fevers
- Diarrhoea
- Dysenteries
- Cholera
- Gastroenteritis
- Amoebiasis
- Anthrax
- Trachoma
- Poliomyelitis
- Yaws

Housefly mouth part

— Haustellum —

— Mouth —

Sand fly

Sand fly:
- Kala azar
- Visceral leishmaniasis
- Sandfly fever
- Oriental sore

— Dappled wing —

Sand flies are small insects light or dark brown in colour

Bed bug
(Cimex lectularius)

Bed bug:
- Skin rash
- Skin blister
- Allergy

Bed bug is a parasitic insects that feed exclusively on blood

Source for the macroscopic images is https://pixnio.com.

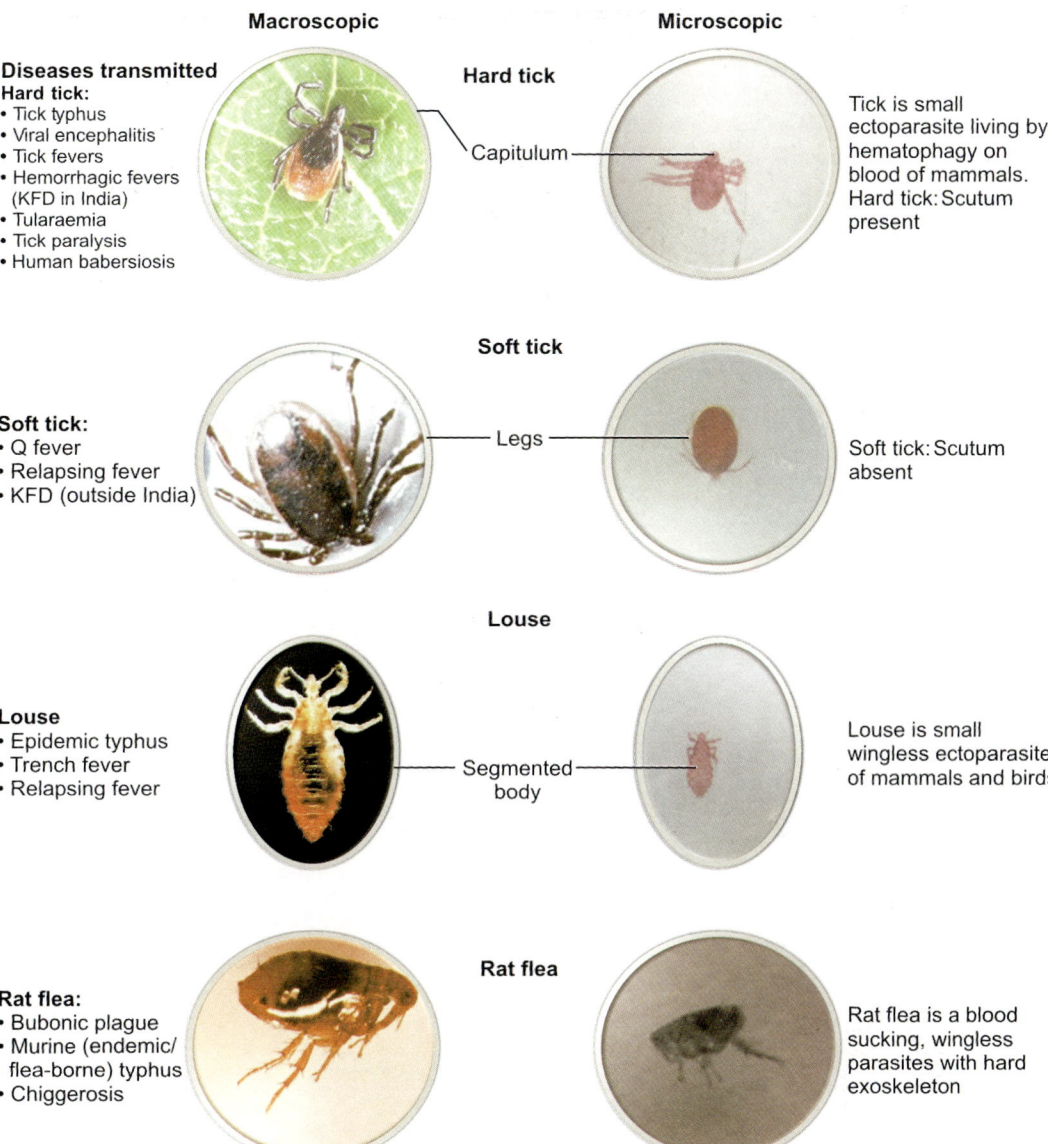

Others

Macroscopic   **Microscopic**

Diseases transmitted
Hard tick:
• Tick typhus
• Viral encephalitis
• Tick fevers
• Hemorrhagic fevers
  (KFD in India)
• Tularaemia
• Tick paralysis
• Human babersiosis

Hard tick

Capitulum

Tick is small ectoparasite living by hematophagy on blood of mammals. Hard tick: Scutum present

Soft tick

Soft tick:
• Q fever
• Relapsing fever
• KFD (outside India)

Legs

Soft tick: Scutum absent

Louse

Louse
• Epidemic typhus
• Trench fever
• Relapsing fever

Segmented body

Louse is small wingless ectoparasite of mammals and birds

Rat flea

Rat flea:
• Bubonic plague
• Murine (endemic/ flea-borne) typhus
• Chiggerosis

Rat flea is a blood sucking, wingless parasites with hard exoskeleton

Source for the macroscopic images is https://en.wikipedia.org.

SYMBOLS

'Smiling sun' logo, a voluntary certification of iodized salt

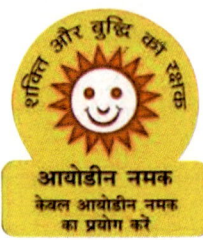

Biohazard symbol

Cytotoxic hazard symbol

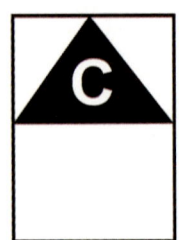

An inverted red triangle is the symbol for family planning health and contraception services in India

DOTS for tuberculosis

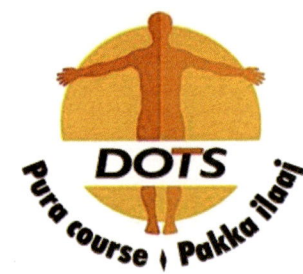

Epidemiological triangle

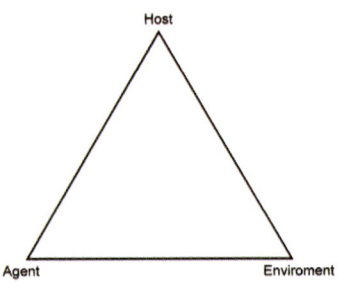

Red ribbon logo for HIV/AIDS

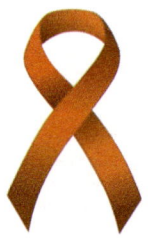

White ribbon symbolize lung cancer

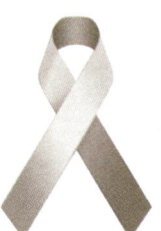

Pink ribbon symbolize breast cancer

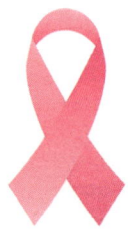

Purple ribbon represents pancreatic cancer, domestic violence

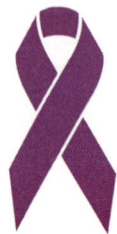

Green ribbon represents childhood depression

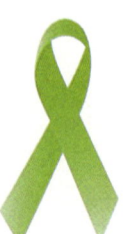

Orange represents kidney cancer, multiple sclerosis, hunger

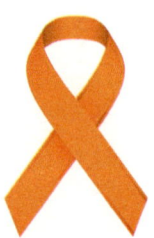

Family/Case

INTRODUCTORY FAMILY/CASE VIVA

Nitika

Q 1. Define family.

A group of persons united by the ties of marriage, blood, or adoption, constituting a single household and interacting with each other in their respective social positions, usually those of spouses, parents, children, and siblings.

The family should be distinguished from a household, which may include boarders and roomers sharing a common residence.

Q 2. What is a nuclear family?

A nuclear family is a family consisting of the marital pair living with their offspring in a separate dwelling. A mother, father and one or more children (biological or adopted).

Advantages
   a. Two people share parenting responsibilities
   b. Financial responsibilities shared

Disadvantage
Only one parent stays home for a major part of time

Q 3. What is an extended family?

An extended family is where blood relatives, often spanning three or more generations, lives together. It is the horizontal extension of the family.

Advantages
   a. More to help with responsibilities
   b. More support   c. More money

Disadvantages
   a. Less room   c. Less privacy
   b. Difficulty getting along

Q 4. What is a joint family?

The typical joint family consists of a number of married couples and their children who live together in the same household. All the men are related by blood and the women of the household are their wives, unmarried girls, and widows of the family. All the property is held in common.

The familial relations enjoy primacy over marital relations.

Advantages
   a. Mainly based on the motto: "Union is strength"
   b. There is sharing of responsibilities practically in all matters which gives the family a greater economic and social security.
   c. It provides economic and social security to the old, the helpless and the unemployed.

Q 5. What is a three-generation family?

It tends to be a household where there are representatives of three generations. It occurs when a young couple is unable to find separate housing accommodation and continue to live with their parents and have their own children.

Q 6. What is a single parent family?

Only one parent and one or more children.

Advantages
   a. Learn responsibility
   b. Independence
   c. Can be more stable

Disadvantages
   a. No one else to help
   b. Less free time
   c. Less money
   d. Need role models

Q 7. What is a blended family?

Two parents, one or both of whom have children from a previous relationship. Step parents and siblings, half-siblings

Advantage
Adults share responsibilities

Disadvantages
   a. Need more patience
   b. Adjustment to new roles

Q 8. What is a broken family?

It is the one where the parents have separated or where death has occurred of one or both the parents. It has an effect on child development may cause mental deprivation.

Q 9. What is a problem family?

Problem family lags behind from the rest of the community. The standards of life are below the accepted minimum and parents are unable to meet the physical and emotional needs of their children.

Q 10. What are other types of family?

a. New families	:	Under 10 years duration
b. Matrilocal	:	Husband moves to wife's house
c. Patriarchal	:	Male dominated
d. Matriarchal	:	Female dominated
e. Monogamous	:	Single spouse
f. Polygamous	:	Polyandrous/Polygamous
g. Matrilinear	:	Maternal lineage
h. Patrilinear	:	Paternal lineage

Q 11. What is a communal family?

A family where all members are playing role in its management.

Q 12. Who is an urban poor?

These are a group of individuals who have constraints to opportunities, and are living in absolute or relative poverty in urban areas.

Q 13. What do you mean by an organized sector?

This is the part of the economy, which works through legal channels of banking, and tax system, which is a determinant of advanced economies. Presently, organized sector constitutes roughly eight percent of Indian economic activity.

Q 14. What do you mean by an unorganized sector?

This is a part of the economic activity which most of the time runs on hard cash with no accountability and tax liability. This sector constitutes roughly 92% of Indian economic activity.

Q 15. Enumerate different socioeconomic scales.

Urban Area: Modified Kuppuswamy, Modified BG Prasad, Kulshreshtha, Srivastava, Jalota

Rural Area: Udaipareek, modified BG Prasad, Rahudkar, Shirpurkar

Q 16. Describe modified Kuppuswamy scale.

Category Score

A. Education	B. Occupation	C. Family income per month in Rs. 2015 (December)
1 = Illiterate	1 = Unemployed	1 = 2094
2 = Primary school certificate	2 = Unskilled worker	2 = 2095 – 6222
3 = Middle school certificate	3 = Semi-skilled worker	3 = 6223 – 10371
4 = High school certificate	4 = Skilled worker	4 = 10372 – 15557
5 = Intermediate or post high school diploma	5 = Clerical, shop owner, farmer	6 = 15558 – 20743
6 = Graduate or postgraduate	6 = Semi-professional	10 = 20744– 41487
7 = Professors or honours	10 = Professional	12 = 41488

The family income per month is based on the consumer price index of the current year.

Scoring:

Category	Score on scale
Upper (I)	26–29
Upper middle (II)	16–25
Lower middle (III)	11–15
Upper lower (IV)	5–10
Lower (V)	<5

Occupation categorized in Kuppuswamy scale:

Category	Description
Lowest	Unemployed
Unskilled	Work not requiring education/training: Peon, watchman, porter, domestic servant, labourer
Semiskilled	Some training to do routine job efficiently: Factory labourer, workshop laborer, lab attendant
Skilled	Long training in complicated work: Mason, carpenter, mechanic, driver, telephone operator
Semi-professional	Post highschool/college education, jobs of routine nature: Mechanical and electrical engineer, highschool teacher, lecturers in college
Professional	Involved in the decision making, laying down policies and executing them: Doctors, senior administrators. May not be highly educated but have organizational ability controlling a large number of people: Expert musicians, newspaper editors, auditors

Q 17. Describe Udai Pareek Scale.

By Udai Pareek and G Trivedi (1964):
- Attempts to examine the socioeconomic status for the rural population only
- This scale has nine factors which assess the socioeconomic status of the individual
- This scale does not emphasize the economic aspect
- The reliability of the scale was found to be very high ($r = 0.93$).

Land	Occupation
0 = no land	1 = labour
1 = <1 acre	2 = caste occupation
2 = 1–5 acres	3 = business
3 = 5–10 acres	4 = independent profession
4 = 10–15 acres	5 = cultivation
5 = 15–20 acres	6 = service
6 = >20 acres	9 = no occupation

Caste

1 = scheduled

2 = lower

3 = artisan

4 = agricultural

5 = prestige

6 = dominant

Farm Power

1 = no drought animal

2 = 1–2 drought animals

4 = 3–4 drought animals or 1 prestige animal

6 = 5–6 drought animals or tractor

Housing

0 = no house

1 = hut

2 = kutcha house

3 = mixed house

4 = pukka house

5 = mansion

Education

0 = illiterate

1 = can read only

2 = can read and write

3 = primary

4 = middle education

5 = high school

6 = graduate

Material possessions

1 = bullock cart

1 = cycle

1 = radio

1 = chairs

2 = improved agricultural implements

3 = television

Social participation

1 = member of 1 organisation

2 = member of >1 organisation

3 = office bearer

4 = wider public leader

Family type

1 = nuclear

2 = joint

3 = extended

Scoring:

Category	Score on scale
Upper (I)	Above 43
Upper middle (II)	33–42
Middle class (III)	24–32
Lower middle (IV)	13–23
Lower (V)	Below 13

Q 18. What are the minimum wages for various categories of workers?

The following rates are applicable in respect of unskilled, semi-skilled, and skilled categories in all schedules employments except employment in shop and establishment and employment in clubs.

Category	Rates as on 01.04.2015 (rupees)	Dearness allowances (pm) w.e.f 01.10.2015 (rupees)	Rates from (rupees) 01.10.2015	
			Per month	Per day
Unskilled	9048.00	130.00	9178.00	353.00
Semi-skilled	10010.00	130.00	10140.00	390.00
Skilled	10998.00	156.00	11154.00	429.00

The following rates are applicable in respect of clerical and nontechnical supervisory staff in all scheduled employments.

Category	Rates as on 01.04.2015 (rupees)	Dearness allowances 01.10.2015 (rupees)	Rates from (rupees) 01.10.2015	
Nonmatriculates	10010.00	130.00	10140.00	390.00
Matriculates but not graduates	10998.00	156.00	11154.00	429.00
Graduate and above	11986.00	156.00	12142.00	467.00

Q 19. What do you mean by social security?

Social security refers to social programs that provide set of benefits available from the government or civil society. These meet social needs of the individual against socially recognized conditions like infirmity, unemployment, old age, and poverty. These programs may be contributory or noncontributory in nature.

The various social welfare programmes in India may be broadly categorized under six heads:
  a. Programmes for the welfare of women
  b. Programmes for the welfare of children
  c. Programme for marginalized group
  d. Food security schemes
  e. Health insurance schemes
  f. Employment related programmes

Q 20. What is health insurance?

Health insurance is a method to finance healthcare. The ILO defines health insurance as the reduction or elimination of the uncertain risk of loss for the individual or household by combining a larger number of similarly exposed individuals or households who are included in a common fund that makes good the loss caused to any one member.

Q 21. What are the types of health insurances?

There are three types of health insurances:

a. Social health insurance: A compulsory health insurance, usually for the formal sector. For example, CGHS, ESI, and others.

b. Private health insurance: A voluntary health insurance wherein people can enroll and purchase the insurance product of their choices. For example, LIC and others.

c. Community health insurance: A voluntary but not-for-profit health insurance scheme and targeting the informal sector. For example ACCORD: Provider model, RAHA: Mutual model, Karuna: Linked model and others.

Q 22. Discuss briefly various schemes for marginalized population.

National Social Assistance Schemes:

Indira Gandhi National Old Age Pension Scheme (IGNOAPS):

It was launched by Ministry of Rural Development. All persons of 60 years and above (revised downwards from 65 in 2011) and belonging to below poverty line category, according to the criteria prescribed by the Government of India time to time are eligible to be a beneficiary of the scheme.

The pension amount, as in Union budget 2012–13, is INR 200 per month per person from 60 to 79 years and INR 500 per month per person for 80 years and above and states are supposed to contribute an equal amount vis-à-vis the scheme.

Indira Gandhi National Widow Pension Scheme:

A pension of Rs 300 per month to be granted to a widow aged between 40 and 79 years, belonging to below poverty line.

Indira Gandhi National Disability Pension Scheme

A pension of Rs. 300 per month (From fiscal 2012-13) to be granted to physically/mentally handicapped individuals aged 18–79 years, living below poverty line, previously age limit was 59 years with minimum 80% disability.

National Family Benefit Scheme (NFBS):

In case of the death of the "primary breadwinner" of a household living below poverty line conditions, a lump sum grant of Rs. 20,000 (from fiscal 2012-13) is provided to the household. The primary breadwinner as specified in the scheme, whether male or female, had to be a member of the household whose earning contributed substantially to the total household income. The death of such a primary breadwinner occurring whilst he or she is in the age group of 18 to 64 years, i.e. more than 18 years of age and less than 65 years of age, makes the family eligible to receive grants under this.

Q 23. What are the different insurance schemes by the Government of India?

Rashtriya Swasthya Bima Yojana (RSBY): It was launched in 2008. The below poverty line population was entitled to all hospitalization episodes (except certain specified exclusions) restricted by package limits and subject to an annual ceiling of Rs. 30,000 per family.

Employees' State Insurance (ESI) Scheme: It was launched in 1952. All employees from any firm having more than 10 employees and earning up to Rs. 15,000 per month.

Dependents are also covered. The Scheme has been extended to shops, hotels, restaurants, cinemas including preview theatres, road-motor transport undertakings and newspaper establishments employing 20 or more persons.There is no limit on the maximum care which can be availed.

Central government health scheme (CGHS): It was launched in 1954. Employees and pensioners of the central government, certain autonomous, semi-autonomous government organizations, members of parliament, state governors, accredited journalists and their dependents are the beneficiaries. It provides comprehensive medical care, including ambulatory, inpatient, home care, and medicines and diagnostic services. No limit on maximum care.

Q 24. Discuss briefly National Food Security Act, 2013/National Food Security Bill, 2013.

National Food Security Bill, 2013 covers whole of India, received assent from President on 10 Sep 2013. It entitles the priority households 5 kg of food grains per person per month, and 2.43 crore Antyodaya households to 35 kg per household per month. The eligible/priority households are combined coverage of Priority and Antyodaya households. The bill does not distinct between BPL and APL.

Q 25. What is Anthyodaya Anna Yojna?

Under this scheme families whose total household income from all sources is less than Rs. 24,200/- are identified as Poorest of Poor and entitled to the following benefits.

Wheat	25 kg	Rs. 2.00/kg
Rice	10 kg	Rs. 3.00/kg
Kerosene oil	22 litres	Rs. 9.09/litre per card
Sugar	13.50 kg	Rs. 6.00/kg per card

Q 26. What is Annapurna Yojna?

Under this scheme, destitute persons more than 65 years of age and not getting any old age pension from any source, are distributed ten kilograms of food grains which are provided free of cost every month.

Q 27. Discuss briefly Mahatma Gandhi National Rural Employment Guarantee Act (MGNREGA).

Mahatma Gandhi National Rural Employment Guarantee Act was launched in 2005 by Ministry of Labour. It has the following salient features:
- 1/3rd women (gender empowerment)
- 100 day/year of employment (50 days extra have been approved for areas receiving deficient rainfall)
- Wages = wage rate of respective state
- Job to be given <5 km from village, if >5 km, then 10% of salary is to be given as travel allowance
- Conditional cash transfer
- Volunteer to do unskilled manual work

- Job card (valid for 5 years)
- Work to be given within 15 days (otherwise allowance)

Environment

Q 28. What is the WHO term for housing and define it?

Housing is a residential environment. It is the physical structure that man uses and the environs of the structure including all necessary services, facilities, equipment and devices needed or desired for the physical and mental health and social well-being of the family and individual.

Q 29. What are the various housing standards?

The various housing standards are:

a. It should be elevated

b. Open space left all-round the house for proper lighting and ventilation.

c. In rural areas, the built does not exceed one-third of total area and in urban areas, the built-area may be up to two-thirds.

d. Walls and floors should be pucca and impermeable, free from crevices and cracks, damp proof

e. Roof height should not be less than 10 feet.

f. At least two windows on opposite walls should be 1/5th of floor area.

g. A separate kitchen should be present

h. Safe water supply

i. Sanitary privy should be accessible

Q 30. What are health consequences of *kutcha* house?

Poor housing conditions in *kutcha* house predispose to the following health conditions like common cold, TB, diphtheria, influenza, whooping cough, scabies, ringworm, impetigo, leprosy, plague, and others.

Q 31. Define overcrowding. What are the diseases likely to occur due to over-crowding?

More people living in a single dwelling than there is space for, so that movement is restricted, privacy secluded, hygiene impossible, rest and sleep difficult.

Overcrowding is a health problem and it may promote spread of infectious diseases like respiratory diseases. For example, TB, influenza, diphtheria. Psychosocial health is also compromised, which can lead to psychosomatic and mental diseases.

Q 32. What is the optimum floor area for occupancy of a single person?

For occupancy of a single person, optimum area is 100 sq ft.

Q 33. What do you mean by sex separation?

Overcrowding is considered to exist if two persons who are more than 9 years age of opposite sex, not husband and wife, and obliged to sleep in the same room.

Q 34. What do you mean by adequate lighting?

A room is said to be adequately lighted when one is able to read in the center of the room without the help of artificial light during daytime.

Q 35. What is indoor air-pollution and its consequences?

The major sources of indoor pollution include combustion of solid fuels, tobacco smoking, outdoor air pollutants, emission from construction materials and furnishings and improper maintenance of ventilation or air-conditioning system. These predispose to ischemic heart disease, COPD, nasopharyngeal and laryngeal cancers, TB, cataract and low birth weight.

Q 36. What is WaSH?

WaSH is the collective term for water, sanitation, and hygiene.

Q 37. What is safe drinking water?

Safe and wholesome water is water free from the pathogenic organism, harmful chemical substances, colour, and odour.

Q 38. What are methods of water purification at the household level?

Household purification of water:
  a. Boiling: Rolling boiling for 10–20 minutes is effective in killing bacteria, spores, cysts, and ova. It removes temporary hardness as well.
  b. Chemical disinfection: Chlorination
  c. Filtration: Filter, RO

Q 39. What is an appropriate method of water retrieval?

The purified water should be retrieved with the help of the ladder.

Q 40. What is sanitary latrine?

Sanitary latrine is one in which there is a water seal trap and flush. The excreta should not contaminate the ground or surface water, and soil. The excreta should not be accessible to flies, etc.

Q 41. What are appropriate methods for refuse disposal?

The choice of waste disposal depends upon local factors like cost and availability of land and labour. The principal methods of refuse disposal are dumping, controlled tipping, burial, in municipal waste and others.

Q 42. What are the diseases due to poor WaSH practices?

The diseases due to poor WaSH practices are diarrhoea, cholera, intestinal nematode infection, lymphatic filariasis, trachoma, schistosomiasis, malaria, other infectious diseases.

Q 43. A 10-year-old child with history of unprovoked dog bite comes to you. What is the treatment?

Approach to dog bite:

Category	Site	Treatment
I	Licks on unbroken skin Touching/feeding animals	None
II	Nibble, cuts, scratches without oozing of blood	Anti-rabies vaccine Local treatment of wounds
III	Licks on mucous membrane or broken skin Bites with breach of skin, bleeding	Anti-rabies vaccine Rabies immunoglobulin Local treatment of wounds

Q 44. A 20-year-old female presents to the hospital with the history of rat bite. What is the treatment?

A case of rat bite is treated as category I of dog bite.

Q 45. A 30-year-old male during a visit to jungle was bitten by monkey. What is the treatment?

A case of monkey bite or any wild animal is treated as category III of dog bite.

Q 46. What is the causative organism for leptospirosis? How does it spread to humans?

Leptospirosis is a bacterial infection caused by Leptospira. The disease is associated with fields, lakes and rivers contaminated with rodent urine commonly.

Q 47. What are the clinical features of leptospirosis? How will you manage the case of Leptospirosis?

Leptospirosis causes wide range of symptoms and without treatment can lead to kidney damage, meningitis, liver failure, respiratory distress, and even death. Leptospirosis is treated with antibiotics, such as doxycycline or penicillin.

UNDER-FIVE CHILDREN

Arun Padmanandan

MALNUTRITION

Introduction

Q 1. Define under-nutrition.

According to WHO, under-nutrition is defined by poor anthropometric status as a consequence of inadequate dietary intake, leading to frequent infections and thus resulting in the deficiency of calories, proteins, vitamins, and minerals.

Q 2. Define over-nutrition.

According to WHO, it is a condition which is caused as a result of excessive intake of specific nutrients.

The term malnutrition refers to both under-nutrition and over-nutrition.

Q 3. What are the indicators of under-nutrition?

Stunting, wasting and underweight are the indicators of under-nutrition.

Q 4. Define stunting.

It is defined as low height for age. It is an indicator of chronic malnutrition.

Q 5. Define wasting.

It is defined as low weight for height. It is an indicator of acute malnutrition.

Q 6. Define underweight.

It is defined as low weight for age. It is a combined indicator of acute and chronic malnutrition.

Q 7. Define WHO classification of malnutrition.

WHO recommends the use of Z scores or standard deviation scores (SDS) for evaluating the anthropometric status.

Z scores/SDS score of < -3 SD indicate severe malnutrition

Z scores/SDS score of < -2 to -3 SD indicate low malnutrition

Z scores/SDS score of $> +1$ SD indicate overweight.

Q 8. Define Indian Academy of Pediatrics classification of malnutrition.

Grade of malnutrition	Weight for age of standard (%)
Normal	>80%
1st grade	71–80% (mild malnutrition)
2nd grade	61–70% (moderate malnutrition)
3rd grade	51–60% (severe malnutrition)
4th grade	<50% (very severe malnutrition)

Q 9. What are the age-independent indices to diagnose under-nutrition?

Kanawati and McLaren index, Rao and Singh index, Dugdale index, Quaker Arm Circumference measuring stick (QuAC stick), Jeliffe ratio.

Kanawati and McLaren Index: The ratio of mid-arm circumference to head circumference. The cut-offs recommended are

MAC/HC ratio >0.310 = nutritionally healthy

MAC/HC ratio 0.310 – 0.280 = mild protein energy malnutrition

MAC/HC ratio 0.279 – 0.250 = moderate protein energy malnutrition

MAC/HC ratio <0.250 = severe protein energy malnutrition

Rao and Singh Index: It measures the ratio between weight in kg divided by height square in cm multiplied by 100. A ratio of <0.14 is indicative of malnutrition.

QuAC Stick: QuAC stands for Quaker Arm Circumference measuring stick. It is simply a height measuring stick which is marked off in arm circumference measurements.

Jeliffe's ratio: It is defined as the ratio of head circumference to chest circumference. At one year of age, the head circumference and chest circumference are equal. If the ratio is <1 at 1 year of age, it denotes malnutrition.

Burden

Q 10. What is the burden of hunger in India?

With >200 million hungry people, India has the largest number of hungry in the world. On Global Hunger Index, India ranks 66th out of 68 countries.

In the Index, all Indian states are at a serious level of hunger and 12 states fall in the alarming category.

Madhya Pradesh is India's most malnourished state.

Q 11. What is nutrition statistics of India?

The Government of India is in the process of releasing its 2013-14 Rapid Survey on Children (RSOC). This new national survey, covering all 29 states in India, relies on data collected by the Ministry of Women and Child Development in partnership with UNICEF, India.

Indicator	2005-06 NFHS-3	2013-14 RSOC	2015-16 NFHS-4
Under-five underweight	35.7%	29.4%	42.5%
Under-five stunting	47.9%	38.8%	38.4%
Under-five wasting	19.8%	15%	21.0%
Exclusive breastfeeding of infants under 6 months old	46.4%	71.6%	54.9%

Q 12. What is Global Nutrition Report (GNR)?

GNR is a report card on the world's nutrition globally, regionally, country by country and efforts taken to improve it. It assesses the progress in meeting global nutrition targets established by the world's health assembly.

Q 13. What are the Global Nutrition Targets 2025?

- Achieve 40% reduction in the number of under-five children who are stunted.
- Achieve 50% reduction of anaemia in women of reproductive age group.
- Achieve 30% reduction of low-birth weight.
- Ensure that there is no increase in childhood overweight.
- Increase the rate of exclusive breastfeeding in the first 6 months up to at least 50%.
- Reduce and maintain childhood wasting to <5%.

Risk Factor

Q 14. What are the immediate causes of malnutrition?

Low dietary intake, low birth weight, and infection.

Q 15. What are the basic determinants that influence the nutritional status?

They include political and economic structure, sociocultural environment.

Clinical Features

Q 16. What are the signs of protein-energy malnutrition in young children?

The signs of protein-energy malnutrition in young children include: Oedema, depigmented hair, easily pluckable hair, thin sparse hair, straight hair, muscle wasting, diffuse skin depigmentation, psychomotor changes, moon-like facies, hepatomegaly, and flaky paint dermatosis.

Q 17. What is head to toe examination of an under-five child?

Head to toe examination is the general physical examination of an under-five child. It is as follows:

Physical examination	Finding	Probable diagnosis
Skin	Tugor	Anaemia
	Flaky paint appearance	Jaundice
		Dehydration
Hair	Red flag sign	Kwashiorkor
	Louse infestation	Pediculosis capitis
Scalp	Ping-pong	Rickets
	Raised anterior fontanel	Intracranial tension
Forehead	Frontal bossing	Acromegaly
Eyebrows	Loss of eyebrows	Leprosy
Eyes	Discharge	Conjunctivitis
Eyelid	Papule	Stye
Eyelashes	Trichiasis	Trachoma
Conjunctiva	Icterus	Jaundice
Upper palpebral	Pallor	Anaemia
Lower palpebral	Xerosis	Vitamin A deficiency
Lateral bulbar		
Cornea	Ulcer	Vitamin A deficiency
Nose	Bleeding	Pricking or foreign body
Lips	Blue	Cyanosis
	Cleft	Cleft lip
	Chelitosis	Vitamin B deficiency
Gingiva	Bleeding	Scurvy
Teeth	Black, distorted	Caries
Tongue	Pallor	Anaemia
	Whitish coat	Candida
	Glossitis	Vitamin B_{12} deficiency
Tonsils	Enlarged with white exudates	Tonsilitis
Palate	Split palate	Cleft palate
Floor of the mouth	Bluish frog like swelling	Plunging ranula
Ears	Discharge	Otitis media
	Wax	Impacted wax
Neck	Lymph nodes	Infections
	Diffuse thyroid swelling	Goitre
	Web neck	Turner syndrome

(Contd.)

Physical examination	Finding	Probable diagnosis
Chest	Pigeon chest	Rickets
	Rosary	Rickets
	Chest indrawing	Pneumonia
Hands	Widen wrist	Rickets
Palm	Pallor	Anaemia
Nails	Spoon-shaped	Anaemia
	White lines	Hypoproteinemia
Spine	Bending	Scoliosis
Genitalia	Lack of scrotal congruity in male	Sexual immaturity
	Wide part labia minora in female	Sexual immaturity
Legs	Bow legs	Rickets

Q 18. What is the importance of weight in anthropometric measurement and how will you measure it?

The measurement of weight is the most reliable criteria of assessment of health and nutritional status of children.

Different types of weighing scales are available. They are
  a. Beam balance scales
  b. Spring scales
  c. Electronic weighing scales
  d. Bathroom type of mechanical scale (very unreliable)

Beam balance scales are preferred as they are less inaccurate. Spring scales must be avoided because they get stretched and become inaccurate due to frequent usage, or the spring can expand itself in very hot weather conditions.

Q 19. How will you measure the height/length in the community?

Children >2 years of age a vertical measuring rod or scale fixed to a wall/stadiometer can be used.

After removing the shoes, the subjects should stand on a flat floor by the scale, with feet parallel and heels, buttocks, shoulders, and back of the head touching the upright.

The head should be erect with the lower border of the orbit in the same horizontal plane as the external auditory meatus. The arms must be hanging by the sides.

The headpiece, which can be a metal bar or wooden block, should be lowered slightly crushing the hair making adequate contact with the top of the head.

Children <2 years of age crown-heel length is measured. This is carried out with the help of wooden length-board/infantometer.

Q 20. How will you measure the head circumference in the community?
Head circumference is usually measured by using a fibreglass tape. Cloth tapes must be avoided because they stretch on repeated use. The child head must be steady and the greatest circumference is measured by placing the tape firmly around the frontal bones just superior to the supra-orbital ridges, passing it around the head at the same level on each side and laying it over the maximum occipital prominence at the back of the head. Measurement is made to the nearest 0.1 cm.

Q 21. How will you measure the chest circumference in the community?
A fibreglass, the non-stretchable tape must be used at the level of nipples during mid-inspiration.

Q 22. How will you measure the mid-upper arm circumference (MUAC) in the community?
Before measuring MUAC, the age of the child must be asked from the mother because MUAC is not measured in infants below 6 months of age.

First MUAC is preferably carried out in left arm usually bent at right angles, then the mid-point of the arm is marked between the tip of the shoulder and olecranon process of the elbow.

Then, the MUAC is measured by placing the tape around the arm.

MUAC of 12.5–13.5 cm is indicative of moderate malnutrition and < 12.5 cm is indicative of severe malnutrition.

Mid-upper arm circumference can be measured using:

Bangle test: A fibreglass ring of 4 cm internal diameter is slipped up the arm if it passes the elbow, it means the upper arm is <12.5 cm and the child is malnourished.

Shakir's tape*:* Fibreglass tape with colour markings.
a. Red indicates MUAC of <12.5 cm
b. Yellow indicates MUAC of 12.5–13.5 cm
c. Green indicates MUAC of >13.5 cm.

Q 23. How will you measure the skin fold thickness in the community?
In practice, three instruments can be used to measure skin fold thickness:
a. Harpenden's caliper: Most commonly used
b. Lange caliper
c. United States Army Medical Research and Nutrition caliper.

The most common sites used for measuring skin fold thickness are triceps and subscapular skin folds.

A length-wise skin fold is firmly grasped and slightly lifted up between the thumb and index finger of left hand. Extreme care should be taken to avoid the muscle being included.

The caliper is then applied 1 cm below the examiner's hands at a depth equal to the skin fold while the skin fold is still gently held throughout the measurement.

Average of three measurements must be taken

Q 24. Define growth chart. How do you interpret a growth chart?
Growth charts are a visible display of a child's growth and development.

It was first designed by David Morley. The growth charts evolved as follows:

  a. NCHS (National Centre for Health Statistics) 1977 growth charts
  b. CDC (Centers for Disease Control and Prevention) 2000 growth charts
  c. WHO (World Health Organization) growth charts 2006. [Annexure 1 to 6]

The WHO undertook the Multicentre Growth Reference study between 1997 and 2003 to generate new curves for assessing the growth and development of the child. The MGRS collected primary growth data and related information from approximately 8500 children from widely different ethnic and cultural backgrounds (Brazil, Ghana, India, Norway, Oman, and USA). In India, New Delhi was selected as a study site for MGRS and sample was drawn from 58 affluent neighbourhood in South Delhi.

Plotting in growth charts:

X-axis: Some graphs have X-axis showing age and some have length/height. The plot on vertical lines corresponding to complet age or length/height to the nearest whole centimeter.

Y-axis: Y-axis shows length/height, weight or BMI. The plot on horizontal lines corresponding to length/height, weight or BMI as precisely as possible.

Plotted point: The point on a graph where a line extended from a measurement on X-axis intersects with a line extended from a measurement on Y-axis.

Interpret the plotted graph according to the indicators.

India has adopted the new WHO child growth standards (2006) in February 2009.

Z score	Length/height for age	Weight for age	Weight for length/height	BMI for age
>3	Very tall. Refer	Growth problem, better assessed by weight for length or BMI for age	Obese	Obese
>2	Normal	-do-	Overweight	Overweight
>1	Normal	-do-	Possible risk of overweight	Possible risk of overweight
0 (median)	Normal	Normal	Normal	Normal
< – 1	Normal	Normal	Normal	Normal
< – 2	Stunted	Underweight	Wasting	Wasting
< – 3	Severely stunted	Severely underweight	Severe wasting	Severe wasting

WHO Anthro provides the standards which are available for both boys and girls below 5 years of age.

WHO Anthro Plus provides the standards which are available for both boys and girls 5 to 18 years of age [Annexures 8–12].

Mother and child protection card provide the growth chart along with family identification and registration, birth record, pregnancy record, institutional identification, care during pregnancy, preparation for delivery, registration under JSY, detail about immunization, breastfeeding, introduction of supplementary food and milestones of the baby (Annexure 13).

Q 25. Define marasmus.

Marasmus is a condition that occurs as a result of rapid deterioration in the nutritional status. Acute starvation or acute illness over a borderline nutritional status could precipitate marasmus. It is characterized by marked wasting of muscle and fatty tissues.

Q 26. What are the clinical features of marasmus?

The main clinical sign is severe wasting. The child appears very thin and has no fat. There is severe wasting of shoulders, arms, buttocks, and thighs.

The loss of buccal pad of fat creates the aged or wrinkled appearance. Baggy pants appearance refers to the loose skin of the buttocks hanging down. The axillary pad of fat may also be diminished.

Affected children may appear to be alert in spite of the condition. There is no oedema.

Q 27. Define kwashiorkor.

It usually affects children between aged 1 and 4 years. The main sign is pitting oedema, starting in the legs and feet and spreading to the hands and face.

Q 28. What are the clinical features of kwashiorkor?

The child may have a fat sugar baby appearance.

Oedema is present. Muscle wasting is always present. The child is weak, hypotonic and unable to stand or walk.

Skin lesions consist of increased pigmentation, and desquamation. Pigmentation may be confluent resembling flaky paint or enamel spots. The distribution is typically on buttocks, perineum, and upper thigh.

Smooth tongue, cheilosis, and angular stomatitis are common.

Hair changes include loss of curls and sparseness over the temple and occipital regions. Hairs lose their lustre and are easily pluckable. FLAG sign, which is the alternate bands of hypopigmented and normally pigmented hair pattern, is seen when the growth of the child occurs in spurts.

Mental changes include unhappiness, irritability, and intermittent cry. No signs of hunger and difficult to feed them.

Q 29. Define marasmic kwashiorkor.

It is a mixed form of protein energy malnutrition and manifests as oedema occurring in children who may or may not have other signs of kwashiorkor and have varied manifestations of marasmus.

Q 30. Define severe acute malnutrition (SAM).

According to WHO, SAM is defined by a very low weight (below 3 standard deviation score of the median growth standards), by visible severe wasting or by the presence of severe nutritional oedema.

Q 31. Define the WHO diagnostic criteria for severe acute malnutrition in children.

Indicator	Measure	Cut-off
Severe wasting	Weight for height	<– 3 SD
Severe wasting	Mid-upper arm circumference	<115 mm
Bilateral oedema	Clinical sign	

Severe wasting, bilateral oedema are independent indicators of severe acute malnutrition that require urgent action.

Management

Q 32. How do you classify malnourished children according to IMNCI guidelines? What is F-IMNCI and mention its facilities?

IMNCI stands for Integrated Management of Neonatal and Childhood Illness. Its strategy is one of the main interventions in RCH II and NHM. It encompasses a range of interventions to prevent and manage the commonest major childhood diseases.

F-IMNCI stands for facility-based IMNCI. It basically integrates facility-based care with the IMNCI strategy so as to empower the health personnel with the skill to manage newborn and childhood illness at the community level as well as at the health facility.

It focuses on providing appropriate inpatient management of the major causes of neonatal and childhood mortality like asphyxia, severe malnutrition, diarrhoea, pneumonia, low birth weight, sepsis, malaria, meningitis. The newborn care facilities at different levels of health care are:

At PHC/subcentres which are MCH level 1: All the newborns at birth are given care at newborn care corner in labour rooms. The sick newborns are referred to higher centres.

At CHC/first referral units which are MCH level 2: All newborns at birth are given care at newborn care corner in labour rooms and also in operation theatre. The sick newborns are referred to newborn stabilization unit.

At district hospital which is level 3: All newborns are given care at newborn care corner in labour rooms and also in operation theatre. The sick newborns are referred to special newborn care unit.

Q 33. How do you manage mild and moderate malnutrition?

The mainstay of treatment is the provision of adequate amounts of protein and energy; at least 150 kcal/kg/day. In order to achieve these high energy intakes, frequent feeding up to seven times a day is often necessary.

A protein intake of 3 g/kg/day is sufficient. Milk is the most frequent source of the protein used in therapeutic diets, though other sources, including vegetable protein mixtures, have been used successfully.

The best measure of the efficacy of treatment of mild and moderate malnutrition is weight gain.

Q 34. How do you manage severe acute malnutrition (SAM)?

Step 1:   Treat/prevent hypoglycemia

Step 2:   Treat/prevent hypothermia

Step 3:   Treat/prevent dehydration

Step 4:   Correct electrolyte imbalance

Step 5:   Treat/prevent infection

Step 6:   Correct micronutrient deficiencies

Step 7:   Initiate re-feeding

Step 8:   Achieve catch-up growth

Step 9:   Provide sensory stimulation and emotional support

Step 10:   Prepare for follow-up after recovery

Q 35. When nutritional rehabilitation centres for SAM babies was launched?

The nutritional rehabilitation centre was launched under the collaboration of UNICEF and GoI. It helps in restoring the severe acute malnourished children back to good health and providing nutritional education to mothers.

The services provided by these centres are:
   a. Patient admission, treatment, and management.
   b. Nutritional support to admitted inpatients
   c. Capacity building of the primary caregivers on how to prepare low cost nutritious diet

Admission criteria in nutritional rehabilitation centre:
   a. Weight for height/length <3 SD and/or
   b. Mid-upper arm circumference <11.5 cm and/or
   c. Presence of bilateral pitting pedal oedema.

Q 36. What is F-75 diet?

F-75 diet is a starter diet given for malnourished children that provides 75 kcal energy, 0.9 g of protein and 1.2 g of lactose.

   It can be prepared at home by adding 30 ml of cow milk, one level teaspoon of sugar approx. 9 g, powdered puffed rice of about 2.5 g, one level teaspoon of vegetable oil 2 g, 100 ml of water.

Q 37. What is F-100 diet?

F 100 diet is a catch-up diet, which is given for malnourished children. Once appetite returns, starter F-75 diets are gradually replaced with feeds, which have a higher calorie density. F-100 that provides 100 kcal energy, 2.9 g protein, and 3.8 g of lactose.

It can be prepared at home by adding 75 ml of toned dairy milk, half-teaspoon sugar 2.5 g, 7 g of powdered puffed rice, 2 g of vegetable oil, 100 ml of water.

Q 38. What is RUTF (ready to use therapeutic food)?

RUTF is oil-based paste and as such can be stored at home unrefrigerated with a little risk of microbial contamination for several months. The child should continue to receive other foods and breastfeeding during medical nutrition therapy with RUTF.

Q 39. What is community-based therapeutic care (CTC)?

CTC combines facility or inpatient management of severe acute malnutrition with complications and community-based management of severe acute malnutrition without complications or mild to moderate malnutrition.

Prevention

Q 40. What are the preventive measures for malnutrition?

Primary prevention: Health promotion and specific protection.
Health promotion: Nutrition education, promotion of breastfeeding, development of low cost weaning foods, measures to improve family diet, family planning, and birth spacing.

Specific promotion: Diet must contain protein and energy rich foods. Milk, eggs and fresh fruits to be given, immunization and food fortification.

Secondary prevention: Early diagnosis and treatment
Early diagnosis of any lag in growth, treatment of infections and diarrhoea, deworming, development of rehydration programmes for diarrhoea, development of supplementary feeding programmes.

Tertiary prevention: Rehabilitation
Nutritional rehabilitation services, hospital treatment and follow-up care

Action at Family Level

a. Education on the selection of right kind of foods to both husband and wife of a family.
b. Education on food expenditure and budgets
c. Promotion of breastfeeding and improving infant and child feeding practices
d. Nutrition education, planning a kitchen garden or poultry

Action at Community Level

a. Diet and nutrition surveys in the representative population using standardized methods
b. Supplementary feeding programmes, mid-day school meals, vitamin A prophylaxis programme
c. Enrollment of vulnerable population in ICDS
d. Health education

Action at National Level

a. Rural development
b. Increasing agricultural production
c. Population stabilization
d. Nutrition intervention programmes
e. Nutrition related health activities

Q 41. What are the various Government of India programmes to address under nutrition?

Target group	Schemes
Pregnant and lactating mothers	ICDS, IGMSY, RCH2, NHM, JSY
Children between 0 and 3 years	ICDS, RCH 2, NHM, RGNCS
Children between 3 and 6 years	ICDS, RCH 2, NHM, RGNCS, TSC/NBA, NRDWP
School going children 6 to 14 years	Mid-day meals, Sarva Siksha Abhiyan
Adolescent girls 11 to 18 years	RGSEAG, KSY, NHM, TSC/NBA, NRDWP
Adults and communities	MNREGS, SDM,WWSP, ALP, TPDS, AAY, NRDWP, TSC/NBA, NFSM, NHM, RKVY, ISOPOM, AAH, DAF

ICDS: Integrated Child Development Services

IGMSY: Indira Gandhi Matritva Sahyog Yojna

NHM: National Health Mission

RGNCS: Rajiv Gandhi National Creche Scheme

TSC/NBA: Total Sanitation Campaign/Nirmal Bharat Abhiyan

RGSEAG: Rajiv Gandhi Scheme for Empowerment of Adolescent Girls

KSY: Kishori Sakthi Yojana

NRDWP: National Rural Drinking Water Supply Programme

SDM: Skill Development Mission

WWSP: Women Welfare and Support Programme

ALP: Adult Literacy Programme

NFSM: National Food Security Mission

ISOPOM: Integrated Scheme of Oilseeds, Pulses, Oilpalm and Maize

AAH: Augmenting Animal Husbandry

DAF: Dairying and Fisheries

PNEUMONIA

Introduction

Q 1. Define pneumonia.

Pneumonia is an acute respiratory infection that fills the alveoli in the lungs with pus and fluid making breathing painful and limiting oxygen intake. Infection is due to viruses or bacteria, less commonly by other micro-organisms.

Burden

Q 2. What is the burden of pneumonia?

Pneumonia is the single largest infectious cause of death in children worldwide. Pneumonia accounted for 16% of all deaths of children under five years old in the year 2015.

Risk Factor

Q 3. What are the causes of pneumonia?

The common causes of pneumonia are:

a. *Streptococcus pneumoniae* is the most common bacterial cause of pneumonia

b. *Haemophilus influenzae* type b (Hib)

c. Respiratory syncytial virus is the most common viral cause of pneumonia

d. *Pneumocystis jiroveci* is one of the most common causes of pneumonia in HIV positive infants

Q 4. What are the risk factors for pneumonia?

The risk factors for pneumonia are

a. Immuno-compromised children

b. Malnutrition

c. Lack of exclusively breastfed

d. Commodity symptomatic HIV infections, measles

e. Indoor air pollution

f. Overcrowding

g. Parental smoking

h. Poor WaSH practices

Clinical Features

Q 5. What are the presenting symptoms of pneumonia?

The symptoms of viral pneumonia are more compared to bacterial pneumonia. The various presenting symptoms of pneumonia are the combination of the following:

a. Cough

b. Difficult breathing

c. Fever

d. Fast breathing

e. Chest wall indrawing

Q 6. What are the danger signs of pneumonia?

The danger signs of pneumonia are:

a. Lethargy or unconsciousness

b. Abnormally sleepy

c. Inability to drink or breastfeed

d. Persistent vomiting

e. Central cyanosis

f. Severe respiratory distress

g. Convulsions

h. High fever

i. Hypothermia

j. Stridor in calm child

Q 7. What are the first five signs to be assessed in the child suspected of pneumonia?
The first five signs looked in the child suspected of pneumonia are:

a. Count breathing
b. Chest indrawing
c. Nasal flaring
d. Grunting
e. Bulging fontanelle

Q 8. What is fast breathing?
Fast breathing is present when respiratory rate is

a. >60 per min in a child 0–2 months
b. >50 per min in a child 2–12 months
c. >40 per min in a child 12 months–5 years

Q 9. What is chest indrawing?
Chest indrawing is when lower chest wall moves in or retracts during inhalation (in a healthy person, the chest expands during inhalation).

Q 10. What is an intercostal indrawing or intercostal retraction?
An intercostal indrawing or intercostal retraction is when only the soft tissue between the ribs goes in during inspiration.

Q 11. What is nasal flaring?
Nasal flaring is widening of the nostrils of the young infant inspiration.

Q 12. What is grunting?
Grunting is the soft, short sounds a young infant has during expiration.

Q 13. What is stridor?
Stridor is a harsh noise which is produced when the child breathes in. It is produced as a result of inflammation of larynx, trachea, epiglottis. Put your ear near the calm child's mouth as stridor can be difficult to hear.

Management

Q 14. How do you classify and manage pneumonia in a child aged 2 months up to 5 years?

Classification	Very severe disease	Severe pneumonia	Pneumonia	No pneumonia/ cold or cough
IMNCI classification	Very severe disease/severe pneumonia		Pneumonia	No pneumonia
Signs and symptoms present	Danger signs Chest indrawing Fast breathing	Chest indrawing Fast breathing Others	Fast breathing	Cold cough

(Contd.)

(Contd.)

Treatment	Hospitalize Oxygen therapy for first 48 hours Inj chloramphenicol		Hospitalize For first 48 hours IM Inj benzyl penicillin/ IM Inj chloramphenicol/ IM Inj Ampillicin		Tab/syp Cotrimoxazole		Assess for ear and sore throat
	Assess after 48 hours		Assess after 48 hours		Assess after 48 hours		
	Improves	Do not improve/ worsen	Improves	Do not improve/ worsen	Impro-ves	Do not improve/ worsen	
	Oral Ampi-cillin/ amoxi-cillin for 10 days	Injection cloxacillin and Gentamy-cin	Oral Ampicillin/ Amoxi-cillin/ Chloram-phenicol/ Inj prociane penicillin	Injection cloxacillin and Gentamy-cin	Con-tinue for 3 days	Refer	

Symptomatic treatment, continue breastfeeding, keep the child warm, prevent low blood sugar

Inj chloramphenicol (25 mg/kg/dose) 6 hourly intramuscular, Inj gentamycin (2.5 mg/kg/dose) 8 hourly intramuscular, Inj cloxacillin (25 mg/kg/dose) 6 hourly intramuscular, Inj ampicillin (50 mg/kg/dose) 6 hourly intramuscular, Inj benzyl penicillin (50000 IU/kg/dose) 6 hourly intramuscular, Inj procaine penicillin (50000 IU/kg/dose) 6 hourly intramuscular

Q 15. How do you classify and manage pneumonia in a child up to 2 months of age?

Classification	Very severe disease	Severe pneumonia	No pneumonia/Cold or cough
IMNCI classification	Possible serious bacterial infection		
Signs and symptoms present	Danger signs Chest indrawing Fast breathing	Chest indrawing Fast breathing others	Cold Cough
Treatment	Hospitalization Give the first dose of Inj benzyl penicillin (50000 IU/kg/dose) 6 hours IM Inj gentamycin (2.5 mg/kg/dose) 8 hours IM Inj ampicillin (50 mg/kg/dose) 6 hours IM		Assess for ear and sore throat

Symptomatic treatment, continue breastfeeding, keep the child warm, prevent low blood sugar

Prevention

Q 16. What are the vaccines available for prevention of pneumonia?

Measles vaccination at 9 and 15 months can protect a child from pneumonia.

Hib vaccine: *Haemophilus influenzae* type b vaccine, Schedule: 6, 10, 14 weeks, booster at 18 months.

Pneumococcal vaccines:

PPV23: Polysaccharide nonconjugate vaccine contains capsular antigens of 23 serotypes. Recommended for adults, children above 2 years of age, patient undergone splenectomy or sickle cell disease, chronic diseases of heart, lung, and liver, organ transplants, malignancies etc. Dosage: 0.5 ml

PCV: It is a conjugate vaccine and two conjugate vaccines are available: PCV10 and PCV13. WHO recommends 3 primary doses at 6, 10, 14 weeks.

Q 17. What is the global action plan for pneumonia and diarrhoea (GAPPD)?

The World Health Organization and UNICEF released the global action plan for pneumonia and diarrhoea (GAPPD). It aims to expedite pneumonia control in children with three actions. They are:

  a. Protect children from pneumonia by promoting exclusive breastfeeding and adequate complementary feeding.
  b. Prevent pneumonia with vaccinations, hand hygiene, reducing indoor air pollution, HIV prevention and cotrimoxazole prophylaxis for HIV patients.
  c. Treat pneumonia.

Q 18. What is IMNCI?

IMNCI is Integrated Management of Neonatal and Childhood Illness.

Q 19. What is IMCI?

IMCI is Integrated Management of Childhood Illness.

Q 20. What is F-IMNCI?

Facility-based IMNCI (Integrated Management of Neonatal and Childhood Illness)

Q 21. What is the rationale for adaption of IMCI to IMNCI in India?

The rationale for IMNCI is large proportion of neonatal deaths occur in India. Therefore, neonate was added as a separate entity.

Q 22. Under IMNCI what does the colours pink, green and yellow signify?

  a. Pink urgent referral
  b. Yellow treatment at outpatient health facility
  c. Green home management

DIARRHOEA

Introduction

Q 1. Define diarrhoea.

Diarrhoea is defined as a change in consistency and frequency of stools, i.e. liquid or watery stools, that occurs more than three times a day.

Q 2. What are the types of diarrhoeal diseases?

Persistent diarrhoea is diarrhoea for 14 days or more

Chronic diarrhoea is diarrhoea for 28 days or more

Bloody diarrhoea is presence of blood in the stools; also called dysentery

Burden

Q 3. What is the burden of diarrhoea?

Diarrhoea is a global killer. It kills 2195 children everyday. This burden is more than AIDS, malaria, and measles combined. Diarrhoea is the second leading cause of death among children under the age of five.

Risk Factor

Q 4. What are the causes of acute diarrhoea?

Bacterial: *E. coli*, Shigella, *Vibrio cholerae*, Salmonella, Campylobacter spp., others

Viral: Rotavirus, Norwalk virus, Calicivirus, Astrovirus, Enterovirus, etc

Parasitic: Giardia, *Cryptosporidium parvum, Entamoeba histolytica*, Cyclospora and *Isospora belli*.

Q 5. What are the risk factors of diarrhoea?

Poor sanitation, poor personal hygiene, nonavailability of safe drinking water, unsafe food preparation practices, low rates of breastfeeding and immunization, malnutrition.

Clinical Features

Q 6. How will you assess a child with acute diarrhoea?

History: Includes information on:

    a. Onset of diarrhoea, duration, and number of stools per day

    b. Blood in stools

    c. Number of episodes of vomiting

    d. Presence of fever, cough or other significant symptoms

    e. Type and amount of fluids taken during illness and pre-illness

    f. Drugs taken

    g. Immunization history

Q 7. What are the danger signs of dehydration?

    a. Continuous diarrhoea beyond 3 days

    b. Increased volume/frequency of stools

    c. Repeated vomiting

    d. Increasing thirst and refusal to feed

    e. Fever or blood in stools

Q 8. How do you assess dehydration in a child and what are the types of dehydration?

		Look at	
Appearance	Well alert	Restless, irritable	Lethargic, unconscious
Eyes	Normal	Sunken	Very sunken
Tears	Present	Absent	Absent
Mouth and tongue	Moist	Dry	Very dry
Thirst	Not thirsty	Drinks eagerly	Not able to drink
Breathing	Normal	Rapid	Very rapid
		Feel	
Skin pinch	Goes back quickly	Goes back slowly	Goes back very slowly
Anterior fontanelle	Normal	Depressed	Markedly depressed
Assess			
Pulse	Normal	Rapid and low volume	Feeble or imperceptible
Urine	Normal	Dark	Scanty
Weight loss	<5%	6–9%	10% or more
Decide:	No dehydration	If 2 or more signs present, then it is: Some dehydration	If 2 or more signs present, then it is: Severe dehydration
Treat:	Plan A	Plan B	Plan C

Q 9. How do you know about the lethargic child?
A lethargic child is not simply asleep. The child cannot be fully awakened. The child has a dull mental state and the child may appear to be drifting into unconsciousness.

Q 10. How will you assess the dryness of mouth and tongue in a child?
Dryness of mouth and tongue can be palpated with a clean finger. The mouth may be dry in a child who habitually breathes through the mouth. The mouth may be wet in a dehydrated child owing to recent vomiting or drinking.

Q 11. How to check skin pinch in a child?
  a. Ask the mother to place the child on the examining table with a flat back, arms at his sides and straight legs
  b. Use your thumb and first finger to locate the area on the child's abdomen halfway between the umbilicus and the side of the abdomen.
  c. Pick up all the layers of skin and the tissue underneath them.
  d. Hold the pinch for one second. The skin pinch goes back very slowly if more than two seconds, slowly if less than 2 seconds, but not immediately, or immediately.

Management

Q 12. What are the principles of management of acute diarrhoea?

a. Rehydration and maintaining hydration
b. Ensuring adequate feeding
c. Oral supplementation of zinc
d. Early recognition of danger signs and treatment of complications

Q 13. What is the treatment for cases with NO dehydration?

Treatment Plan A

a. Treat at home after explaining the danger signs to the mother/caregiver.
b. Give the mother WHO ORS.

Q 14. What is ORS?

ORS is oral rehydration solution

Q 15. What is the composition of new WHO ORS?

Constituent	Grams per litre	Osmolar or ion	mmol/l
Sodium chloride	2.6	Sodium	75
Glucose, anhydrous	13.5	Chloride	65
Potassium chloride	1.5	Glucose, anhydrous	75
Trisodium citrate, dihydrate	2.9	Potassium	20
		Citrate	10
Total	20.5	Total	24

Q 16. What is the composition of WHO ORS?

Constituent	Grams per litre	Osmolar or ion	mmol/l
Sodium chloride	3.5	Sodium	90
Glucose, anhydrous	20	Chloride	80
Potassium chloride	1.5	Glucose, anhydrous	111
Sodium bicarbonate/citrate	2.5/2.9	Potassium	20
		Bicarbonate/citrate	30/10
Total	27.5/27.9	Total	24

Q 17. Why is new WHO ORS recommended for diarrhoea?

New WHO ORS because of improved effectiveness of reduced osmolarity

a. Decrease in stool output by 25%
b. Decrease vomiting by 30%
c. Decrease need for IV fluids.
d. Decrease both sodium and glucose results in the decrease in osmolarity.

Q 18. What is ReSoMal?

ReSoMal is rehydration solution for malnourished children. Its composition is one WHO ORS packet, 2 litres of water, 50 grams of sugar and 40 grams of electrolytes.

Q 19. How will you teach the mothers to prepare ORS?

The steps for making ORS are:

   a. Wash your hands with soap and water
   b. Pour all the powder from one packet into a clean container
   c. Measure 1 litre of clean drinking water. It is best to boil and cool the water
   d. Pour the water into the container
   e. Mix well until the powder is completely dissolved
   f. She should keep the container covered.
   g. She should throw away any solution remaining after 24 hours.

Q 20. What is the mechanism of action of ORS?

Glucose promotes/increases the absorption of sodium and water from the intestine with the help of SGLT-1 transporter in the intestine.

Q 21. How do we prepare homemade ORS solution?

   a. Clean water: 1 litre (5 cups each cup of about 200 ml)
   b. Sugar: 6 level teaspoons (each teaspoon measuring about 5 grams)
   c. Salt: Half level teaspoon
   d. Stir the contents well until the sugar dissolves
   e. Do not add too much sugar as it will make diarrhoea worse and too much salt will be harmful to the child as well.
   f. Do not store the ORS for more than 24 hours because of the risk of bacterial contamination.

Q 22. What are the home available fluids for acute diarrhoea?

   a. Fluids that contain salt (preferable) like salted rice water, salted yogurt drink, vegetable or chicken soup.
   b. Fluids that do not contain salt (acceptable) are plain water, unsalted rice water, unsalted soup, and yogurt without salt, green coconut water, weak unsweetened tea, and unsweetened fresh fruit juice.
   c. Fluids that must be avoided are commercial carbonated beverages, commercial fruit juices, and tea.

Q 23. What are the advantages of rice-based ORS?

   a. Rice-based ORS has starch instead of glucose, therefore, decrease diarrhoea by adding more substrate to the gut lumen without increasing osmolality.
   b. Tastes better
   c. Provides more calories than the glucose-based.
   d. Shortens the duration of diarrhoea in cholera

Q 24. What is super ORS?

Super ORS contain more complex sugars instead of glucose. They may be food-based (as rice-based) or starch free (glycine/alanine based).

Q 25. What is super super ORS?

Super super ORS is addition of zinc to super ORS.

Q 26. What is the Treatment Plan A?

Treatment Plan A: ORS, breastfeeding for children below 6 months of age, homemade fluids

Age	Amount of ORS or other culturally appropriate ORT fluids to give after each loose stool	Amount of ORS to provide for use at home
<24 months	50–100 ml	500 ml per day
2–10 years	100–200 ml	1000 ml per day
>10 years	Ad lib	2000 ml per day

a. Explain the use of ORS, i.e. the amount to be given, how to mix.
b. Give a teaspoonful every 1–2 min for a child under 2 years.
c. Give frequent sips from a cup for an older child.
d. If the child vomits, wait for 10 min. Then give the solution more slowly (a spoonful every 2–3 min).
e. If diarrhoea persists after the ORS packets are used up, tell the mother to give other fluids as described or return for more fluids.

Q 27. What is the treatment plan for some dehydration?

Treatment Plan B:

All cases with signs of dehydration needed to be treated in a health center or hospital provided oral fluid therapy must be commenced properly and continued through the transport.

1. The daily fluid requirements in children are
   Up to 10 kg = 100 ml per kg
   10–20 kg = 50 ml per kg
   >20 kg = 20 ml per kg
2. Rehydration therapy is calculated as 75 ml per kg of ORS, to be given over 4 hours.

Age	<4 months	4–11 months	12–23 months	2–4 years	5–14 years	≥15 years
Weight (kg)	<5	5–8	8–11	11–16	16–20	>30 kg
ORS (ml)	200–400	400–600	600–800	800–1200	1200–2200	>2200
No. of glasses	1–2	2–3	3–4	4–6	6–11	12–20

Approximate amount of ORS required (ml) = the patient's body weight (kg) × 75

If body weight is not known, the approximate amount to be given in the first 4 hours is according to age.

3. Maintenance therapy to replace fluid losses with ORS in volumes equal to diarrhoeal losses, usually to a maximum of 10 ml/kg/stool. Continue breastfeeding and semi-solid foods to be continued and plain water can be offered in between.

Q 28. What is the treatment plan for children with severe dehydration?

Treatment Plan C:
IV fluids should be started immediately using Ringer lactate with 5% dextrose.
ORS should be started simultaneously if the child can take orally.
IV fluids a total of 100 ml per kg is given over 6 hours in children <12 months and over 3 hours in children >12 months.

Age	30 ml/kg	70 ml/kg
<12 months	1 hour	5 hours
>12 months	30 min	2½ hours

Prevention

Q 29. What is the nutritional management of diarrhoea?
  a. Continue exclusive breastfeeding
  b. Start optimally energy dense foods
  c. Staple foods should be enriched with fat or oil and sugar, e.g. khichri with oil, rice with milk, curd, and sugar, mashed banana with milk or curd, mashed potatoes with oil and lentil.
  d. High fiber content foods
  e. In non-breastfed infants, cow or buffalo milk can be given undiluted after correction of dehydration together with semi-solid foods
  f. Milk cereal mixtures, e.g. dalia, sago or milk-rice mixture is preferable

Q 30. What is the role of zinc supplementation in diarrhoea?
Zinc supplementation is helpful in decreasing the severity and duration of diarrhoea and the risk of persistent diarrhoea.
  Dose is 20 mg of elemental zinc per day for children >6 months for a period of 14 days (10 mg for children 2 months to 6 months).

Q 31. How do you prevent diarrhoea?
  a. Adequate nutrition
  b. Good WaSH Practices
  c. Vaccination
  d. Health education
  e. Proper child rearing practices
  f. Others

Q 32. Name the vaccines available for cholera.

There are three WHO pre-qualified oral cholera vaccines: Dukoral, Shanchol, and Euvichol. All three vaccines require two doses for full protection.

Q 33. What is the national program for diarrhoea control in our country?
National Diarrhoeal Disease Control Programme, since 2003 is included in Integrated Management of Neonatal and Childhood Illness which includes national guidelines on diarrhoea, ARI, malaria, anaemia, vitamin A supplementation and immunizations.

Q 34. Is diarrheoa under Integrated Disease Surveillance Project (IDSP) reporting?
Acute diarrhoeal disease (including acute gastroenteritis) is under Form P of IDSP.

Q 35. What are the various forms under IDSP? [Annexures 14 to 16]
   a. Form S: For Syndromic Surveillance (Suspect Cases)
   b. Form P: For Presumptive Surveillance (Probable Cases)
   c. Form L1: For Peripheral Laboratories (L1)
   d. Form L2: For District and Private Laboratories (L2)
   e. Form L3: For Medical College and Reference Laboratories (L3 and L4 laboratories)
   f. Form W: For Water Quality Monitoring

Q 36. Is cholera under Integrated Disease Surveillance Programme (IDSP) reporting?
Cholera is under Form L of IDSP.

Q 37. Brief about the WHO cholera kits.
WHO revised the cholera kits in 2016. Each treatment kit provides enough material to treat 100 patients. In total there are 6 kits:
   a. 1 for investigation
   b. 1 with laboratory supplies for confirmation
   c. 3 for the community, peripheral and central levels
   d. 1 support kit with logistical materials

Q 38. What are the diseases under International Health Regulations (IHR 2005)?
Group 1: A single case of smallpox, poliomyelitis due to wild type poliovirus, human influenza caused by a new subtype and severe acute respiratory syndrome (SARS) must be immediately notified to WHO, irrespective of the context in which it occurs.
Group 2: Events involving epidemic-prone diseases of special national or regional concern, which "have demonstrated the ability to cause serious public health impact and to spread rapidly internationally" must always, be assessed using the decision instrument but only notified when fulfilling the requirements of the algorithm.

SICK NEONATE

Introduction

Q 1. Define neonatal period.
Neonatal period is defined as the period from birth to under four weeks (<28 days) of age.

The first week of life (<7 days) is known as early neonatal period and late neonatal period extends from 7th to 28th day of life.

Q 2. Define postneonatal period.
It is the period of infancy extending from 28 days of life up to one year of age.

Q 3. Define perinatal period.

It is the period that extends from 22nd week of gestation to less than 7 days of life.

Q 4. Define neonatal mortality rate.

It is defined as deaths of infants under the first 28 days of life per 1000 live births per year.

Q 5. What is intrauterine growth restriction (IUGR)?

Intrauterine growth restriction results when the foetus does not grow as per the normal foetal growth trajectory. There are two types of IUGR:

a. Symmetric IUGR: The size of the head, body weight, and length are equally reduced. Causes include genetic and chromosomal disorders or TORCH infections.

b. Asymmetric IUGR: Head circumference is preserved compared to length and weight. Causes include placental insufficiency, pregnancy-induced hypertension or medical diseases.

Q 6. What is small for gestational age (SGA)?

It is a statistical definition and denotes weight of the infant is less than two standard deviation or less than the tenth centile of the population norms (plotted on the intrauterine growth chart).

Burden

Q 7. What is the neonatal mortality rate of India?

According to the WHO Global health observatory report on India statistics, the NMR for the year 2015 was 27.7 per 1000 live births.

According to the World Health Bank report, the neonatal mortality rate for the year 2015 was 28 per 1000 live births.

Risk Factor

Q 8. What are the causes of neonatal deaths?

The causes of under-five child deaths in India 2010 [CHERG 2012: Child health epidemiology reference group funded by Bill and Melinda Gate foundation] are:

a. Preterm: 36%
b. Asphyxia: 10%
c. Pneumonia: 8%
d. Sepsis: 8%
e. Congenital disorders: 5%

Q 9. What are the causes of under-five deaths?

The causes of under-five child deaths in India 2010 [CHERG 2012] are:

a. Pneumonia: 23%
b. Preterm: 18%
c. Diahrroea: 12%
d. Asphyxia: 10%
e. Sepsis: 8%

Q 10. Who are "at-risk" infants?

At-risk babies include:

  a. Artificial feeding
  b. Birth order >5
  c. Low birth weight
  d. Failure to thrive (failure to gain weight in 3 successive months)
  e. Severe malnutrition
  f. Twins
  g. Working mother/single parent

Clinical Features

Q 11. When is the first examination done for a newborn?

The first examination is done as soon after birth and preferably in the delivery room. The examination looks for whether the baby has not suffered injuries during the birth process and to detect malformations and finally to assess maturity.

Q 12. When is the second examination done for a newborn?

A specialist does this preferably within 24 hours of birth. It is a detailed examination conducted from head to toe in good light. The following things will be seen:

  a. **Head and face:** Hydrocephalus, large fontanelles, prominent scalp vein, cataract, coloboma, conjunctivitis, accessory auricles, pre-auricular pits, harelip, cleft palate.
  b. **Skin:** Look for cyanosis of lips and skin, jaundice, pallor in the palmar crease and lower bulbar conjunctiva, erythema, vesicles, and bullae.
  c. **Central nervous system:** Neck rigidity, hyperextension, and hyperflexion of limbs, asymmetrical posture, tendon reflexes, and abnormal movements.
  d. **Cardio-respiratory system:** Pulse, cardiac murmurs, respiratory rate, subcostal retractions, crepitations, wheeze, stridor.
  e. **Gastro-intestinal system:** Abdominal distension, mass abdomen, congenital hernia, imperforate anus.
  f. **Genital system:** Hypospadias, undescended testis, hydrocele, fused labia, enlarged clitoris.
  g. **Limbs and Joints:** Joint deformities, congenital dislocation of hip, extra digits.
  h. **Spine:** Neural tube defects.
  i. **Body size:** Body weight, length, head circumference, chest circumference.
  j. **Body temperature**

Management

Q 13. What is Level 1 (L1) health facility?

Level 1 includes all sub-centres and non-24 × 7 PHC where deliveries are conducted by a skilled-birth attendant (SBA).

Q 14. What are the facilities for newborn care at L1 health facility?

L1 health facility has a newborn care corner (NBCC).

Q 15. What are the services given in newborn care corner (NBCC)?

The services given in newborn care corner are:

a. Essential newborn care including resuscitation

b. Zero day immunization (OPV, BCG, Hep B)

c. Inj vitamin K

d. Care of normal and sick newborn

e. Referral services

Q 16. What is level 2 (L2) health facility?

Level 2 health facility includes all 24 × 7 facilities PHC, non-FRU CHC and others providing BEmOC services.

Q 17. What facility does L2 health facility has for newborn care?

Level 2 has either a NBCC or newborn stabilization unit (NBSU).

Q 18. What are the services given at newborn stabilization unit (NBSU)?

The services given in newborn stabilization unit are:

a. Essential newborn care including resuscitation

b. Zero day immunization (OPV, BCG, Hep B)

c. Inj vitamin K

d. Care of normal and sick newborn

e. Identification and management of LBW infants ≥1800 g with no other complications

f. Referral services

Q 19. What is Level 3 (L3) health facility?

Level 3 health facility includes all FRU-CHC, sub-district hospital, district hospital and tertiary care hospitals where complications are managed including C-section and blood transfusion.

Q 20. What facility does L3 health facility has for newborn care?

Level 3 has newborn stabilization unit (NBSU) at CHC, sub-district hospital and others or special newborn care unit (SNCU) at the district hospital and tertiary care hospitals.

Q 21. What are the services given at special newborn care unit (SNCU)?

The services given in newborn stabilization unit are:

a. Essential newborn care including resuscitation

b. Zero day immunization (OPV, BCG, Hep B)

c. Inj vitamin K

d. Care of normal and sick newborn

e. Identification and management of LBW infants <1800 g

Q 22. What is essential newborn care?

The essential newborn care includes:

a. Prevention of infection

b. Provision of warmth

c. Resuscitation

d. Early initiation of breastfeeding

e. Weighing the newborn

Q 23. What is care of a normal newborn?
a. Breastfeeding/feeding support
b. Immunization

Q 24. What is care of the sick newborn?
At NBCC
Identification and prompt referral of at-risk and sick newborn
At NBSU
a. Identification and prompt referral of at-risk and sick newborn
b. Phototherapy for newborns with hyperbilirubinemia
c. Management of newborn sepsis
d. Referral services

At SNCU
a. Managing all sick newborns (except those requiring mechanical ventilation and major surgical interventions)
b. Follow-up of all babies
c. Referral services

Q 25. What immediate care do you give to a newborn?
The immediate care to newborn includes:
a. Clearing the airway
b. APGAR score
c. Care of the cord
d. Care of the eyes
e. Care of the skin
f. Maintenance of body temperature
g. Breastfeeding

Q 26. What is Apgar score and what is its importance?
Apgar score is an objective method of evaluating the newborn's condition. It is performed at 1 minute and again at 5 minutes after birth. Apgar score should be obtained every 5 minutes for up to 20 minutes if the 5 minutes score is less than seven.

Apgar score			
Signs	**0**	**1**	**2**
Heart rate	Absent	Slow (<100 beats/min)	Normal (>100 beats/min)
Respiration	Absent	Weak cry	Good strong cry
Muscle tone	Limp	Some flexion	Active movements
Reflex irritability	No response	Grimace	Cough or sneeze
Colour	Blue or pale	Body pink, extremities blue	Completely pink

A normal score is 8 to 10, a score less than 7 needs action

Q 27. What is routine care given during delivery for healthy newborn?

The routine cares given during delivery for healthy newborn are:

    a. Personnel and equipment to be available during delivery
    b. Standard precautions and asepsis at birth
    c. Clean hands, clean surface, clean blade, clean tie, nothing to be applied to the cord
    d. Prevention and management of hypothermia
    e. Delayed clamping of the umbilical cord
    f. Cleaning of the baby
    g. Clamping of the cord
    h. Placement of identity band

Q 28. What care will you provide to the baby in the initial few hours after birth?

The care provided to the baby in the initial few hours after birth is:

    a. Recording of weight
    b. Head to toe examination
    c. Initiation of breastfeeding
    d. Administration of vitamin K
    e. Communicating with the family members
    f. Rooming in

Q 29. What is rooming in?

Keeping the baby's crib by the side of the mother's bed is known as rooming in. In the initial few hours of life, the baby is very active and the closeness of the baby to the mother will facilitate early breastfeeding and bonding.

Q 30. What are the common parental concerns regarding the health of the neonate which are considered usually normal by the health professionals?

The common parental concerns are:

    a. Weight loss in the first week
    b. Crying during micturition
    c. Bathing
    d. Applying cosmetics which must be discouraged
    e. Regurgitation
    f. Frequent stools
    g. Breast engorgement
    h. Rashes and skin peeling
    i. Diaper rash

Q 31. How do you prevent hypothermia in a newborn child?

Prevention of hypothermia is by:

    a. Warm chain
    b. Incubators and radiant warmers

Q 32. What do you mean by warm chain?

Warm chain is a set of ten steps aimed at decreasing heat loss, promoting heat gain

    a. Warm delivery room
    b. Warm resuscitation

   c. Immediate drying

   d. Skin to skin contact

   e. Breastfeeding

   f. Bathing postponed

   g. Appropriate clothing

   h. Mother and baby together

   i. Professional alertness

   j. Warm transportation

Q 33. What are the common congenital malformations in a neonate?

The common congenital malformations in a neonate are:

   a. Tracheoesophageal fistula

   b. Anorectal malformation

   c. Anencephaly, congenital hydrocephalus, myelomeningocele

   d. Cleft lip and cleft palate

   e. Diaphragmatic hernia

   f. Others

Q 34. What protocol will you follow while transporting sick neonates?

The protocol while transporting sick neonates is:

   a. Determine the indication for transport: Like birth weight <1200 gram or <30 weeks of gestation, severe respiratory distress, severe jaundice, major malformations, and refractory seizures.

   b. Prepare for transport: Stabilize the baby like maintain temperature, airway, breathing, circulation, and blood sugar, counsel the parents, communicate with the referral facility, arrange supplies, equipment and transport vehicle.

   c. Care during transport: Monitor frequently temperature, airway, breathing, circulation, and blood sugar. Ensure the baby receives feeds or fluids, stop the vehicle if necessary to manage problems.

   d. Feedback after transport: Communicate with referral team for the condition at arrival and outcome.

Prevention

Q 35. What is infant and young child feeding?

Infant and young child feeding is recommendations for appropriate feeding of newborn and children under two years. It includes:

   a. Initiation of breastfeeding immediately after birth

   b. Exclusive breastfeeding for the first six months

   c. Adequate complementary feeding

Q 36. What do you mean by exclusive breastfeeding (EBF)?

Exclusive breastfeeding is when an infant receives only breast milk, without any additional food or fluids, other than ORS, vitamins, and medicine, until 6 months of age.

Q 37. When to start breastfeeding to newborn?

Start breastfeeding as early as possible. It is recommended within half an hour after normal delivery and within 4 hours of birth after cesarean section.

Q 38. What are the benefits of breastfeeding?

The benefits of breastfeeding are:
a. Benefits to the baby: Less infections, easily digested, better bonding, better cognitive development
b. Benefits to the mother: Involution of uterus, delays pregnancy, lower risk of breast cancer
c. Benefits to the family/society: Cost safer, child survival

Q 39. What is pre-lacteal feed?

A pre-lacteal feed is any food other than mother's milk given to a newborn before initiating breastfeeding. For example, honey.

Q 40. What is colostrum?

Colostrum is mother's first breast milk rich in immunoglobulin.

Q 41. What are the signs of good attachment of the baby to the mother's breast?

The four signs of good attachment are:
a. Chin touching breast (or very close)
b. Mouth wide open
c. Lower lip turned outward
d. More areola visible above than below the mouth

Q 42. What are the signs of the good position of the baby to the mother's breast?

The signs of the good position of the baby to the mother's breast are:
a. The child's whole body should face the mother and be close to her
b. The child's head and neck should be supported, in a straight line with his body, to face the breast
c. The child's abdomen should touch mother's abdomen, to be as close as possible to his mother

Q 43. What are the recommendations for breastfeeding?

The recommendations for breastfeeding are:
a. Exclusive breastfeeding up to 6 months
b. Breastfed as often as the child wants, at least 8 times in 24 hours.
c. Breastfed when the child shows signs of hunger, e.g. sucking fingers, or moving the lips.
d. Breastfed at least 10 minutes on each breast every time

Q 44. When does weaning/complementary feeding start in infants?

Weaning/complimentary feeding started in infants at 6 months of age.

Q 45. What are the recommendations for complementary feeding?

The recommendations for complementary feeding are:
a. Breastfeed as often as the child wants 6 months up to 23 months
b. Give adequate servings of complementary foods, 3 times per day if breastfed and 5 times if not breastfed, with 1–2 nutritious snacks, as desired, from 9 to 23 months.
c. Give small chewable items to eat with fingers.
d. Allow the child to try to feed self with help.

Q 46. What are the eligibility criteria for Kangaroo mother care?

All stable LBW babies are eligible for KMC. However, very sick babies needing special care should be cared under radiant warmer initially.

    a. Birth weight > = 1800 grams KMC starts at birth

    b. Birth weight 1200–1799 grams KMC starts after a few days

    c. Birth weight <1200 grams starts after a few days to weeks

Q 47. What are components of KMC?

The components of KMC are:

    a. Skin to skin contact

    b. Exclusive breastfeeding

Q 48. What are pre-requisites of KMC?

The pre-requisites of KMC are:

    a. Support to the mother

    b. Postdischarge follow-up

Q 49. What are the benefits of KMC?

The benefits of KMC are:

    a. Thermal control

    b. Increased breastfeeding

    c. Early discharge from hospital

    d. Better infant bonding

Q 50. How to provide Kangaroo mother care (KMC)?

To provide Kangaroo mother care (KMC):

    a. Request the mother to sit comfortably in privacy

    b. Keep the cap, nappy and socks on baby

    c. Place the baby prone on the mother's chest in an upright and extended posture, between her breasts, in skin-to-skin contact

    d. Turn the baby's head to one side to keep the airway clear.

    e. Cover the baby with the mother's blouse, 'pallu' or gown. Wrap both baby and mother with a blanket or shawl

    f. Ask the mother to breastfeed the baby frequently

Q 51. When should KMC be discontinued?

KMC is desirable until the baby weight reaches 2500 gm.

Q 52. What is ENAP?

ENAP is every newborn action plan. Its goals are ending preventable newborn deaths and stillbirths by 2035.

Q 53. What is INAP (Indian newborn action plan)?

The Indian newborn action plan (INAP) is India's committed response to the global every newborn action plan (ENAP), launched in June 2014. It aims at attaining single digit neonatal mortality rate and stillbirth rate by 2030, with all the states to individually achieve this target by 2035.

Q 54. What are the milestones in child survival programmes in India?

The Milestones in Child Survival Programmes in India are:
   a. Child Survival and Safe Motherhood Programme (CSSM)—1992
   b. RCH I—1997
   c. RCH II—2005
   d. National Rural Health Mission—2005
   e. RMNCH+A Strategy—2013
   f. National Health Mission—2013
   g. India Newborn Action Plan (INAP)—2014

Q 55. What are the interventions under National Health Mission focusing on newborns?

   a. Janani Suraksha Yojana 2005
   b. IMNCI at community level and F-IMNCI at health facilities 2007
   c. Navjat Shishu Suraksha Karyakram 2009
   d. Janani Shishu Suraksha Karyakram 2011
   e. Facility based newborn care 2011
   f. Home based newborn care 2011
   g. Rashtriya Bal Swasthya Karyakram 2013
   h. Mission Indradhanush 2014
   i. Mothers' Absolute Affection 2016

Q 56. What is Rashtriya Bal Swasthya Karyakram?

Rashtriya Bal Swasthya Karyakram is a program which aims early identification and early intervention for children from birth to 18 years to cover 4 D that is defects at birth, deficiencies, diseases, development delays including disability.

Q 57. What is Navjaat Shishu Suraksha Karyakram?

Navjaat Shishu Suraksha Karyakram is a programme on basic newborn care and resuscitation is being launched by the Ministry of Health and Family Welfare to target important interventions of care at birth, i.e. prevention of hypothermia, prevention of infection, early initiation of breastfeeding and basic newborn resuscitation.

Q 58. What is Mission Indradhanush?

The Mission Indradhanush is a program which aims to cover all those children who are either unvaccinated or are partially vaccinated against vaccine preventable diseases by 2020.

Q 59. What is mother's absolute affection (MAA) programme?

Mother's absolute affection is a program, which aims to bring undiluted focus on promotion of breastfeeding.

Q 60. What is Integrated Child Development Scheme (ICDS)?

The Government of India and Ministry of Social and Women's Welfare initiated ICDS in 1975 in pursuance of the National Policy for Children.

Under this program, the following services are provided:
   a. Supplementary nutrition
   b. Immunization

c. Health check-up

d. Medical referral services

e. Nutrition and health education for women and

f. Non-formal education of children up to the age of 6 years, and pregnant and nursing mothers in rural, urban, and tribal areas.

ADOLESCENT

(An individual aged 10 to 19 years)   **Ashish Pundhir**

ANAEMIA

Introduction

Q 1. What is the continuum of anaemia among pregnant mothers, adolescents, and children?

A pregnant woman with nutritional anaemia results into the inadequate transport of iron into a foetus, which increases the risk of premature delivery, low birth weight, and reduced capacity for providing care to the infant. A low birth weight infant is at risk of impaired mental development, inadequate growth and increased risk of contracting chronic diseases of an adult. Subsequently, the stunt in growth of child and adolescent stage in conjunction with inadequate food, health and care results to low weight gain during pregnancy (risk of maternal morbidity (anaemia), as well as mortality increased).

Q 2. Mention the public health importance of nutritional anaemia.

Nutritional anaemia can cause cognitive impairment, poor school performance, decreases immunity, and limitation in behavioral and language development. In pregnant women with nutritional anaemia, the risk of premature delivery, foetal and maternal morbidity is increased.

Q 3. What is the requirement of iron in the diet for various age groups?

Iron requirements (mg/1000 kcal)

a. Pregnant women 1.9 in the second trimester, 2.7 the third trimester

b. Infants (1.0)

c. Adolescent girls (0.8)

d. Adolescent boys (0.6)

e. Non-pregnant women (0.6)

f. Preschool and school age child (0.4)

g. Adult men (0.3)

Q 4. What is the WHO classification of anaemia?

The cut off for haemoglobin (gm %) in blood to diagnose anaemia:

a. Mild anaemia: 10 to 11.9

b. Moderate anaemia: 7 to 9.9

c. Severe anaemia: <7

   d. Anaemia in non-pregnant woman (above 15 years of age): <12

   e. Anaemia in pregnant women: <11

Q 5. What is the cutoff of haemoglobin gm/dl to diagnose anaemia in various age groups?

Anaemia-Haemoglobin (g/dl) is less than

   a. 6–59 months ≤11

   b. 5–11 years: 11.5

   c. 12–14 years: 12

   d. 15 years and above: 12

   e. Pregnant women: 11

   f. Men: 13

Q 6. What is the distribution of haemoglobinopathies in India and importance of its exclusion?

The haemoglobinopathies are classified either into thalassemia syndromes (alpha or beta thalassemia) or into structural haemoglobin variants (HbC, HbE, HbS).

   Geographical distribution of haemoglobinopathies:

   a. Alpha thalassemia: Western Rajasthan, Maharashtra

   b. Beta thalassemia: Punjab, Andhra Pradesh

   c. HbS: Assam, Madhya Pradesh

   d. HbD: Assam

   e. HbE: North eastern states, West Bengal

   f. HbF: Kerala

   g. HbJ Meerut: West Bengal

   It is always important to rule out haemoglobinopathies especially in endemic areas to prevent iron load. Further, it is to be noted iron supplements are to be administered only if there is a deficiency of iron, especially in thalassemia and sickle cell disease.

Burden

Q 7. What is the prevalence of anaemia in India?

The prevalence of anaemia as per National Family Health Survey (NFHS-4) was 53% in 15–49 years of age group women and 22.7% in men.

Risk Factor

Q 8. What are the main causes of nutritional anaemia?

Main causes of nutritional anaemia are deficiency of iron or folic acid or vitamin B_{12}.

Q 9. What are the causes of iron deficiency anaemia?

Most common cause of iron deficiency anaemia is nutrition and infectious factors. The various factors are:

   a. Poor dietary intake of iron resulting in the deficiency of iron in the body and thus iron deficiency anaemia.

   b. Low bio-availability of iron-habitual intake of cereal-based diet high in phytate and poor consumption of iron absorption enhancers such as vitamin C.

   c. Dietary deficiency of vitamins such as folic acid, vitamin C, vitamin B_{12}

   d. Malaria

e. Hookworm infestation and schistosomiasis: Unhygienic practices and unsanitary environment promote infections with gastro-intestinal parasites.

f. Menorrhagia

g. Gender bias

h. Post-marital women status

i. Teen marriage and early pregnancy

j. Standard of living of household, literacy and economic status, poverty, illiteracy and poor living standards are usually associated with anaemia.

Q 10. What are the causes of megaloblastic anaemia?

Deficit folic acid or vitamin B_{12} due to dietary deficiency (vegetarian diet), inadequate absorption from intestine due to deficit intrinsic factor, intake of medications which interfere with absorption and metabolism either of folic acid (phenytoin, methotrexate, and trimethoprim) or vitamin B_{12} (metformin, proton pump inhibitors).

Clinical Features

Q 11. What are the clinical features of iron deficiency anaemia?

The clinical features of iron deficiency anaemia are pallor of mucous membranes, fatigue, dizziness and drowsiness, craving for mud, loss of appetite, dysphagia, leg cramps on climbing stairs, glossitis, koilonychia, and others.

Q 12. How would you explain the synonymous use of the terms pallor and anaemia is incorrect?

Pallor is a sign based on colour of skin and mucous membrane which can exist even in absence of anaemia. On contrary, anaemia is qualitative or quantitative diminution of red blood cells and/or haemoglobin concentration in relation to standard age and sex. Pallor without anaemia can be present in the following conditions: (i) Respiratory distress; (ii) Shock; (iii) Skin oedema; (iv) Hypoglycemia; (v) Fair-skinned person.

Q 13. How would clinical examination help in identifying a patient suffering from anaemia?

The colour of the mucous membranes of the mouth and conjunctivae gives a better indication than the colour of the creases of the palm of the hand.

a. Palpebral conjunctiva: Pull the eyelids downward outwards and look for the whiteness of inner side of the lower eyelid.

b. Lip: Look for cracks at the corner of the mouth (angular stomatitis)

c. Tongue: Pale and coarse nature of tongue

d. Nail bed: Look for pallor of the flesh underneath the nails and spoon-shaped nail bed (koilonychia).

e. Palm: Compare it with palm of your own hand

Management

Q 14. What are the investigations done for anaemia?

a. Complete blood counts

b. Examination of peripheral blood smear

c. Blood films to be examined for malaria parasites

d. Stool examination for ova cyst and occult blood

Q 15. What is the treatment of anaemia?

a. Mild anaemia gives 60 mg of elemental iron daily for 3 months, follow-up every month if Hb more than 12 gm/dl or else refer.

b. Moderate anaemia gives 60 mg of elemental iron daily for 3 months, follow-up every 14 days if Hb more than 12 gm/dl or else refers.

c. Severe anaemia requires urgent referral to district hospital (DH)/first referral unit (FRU) for blood transfusion and IV iron therapy.

Q 16. What are the indications for blood transfusion in an anaemic patient?

If haemoglobin level is below and less than or equal to 4 gm/dl

If Hb level 4–6 gm/dl when following conditions are present:

a. Dehydration

b. Shock

c. Impaired consciousness

d. Heart failure

e. Very high level of parasitemia

Q 17. Which food item would you advise not to be consumed along with iron tablets?

Food items advised to be avoided with iron tablets:

a. High fiber foods, such as whole grains

b. Raw vegetables

c. Bran and milk

d. Antacids

e. Caffeine/tea

f. Banana

Q 18. What are the side effects of iron tablets?

Iron tablets intake empty stomach may cause stomach cramps, gastritis, nausea, vomiting, constipation, diarrhoea, black-coloured stools, and others.

Q 19. What is the treatment of megaloblastic anaemia?

Due to deficiency of vitamin B_{12}, inj vitamin B_{12} 250–1000 microgram [children (250–500 microgram)], intramuscular, once weekly until the hematocrit becomes normal. For deficiency of folic acid, give tablet folic acid 5 mg, daily for 3–4 weeks.

Q 20. Which is the single most sensitive tool for evaluating the iron status?

Serum ferritin is the single most sensitive tool for evaluating the iron status.

Q 21. Enumerate some iron preparation available in market.

Tab Autrin and Tab FAA 20.

Q 22. When would you consider the use of parental iron therapy over oral iron therapy?

Parental iron therapy is indicated in case there is non-compliance, mal-absorption, occult bleeding from gastro-intestinal tract, chronic diarrhoea and moderate to severe anaemia in pregnancy.

Q 23. How rapidly does parental iron sucrose therapy in comparison to oral therapy increase the haemoglobin level?

Parental administration of iron does not result in the rapid increase of haemoglobin instead its rise is similar to oral preparation. It is to be noted oral iron therapy is effective as parental iron therapy and safer in comparison.

Q 24. How would you compute the dose for parental iron administration (iron sucrose)?

Iron sucrose is preferred over iron dextran because of fewer side effects

In pregnant women

Required iron dose (mg) = 2.4 × (target Hb – actual Hb) × pre-pregnancy weight (kg) + 500 mg* for replenishment of stores

The computed dose is diluted in 100 ml 0.9% normal saline and then the infusion should be administered over the period of 30 minutes. The computed dose should be administered in divided dose either every day or alternate day with maximum of 200 mg in one dose and maximum of 600 mg per week.

Children

Required iron dose (mg) = 4.1 × (target haemoglobin – actual haemoglobin) × weight

Q 25. What are side effects of parental administration of iron sucrose?

Side effects usually occur when the rate of infusion is either very slow or very fast or being infused with a higher dose. Oedema, nausea, headache, vomiting, dizziness, abdominal, muscle pain and cardiovascular collapse are common side effects. To avoid side effects, infuse 100 ml of diluted iron solution within 30 minutes.

Prevention

Q 26. What iron rich foods would you advise to a patient with iron deficiency anaemia?

There are two forms of iron: Heme iron and non-haeme iron.

The haeme iron has better bioavailability and promotes the absorption of non-haeme iron. Food rich in haeme iron are liver, meat, poultry, and fish.

Foods containing non-haeme iron are of vegetable origin such as:

a. Cereals (wheat, jowar and bajra)
b. Green leafy vegetables (spinach, onion stalk, fenugreek leaves, mint, and mustard leaves)
c. Legumes (including sprouts)
d. Nuts
e. Pulses (red gram, black gram, and soya bean)
f. Sesame
g. Oilseeds
h. Jaggery
i. Dried fruits

---

* In some literature it is mentioned 1000 mg

Q 27. What are the common inhibitors, which impair the absorption of iron?
This is due to the presence of phytates (in legumes and whole grains), tannins (tea), polyphenols (honey, legumes and many fruits), oxalates, carbonates, phosphates, and dietary fibre, which interfere with the absorption of iron.

Q 28. What do you understand by food fortification? What food items are fortified with iron to prevent anaemia?
Fortification is adding vitamins and minerals to foods to prevent nutritional deficiencies. The nutrients regularly used in grain fortification prevent diseases, strengthen immune systems, and improve productivity and cognitive development. Wheat flour with iron and folic acid, milk, sugar and salt (Tata salt plus) with iron have been fortified in India to prevent anaemia.

Q 29. How will you prevent and control anaemia among adolescents?
The following measures should be undertaken:
Primary prevention of anaemia is achieved through well:
a. Balanced diet rich in iron and other vitamins and minerals involved in iron absorption or in the production of RBCs/haemoglobin.
b. Iron supplementation.
c. Screening of target groups for moderate/severe anaemia and referring these cases to an appropriate health facility.
d. Prevention and treatment of hookworm infestation
   i. To prevent hookworm infestation one should maintain personal hygiene and environmental cleanliness.
   ii. One should use sanitary latrine.
   iii. Albendazole 400 mg tablet, six months apart (in Rajasthan and Madhya Pradesh, it is administered once a month because prevalence of soil transmitted helminths is less than 20%).
   iv. Use of safe drinking water can help protect from various infections and diseases.
   v. Washing hands with soap and water before cooking, consuming food, after defecation and after discarding faecal matter of a child

Q 30. What is iron prophylaxis in various age groups?

	Iron prophylaxis				
Group	6–60 months	5–10 years	10–19 years	Pregnant woman and lactating mother	
Elemental iron (mg)	20	45	100	100	100
Folic acid (µg)	100	400	500	500	
Duration	Biweekly	Weekly	Weekly	6 months daily antenatal and postpartum	

Q 31. Enumerate the food (both vegetarian and non-vegetarian) sources of vitamin B_{12} (cobalamin)?
Vegetarian: Fermented soya beans, dairy products like milk and cheese
Non-vegetarian: Eggs, meat, fish, kidney and liver

Q 32. What initiatives have the Government of India undertaken to prevent and control anaemia among adolescents?

a. National Iron Plus Initiative

b. Weekly Iron Folic Acid Supplementation Programme

c. RMNCH+A

d. Rashtriya Kishor Swasthya Karyakram

Q 33. What is National Iron Plus Initiative?

National Iron + Initiative provides a minimum service package for the management of anaemia across life stages and at different levels of care. This initiative brings together existing programmes for iron and folic acid (IFA) supplementation among pregnant and lactating women and children in the age group of 6–60 months and proposes to include new age groups (adolescents, women in reproductive age group).

National Iron Plus Initiative will include adolescents (10–19 years), both in and out of school. Those in school will be reached through weekly iron and folic acid supplementation while out of school children will be reached through anganwadi centres. The iron and folic acid tablet for adolescents is coloured blue (*'iron ki nili goli'*) to distinguish it from red IFA tablet for pregnant and lactating women.

Q 34. What is weekly iron folic acid supplementation (WIFS) programme?

The WIFS programme is implemented in urban and rural areas for adolescent boys and girls in school (10–19 years) through the platform of Government/Government aided/municipal schools. WIFS will also reach out of school girls in the age group 10–19 years through the platform of Anganwadi Kendra.

This strategy involves a "fixed day—Monday" approach for IFA distribution. Teachers and AWWs will supervise the ingestion of the IFA tablet by the beneficiaries.

MENTAL RETARDATION (INTELLECTUAL DISABILITY)

Introduction

Q 1. Define intellectual disability.

US special educational plan, The Individuals with Disabilities Education Act (IDEA) defines mental retardation as "significantly sub-average general intellectual functioning, existing concurrently with deficits in adaptive behavior and manifested during the developmental period that adversely affects a child's educational performance."

Burden

Q 2. What is the burden of mental health problems?

According to WHO estimated, 1% of Indian population is suffering from severe mental disorders and 10% from mild mental disorders.

Risk Factor

Q 3. What are the common causes of intellectual disability?

Prenatal: Consanguinity, maternal age, infections (toxoplasmosis, rubella), poor nutrition for the mother

Perinatal and neonatal: Prematurity, low birth weight

Postnatal: Malnutrition, infection (TORCH, HIV), head injury, child abuse

Clinical Features

Q 4. How would you suspect intellectual disability (mental retardation)?

Intellectual disability is to be suspected in an adolescent:

a. Having difficulties in the social relation with other adolescents.

b. Shows inappropriate sexual behaviour

c. Is unable to learn at the same rate as other students in class

Note: But the above three must be differentially diagnosed from other psychiatric disorders as difficulties in social relationship and inability to learn at the same rate as other students in class may occur in pervasive developmental disorders, i.e. impairment in reciprocal social interactions, communication and the presence of stereotyped behaviour, interest and activities (e.g. autism, Asperger syndrome, Rett syndrome).

Q 5. Elaborate the adaptive behaviour that should be assessed in adolescents suspected of having intellectual disability.

American Association on Intellectual and Developmental Disabilities (AAIDD) classification of adaptive behaviour has addresses the following skills:

a. Conceptual skills: Ability to speak and understand language

b. Social skills: Ability to follow rules, interpersonal skills

c. Practical skills: Daily living activities

d. Occupational skills: Academic performance, duties

e. Maintenance of safe behavior: Not harming self or others

Q 6. What are the milestones of development that would be helpful for a primary care physician to detect mental retardation?

The milestones of development		
Milestones	**Age at which most children achieve this milestone**	**Suspect mental retardation if milestone is delayed beyond**
Responds to name/voice	1–3 months	4th month
Smiles at others	1–4 months	6th month
Holds head steady	2–6 months	6th month
Sits without support	5–10 months	12th month
Stands without support	9–14 months	18th month
Walks well	10–20 months	20th month
Talks in 2–3 word sentences	16–30 months	3rd year
Eats/drinks by self	2–3 years	4th year
Can tell own name	2–3 years	4th year
Is toilet trained	3–4 years	4th year
Avoids simple hazards	3–4 years	4th year

Source: Problems in Childhood and Adolescence. In Patel V. *Where There Is No Psychiatrist: A Mental Health Care Manual.* New Delhi: Voluntary Health Association of India; 2002

Q 7. Is it true to assert that adolescents in whom milestones were delayed (or children with developmental delay) are intellectually disabled?

Delayed milestones do not imply intellectual disability as these individuals can recuperate and achieve normalcy.

Q 8. What are the complications associated with intellectual disability?

The most common deficits are motor impairments, behavioural and emotional disorders, medical complications, and seizures.

Management

Q 9. How will you treat a case of mental retardation?

It is indicated for a specific indication like co-morbid psychosis, depression, anxiety, or hyperactivity. Haloperidol and chlorpromazine have been used to control stereotyped motor abnormalities. Hyperactivity can be managed with methylphenidate and amphetamine while to control aggression and self-injurious behaviour the use of lithium carbonate can be considered.

Prevention

Q 10. What level of prevention should be undertaken in the context of intellectual disability?

Primary Prevention
The primary prevention comprises the following measures
  a. Essential antenatal and postnatal care
  b. Ensure exclusive breastfeeding for six months
  c. Immunization
  d. Adequate nutrition
  e. Care and love for child

Secondary Prevention
The measures in secondary prevention are:
  a. Early detection and treatment
  b. Preventable disorders, e.g phenylketonuria (low phenylalanine diet), hypothyroidism
  c. Sensory, motor or behavioural areas with early remedial measures
  d. Infections
  e. The following guidelines for parents are vital for making the stimulation programme work are:
   i. Praise abundantly
   ii. Talk a lot to the child about what you are doing
   iii. Guide the child's movements with your hands, gradually decreasing support as the child is able to complete the activity on his own.
   iv. Teach by encouraging imitation.
   v. Make learning fun by trying new things
   vi. Involve other children, as they can be the best teachers

Tertiary Prevention
   a. Behaviour modification, positive (reward) and negative reinforcement
   b. Rehabilitation in vocational, physical and social areas
   c. Parental counseling

Q 11. Enumerate the legislation for intellectual disable adolescents?
   a. Persons with Disability Act (1995)
   b. National Trust Act (1999)

Q 12. What is the name of the national program for mental health?
The Government of India launched the National Mental Health Program (NMHP) in 1982, keeping in view the heavy burden of mental illness in the community and the absolute inadequacy of mental health care infrastructure in the country to deal with it.

RHEUMATIC FEVER AND RHEUMATIC HEART DISEASE

Introduction

Q 1. What is rheumatic fever (RF)?
It is a febrile disease affecting connective tissue and joints (painful or swollen knee, elbows, ankles, and wrists joint) initiated by infection of the throat by group A beta hemolytic streptococci.

Q 2. How does rheumatic heart disease (RHD) occur?
A repeated episode of RF leads to RHD.

Risk Factors

Q 3. What is the cause for RF?
RF results from an autoimmune response to infection with group A Streptococcus (GAS).

Q 4. What is the most common age group affected with the RF/RHD?
RF/RHD affects children in age group of 5–15 years.

Q 5. What are the determinants of Rheumatic heart disease and its impact on the disease itself?
Socio economic and environmental determinants: Poverty, under-nutrition, over-crowding, poor housing, unhygienic living conditions, illiteracy, and others
   Health-system determinants: Shortage of resources for health care, inadequate expertise of health care providers, low level awareness of the disease in the community, absence of community or school health awareness programs and others.

Clinical Features

Q 6. When to suspect RF in a child?
A child presenting with a sore throat and swollen and painful joints should be a suspect for RF.

Q 7. What are the clinical features of RF?
The common clinical features of RF are joint pain, swelling, fever, sore throat, jerky movements, and others.

Q 8. What are the clinical features of RHD?

The common clinical features of RHD are tiredness, breathlessness, increased heart rate, swelling in legs, enlarged liver and others.

Q 9. What is the diagnostic criterion for rheumatic heart fever and disease?

As per revised Jones Criteria 2015

Major Criteria: Carditis, monoarthritis or migratory polyarthritis, polyarthralgia, chorea, erythema marginatum, subcutaneous nodules

Minor Criteria: Monoarthralgia, fever (≥38°C), ESR ≥30 mm/hr and/or CRP ≥3 mg/dl, prolonged PR interval

Diagnosis of the first attack of rheumatic fever: 2 major or 1 major plus 2 minor criteria

Diagnosis of recurrent rheumatic fever: 2 major or 1 major and 2 minor or 3 minor criteria

Q 10. What complications are associated with RF RHD?

Severe mitral regurgitation due to acute rheumatic carditis
Severe mitral stenosis due to chronic rheumatic heart disease

Management

Q 11. What investigations will you advise for a suspected patient of rheumatic fever?

The following tests should be advised to confirm the diagnosis of rheumatic fever
   a. C-reactive protein (CRP)
   b. Erythrocyte sedimentation rate
   c. Anti-streptolysin O titre (confirm presence of past GAS throat infection)
   d. Electrocardiogram and echocardiography (if cardiac involvement)

Q 12. What are the barriers to the use of injection penicillin in RF RHD?

   a. Lack of availability on a regular basis
   b. Substandard quality of some brands
   c. Fear of allergic reaction, given only in government supported centres
   d. A ban on injectable penicillin in some states
   e. Painful injection

Q 13. How will you identify penicillin reaction and manage it?

Immediate reaction occurs within 30 seconds to 2 hours after the administration of injection penicillin which are characterized by feeling of fainting, localized or generalized itching, rashes, sudden pain or swelling (particularly on the face or below eyes) and difficulty in breathing.

Delayed reactions occur within 5 to 15 days after the administration of injection of benzathine penicillin, which are characterized by generalized or localized rash, fever, pain in joints, and breathlessness.

Q 14. Management of penicillin reaction.

   a. Lie the patient down and loosen the clothes
   b. Administer 2 ml of injection hydrocortisone intramuscularly
   c. Feel the pulse of the patient. If the volume is low, raise the foot end.

d. Give 2 ml of injection avil (pheniramine) IM (1 ml in children 5–10 years) if itching, rash or breathlessness are dominant features.

e. Injection adrenaline to be administered only if patient condition is deteriorating. The dose is 0.5 ml given subcutaneously. In case of sudden stoppage of breathing or beating of heart, apply external cardio-thoracic resuscitation (thumping on chest with mouth to mouth respiration).

Prevention

Q 15. What steps would you undertake to prevent rheumatic fever and rheumatic heart disease?

Primordial prevention: Prevention of group A streptococcal infection, vaccine

Primary prevention: Prevention of first episode of acute rheumatic fever

a. Oral penicillin for 10 days/single injection of benzathine penicillin

b. Bed rest

Secondary prevention:

a. Prevention of recurrent ARF episodes by regular delivery of benzathine penicillin

b. Secondary prophylaxis: Prevents occurrence of GAS infections

Tertiary prevention: Prevention of heart failure by balloon valvuloplasty, heart valve replacement, and capacity building for treatment

Q 16. Mention the Programmes and how it aims to implement the RF/RHD intervention.

The rheumatic fever and rheumatic heart disease intervention is implemented through the following programmes:

a. Rashtriya Bal Swasthya Karyakram

b. National Programme for Prevention and Control of Cancer, Diabetes, Cardio-vascular Diseases and Stroke

EPILEPSY AND SEIZURES

Introduction

Q 1. What is epilepsy?

Epilepsy is an illness characterized by recurrent and unprovoked seizure (two or more seizure occurring either on separate days, weeks or months in past 12 months with no evidence for acute cause of seizure) due to a chronic underlying disorder.

Q 2. What is seizure?

A seizure is a brief disturbance of electrical activity in the brain and depending on the distribution of discharges, the range of clinical manifestation varies from convulsive (jerky movements), behavioural change to loss of consciousness.

Q 3. What is the classification of epilepsy?

The International League against Epilepsy Classification categorize seizures as

Focal seizures:

a. Focal onset seizures without dyscognition: Typically repetitive flexion/extension movements (clonic) are seen in the limb.

b. Focal onset seizures with dyscognition: In addition to focal onset seizures, patient is unable to respond to verbal/visual command and impairment in awareness.

Generalized seizures:

a. Tonic-clonic generalized seizures: Muscle stiffening followed by jerking

b. Absence seizures brief episodes of staring and lack of responsiveness.

c. Typical absence seizures are characterized by sudden, brief lapses of consciousness without loss of postural control.

d. An atypical absence seizure is characterized by a longer duration of consciousness and is less abrupt in onset and cessation.

e. Myoclonic seizures involve brief jerks of muscles

f. Tonic seizures have generalized muscle stiffening.

g. Atonic seizures involve the sudden loss of muscle tone.

Q 4. What are the common disorders, which can mimic epileptic seizures?

Syncope, breath holding spells, acute psychiatric states (psychogenic seizures, panic attack, and hyperventilation), migraine variants, abnormal movement disorders, paroxysmal disturbances of sleep like night terrors, narcolepsy, and hysteria.

Q 5. Define status epilepticus.

Status epilepticus is a medical emergency. It is defined as continuous seizure activity or recurrent seizure activity without the recovery of consciousness lasting more than 5 minutes.

Risk Factors

Q 6. What are the risk factors and causes for epilepsy?

The most common causes of seizures between ages 12 and 18 years are brain tumour, trauma, infection, idiopathic, genetic disorder, and illicit drug use.

Q 7. Which precipitating factors (that are likely to lower the seizure threshold) would you seek to identify in an epileptic patient?

Precipitating factors such as sleep deprivation, systemic diseases, electrolyte or metabolic derangements, acute infection, drugs that lower the seizure threshold, alcohol or illicit drug use should be identified.

Clinical Features

Q 8. How will you differentiate whether the patient has fainted (syncope) or had a seizure?

A seizure is abrupt in onset with a few minutes' unconsciousness, commonly with convulsion, associated at times with biting of tongue, froth, urine incontinence, cyanosis, headache, and confusion. These symptoms are usually absent in syncope.

Q 9. How would you distinguish epileptic seizure from psychogenic (hysterical) seizure?

The epileptic seizure usually presents with brief duration impairment in consciousness associated at times with tongue bite, cyanosis, frothing, self-injury, and urine incontinence. These symptoms are usually absent in psychogenic (hysterical) seizure.

Management

Q 10. Enumerate the steps in the management of epilepsy and seizure.

The onset of first episode of seizure does not necessitate antiepileptic drug treatment. Start with one medication at lowest dose and administer any of the anti-epileptic drugs in the following dosage (paediatric): 1. Carbamazepine: 5 mg/kg daily in 2–3 divided doses and increase by 5 mg/kg daily each week (max 1400 mg daily). 2. Phenobarbital: 2–3 mg/kg daily in two divided doses and increase weekly by 1–2 mg/kg (Should not exceed 6 mg daily). 3. Phenytoin: 3–4 mg/kg daily in 2 divided doses 4. Valproate: 15–20 mg/kg daily in 2–3 divided doses and increase each week by 15 mg/kg daily (max 15–40 mg/kg daily).

Q 11. When it is advisable to taper anti-epileptic drug?

The anti-epileptic drug should be tapered when the children are free of seizures for at least 2 years. The anti-epileptic drug should be tapered off gradually over a period of 3 to 6 months.

Prevention

Q 12. What suggestion would you give to the patients with epilepsy and their caretakers?

The following should be suggested to the patients and their caretakers:
  a. Epilepsy is a long-term illness and compliance to medication should be ensured.
  b. People with epilepsy should avoid driving unless they had one year without a seizure. In addition, they should refrain from swimming alone or being near heavy machinery.
  c. Non-pharmacological approaches: Ensuring regular sleep, appropriate meals (ketogenic diet characterized by high fat, low carbohydrate diet provides 3–4 grams of fat for every one gram of carbohydrate).
  d. Stress management, meditation, yoga and others.

Q 13. What misconceptions are associated with epilepsy, which gives rise to social stigma against the patient with epilepsy?

The misconceptions associated with epilepsy, which often gives rise to social stigma, are:
  a. It is due to supernatural forces and witchcraft
  b. It is a form of mental illness which should be treated in a lunatic asylum
  c. Women with this disorder should not be married and cannot have children.
  d. It is contagious.

Q 14. Enumerate the psychosocial legal implications of epilepsy in India.

  a. Epilepsy and marriage: The Marriage Law Amendment Act 1999 enactment permits the patient with epilepsy to be married.
  b. Epilepsy and driving: In India, there are now no restrictions on people with epilepsy driving any vehicle.

FEVER (PYREXIA)

Introduction

Q 1. What is the normal body temperature?

In adults, mean temperature is 36.7°C (range 36–37.4°C) minimum at 6 am and peak at 4–6 pm.

In children varying between 36.1° and 37.8° (97°–100°F) on rectal measurement with lowest between midnight and 6 am and maximum between 5 pm and 7 pm.

Q 2. What is fever?

In adults, fever is when the morning temperature is greater than 37.2°C and the evening temperature is greater than 37.7°C.

In children, fever is when oral temperature more than 37.5°C or 99.5°F.

The oral temperature is 0.25°C to 0.5°C (0.5°F to 1°F) lower than the rectal temperature.

Q 3. Define fever of unknown origin (FUO)/pyrexia of unknown origin (PUO).

It is defined as fever of more than 3 weeks duration, documented fevers above 38.3°C on multiple occasions, and lack of specific diagnosis after one week of admission and investigation in a hospital setting.

Burden

Q 4. Name the country in South East Asian Region (SEAR) that WHO has recently certified as 'malaria free'.

In countries where there has been zero indigenous case of malaria for three consecutive years are eligible for WHO certification of malaria. WHO certified Sri Lanka as 'malaria free'.

Q 5. Name the first WHO region to interrupt indigenous malaria transmission.

In April 2016, WHO officially declared Europe to be the first of its region to interrupt indigenous malaria transmission (all 53 countries had zero indigeneous case of malaria).

Risk Factor

Q 6. Enumerate the differential diagnosis of children presenting with fever and rash.

a. Measles: Maculopapular rash, Koplik spots

b. Meningococcal infection: Petechial or purpuric rash, stiff neck.

c. Dengue haemorrhagic fever: Skin petechiae, bleeding from nose or gums or gastro-intestinal bleeding.

d. Chikungunya: Muscle pain, joint pain.

e. Chickenpox: The rash rapidly spreads to the face and extremities while it evolves into papules, clear fluid-filled vesicles, and then into crusted lesions

Q 7. How would you categorize fever on the basis of periodicity and enumerate the probable differential diagnosis?

The fever is categorized as:

Continuous fever: Does not fluctuate more than one degree centigrade in 24 hours, e.g. typhoid fever, urinary tract infection

Intermittent fever: The temperature elevates for a certain period, then returns back to normal, e.g. malaria

a. Quotidia: Fever having a periodicity of 24 hours, e.g. *Plasmodium falciparum* malaria

b. Tertian fever: Fever having a periodicity of 48 hours, e.g. *Plasmodium vivax* and *ovale*

c. Quartan fever: 72 hours periodicity, e.g. Plasmodium malaria

Remittent fever: Temperature remains above normal throughout the day with fluctuations more than one degree centigrade in 24 hours, e.g. infective endocarditis, dengue.

Q 8. What are the causes of FUO/PUO?

The causes of FUO/PUO are the following:

a. Infections:
  i. Bacterial diseases—tuberculosis
  ii. Viral diseases—hepatitis
  iii. Arthropod borne diseases—dengue, chikungunya
  iv. Parasitic diseases—malaria

b. Neoplasm: Hodgkin's lymphoma, non-Hodgkin's lymphoma, and acute leukemia

c. Autoimmune diseases: Systematic lupus erythematosus, and polyarteritis nodosa

Q 9. What is case definition of dengue as per WHO?

Dengue without warning sign: Fever and two of the following

a. Nausea
b. Vomiting
c. Rash
d. Ache and pain
e. Leucopenia
f. Positive tourniquet test

Dengue with warning sign above with any of the following:

a. Abdominal pain or tenderness
b. Persistent vomiting
c. Clinical fluid accumulation
d. Mucosal bleeding
e. Lethargy, restlessness
f. Liver enlargement >2 cm
g. Laboratory increase in haematocrit concurrent with rapid decrease in platelet count

Q 10. What are the symptoms to diagnose a case of severe or complicated malaria?

A patient with severe or complicated malaria in addition to fever, chills, and rigor will have concomitant symptoms of confusion, drowsiness, convulsion, blurring of vision, photophobia, disorientation, jaundice, anaemia and macroscopic hemoglobinuria.

Q 11. What is case definition of severe dengue as per WHO?

Dengue with at least one of the following criteria:

a. Severe plasma Leakage leading to:
  i. Shock (DSS)
  ii. Fluid accumulation with respiratory distress

b. Severe bleeding as evaluated by clinician

c. Severe organ involvement

Management

Q 12. Which sites through which the core body temperature can be measured?
Oral cavity, ear canal, temporal artery, axilla, and rectum.

Q 13. What is the duration of keeping the thermometer in various sites?
Axillary region: 5–6 minutes
Oral region: 3 minutes
Rectal region: 2 minutes

Q 14. When would you consider documenting rectal temperature preferentially over oral temperature in adults?
In patients who are in tachypneic state or breathe through their mouth, the reliability of recording rectal temperature is higher than oral temperature.

Q 15. What laboratory investigation would you likely to suggest to the patient presenting with fever in a community?
The laboratory investigations to be suggested to the fever are:

a. Complete blood count

   i. Leukocytosis indicative of bacterial infections

   ii. Leukopenia indicative of typhoid fever, rickettsiae, malaria, kala-azar

   iii. Thrombocytopenia indicative of dengue

b. Differential leukocyte count

   i. Neutrophilia suggestive of bacterial infections

   ii. Neutropenia suggestive of bacterial infection like typhoid, paratyphoid and miliary tuberculosis; viral infection

   iii. Lymphocytosis suggestive of viral infections

   iv. Basophilia suggestive of chronic myeloid leukemia, leukemia

   v. Eosinophilia suggestive of parasitic and allergic infection

c. ESR: Elevated ESR >30 mm/hr indicates inflammation and need evaluation for infectious disease, autoimmune or malignant disease.

d. Chest X-ray posterior anterior view

e. Urinalysis

   i. Red cell casts indicative of glomerulonephritis

   ii. White cell casts indicative of pyelonephritis, interstitial nephritis

   iii. Waxy casts indicative of chronic kidney disease

f. Rapid diagnostic test or giemsa stain for malaria and others

g. Others

Q 16. What will be your pharmacological approach for a patient presenting with fever?

a. Usually for low grade fever, antipyretic is not necessary.

b. The preferred analgesic is paracetamol as oral aspirin and NSAIDs.

c. The dose of paracetamol is 500–1000 mg (maximum 4 g in 24 hours) 6–8 hourly. In children, paracetamol is prescribed a dose of 10–15 mg/kg/dose, which is repeated at 4 hourly intervals.

d. Antibiotics should be prescribed in the confirmed diagnosis of bacterial infection but never in isolated viral infection cases.

Q 17. You are a medical officer and patient presenting complaints are fever, chills with a periodicity of 48 hours and microscopy as well as rapid diagnostic test confirms *P. vivax*, then what will be your pharmacological approach for the patient?

The patient will be treated with a combined treatment of chloroquine and primaquine (but remember that primaquine is contraindicated in infants, pregnant women, and individuals with G6PD deficiency).

Chloroquine is administered in dose of 25 mg/kg body weight divided over three days, i.e. on first two days (day 1 and day 2) 10 mg/kg and on the third day 5 mg/kg and primaquine to be 0.25 mg/kg body weight daily for 14 days under supervision.

Q 18. You are a medical officer in north-east and patient presenting complaints are fever, chills with periodicity of 24 hours and microscopy as well as rapid diagnostic test confirms *P. falciparum*, then what will be your pharmacological approach for the patient lying in the following age groups (based on the following kg body weight) as well as mention pack size?

In North Eastern states, patient positive for *P. falciparum* are given artemisin-based combination treatment—artemether (20 mg) and lumefantrine (120 mg) at age specific doses.

For infants greater than 5 months and less than 3 years artemether (20 mg) lumefantrine (120 mg) for 3 days

For child more than 3 years till 8 years—artemether (40 mg), lumefantrine (240 mg) for 3 days

For child between age 9 and 14 years—artemether (60 mg), lumefantrine (360 mg) for 3 days

For child more than 14 years—artemether (80 mg), lumefantrine (480 mg) for 3 days

This combination treatment is not recommended during the first trimester of pregnancy and children whose weight is less than 5 kg.

In addition, primaquine at 0.75 mg/kg body weight single dose is to be prescribed on 2nd day (but not in pregnant women and infants).

In states other than North-East India, the artemisin-based combination treatment comprises artesunate and sulphadoxine-pyrimethamine.

Artesunate is prescribed at a dose of 4 mg/kg/body weight for 3 days and on the first day, sulphadoxine and pyrimethamine should be prescribed at a dose of 25 mg/kg/body weight and 1.25 mg/kg/body weight respectively.

Q 19. You are a medical officer and woman with 10 weeks of pregnancy presents with complaints of fever, chills with a periodicity of 24 hours and microscopy as well as rapid diagnostic test confirms *P. falciparum*, then what will be your pharmacological approach for the patient?

The patient is in her first trimester so she should be prescribed quinine at a dose of 10 mg/kg/body weight three times daily for 7 days. Further, she should be cautioned not to take medication on empty stomach and advice to take her meals regularly, otherwise quinine may induce hypoglycemia.

Q 20. What will be the treatment of mixed infections (*P. vivax* + *P. falciparum*) cases?

North-Eastern states: Age specific ACT-AL treatment for 3 days and primaquine 0.25 mg per kg body weight daily for 14 days.

In states other than North-Eastern—age specific SP-ACT treatment for 3 days and primaquine 0.25 mg per kg body weight daily for 14 days.

Q 21. What is the treatment for severe or complicated malaria?

The initial parenteral treatment for at least 48 hours should be one of the following four options: Quinine, artesunate, artemether or arte-ether

Q 22. What does the National Vector Borne Disease Control Programme (NVBDCP) recommend for laboratory diagnosis of confirming dengue infection?

NVBDCP recommends use of ELISA-based antigen detection test (NS1) for diagnosing the cases from first day onwards and antibody detection test IgM capture ELISA (MAC-ELISA) for diagnosing the cases after the fifth day of onset of disease.

Q 23. Which antipyretic contraindicated in dengue fever?

Aspirin/NSAID like ibuprofen should be avoided in patients with dengue.

Q 24. When is platelet transfusion indicated in patient with dengue?

In the following condition, platelet transfusion is indicated:

a. Platelet count less than 10000/cumm in the absence of bleeding manifestations (prophylactic platelet transfusion).
b. Haemorrhage with or without thrombocytopenia.
c. Note: In stance of severe bleeding or coagulopathy, fresh frozen plasma (FFP)/ packed cell transfusion along with platelet may be indicated.

Q 25. When would you advise a patient with dengue fever to be admitted in a hospital?

If a patient with dengue fever presents with the following presentation should be considered for admission in a hospital:

a. Significant bleeding (e.g. epistaxis, gum bleeding, haematemesis and melena)
b. Hypotensive clinical features (cold and sweaty skin, pale face, rapid and weak pulse, person begins to breathe very quickly)
c. Rapid fall of platelet count
d. Sudden drop in temperature

Prevention

Q 26. What non-pharmacological advises would you give to the patient?

The following advises should be given to the patient:

a. Antipyretics are not required in low grade fever
b. Regular intake of cool water to be taken
c. Sponging is indicated if fever is more than 41.1°C and it should be done gently so that the cutaneous vessels dilate and heat is dissipated.

d. Usually, in high grade fever patient should be instructed to wear a thin layer of clothing or even naked but should avoid being over-packed with clothing.

Q 27. What are advantages of insecticide treated mosquito nets over traditional nets?

The mesh is wider compared to traditional nets permitting better ventilation and light, and a long residual effect due to the slow release of insecticides (synthetic pyrethroids) to the fibre surface.

Q 28. What measures are under the vector control methods?

The measures under the vector control methods are:

a. Biological control: Larvivorous fish like Gambusia and Guppy, which are recommended for control of *Aedes aegypti* and Anopheles species in large water bodies.

b. Chemical control: Temephos is a chemical larvicide where diflubenzuron is insect growth regulator.

c. Adult control:

   i. Pyrethrum space sprayer is used in indoor situation

   ii. For outdoor purpose Malathion fogging is used: Cyphenothrin 5%

   iii. Personal protection measures:

      a. Protective clothing

      b. Repellant like mosquito coils

      c. Insecticide treated mosquito net or long-lasting insecticidal nets

      d. Aerosol against mosquitoes

Q 29. Which insecticides are used under the National Vector Borne Disease Control Programme for malaria control?

The insecticides used under the NVBDCP for malaria control

a. DDT (dichloro-diphenyl-trichloroethane) is used only for indoor spraying.

b. Malathion (in areas with DDT resistance)

c. Synthetic pyrethroids (deltamethrin 2.5%, cyflutin, alphacypermethrin and lambdacyhalothrin)

Q 30. What is the name of the vaccine against malaria, which WHO is intending to pilot?

RTS, AS01 vaccine that will act against only *P.Falciparum* but will not protect against *P. vivax*.

Q 31. How would you administer chemo-prophylactic drugs for malaria?

For a traveller who is travelling from non-malarious areas to malarious areas less than 6 weeks: Doxycycline is 100 mg daily in adults beginning 2 days before travel—4 weeks after leaving a malarious area.

For long-term travellers such as military and paramilitary troops: Drug of choice in such cases is mefloquine 250 mg weekly for adults 2 weeks before to 4 weeks after exposure.

Q 32. What is the vision and goal of National Framework for Malaria Elimination?

Vision: The vision of the framework is to eliminate malaria at a national level and contribute to improved health, quality of life, and alleviation of poverty.

Goals:
  a. Eliminate malaria throughout the entire country by 2030 so there would be no indigenous cases.
  b. Maintain malaria-free status in areas where malaria transmission has been interrupted and prevent re-introduction of malaria.

Q 33. What is global technical strategy for malaria (2016–2030)?

Goals	Milestones	Targets	
	2020	2025	2030
Reduce mortality	≥40%	≥75%	≥90%
Reduce incidence	≥40%	≥75%	≥90%
Elimination	≥10 countries	≥2 countries	≥35 countries
Re- establishment	Prevention	Prevention	Prevention

Q 34. What is national framework for malaria elimination (2016–2030)?

Category	Phase	States/UTs
0	Prevention of re-establishment	0 indigenous cases of malaria
1	Elimination	Including some districts with API <1/1000
2	Pre-elimination	Including some districts with API <1/1000 and some with >1/1000
3	Intensified control	States/UTs with an API >1/1000

Q 35. What is the objective of urban vector borne disease scheme 2016?

Urban vector borne disease scheme was earlier known as urban malaria scheme, its objective is to control malaria, and other vector borne diseases by reducing the vector population in the urban areas through recurrent anti-larval measures since the indoor residual insecticidal spray is usually not acceptable to the urban population.

Q 36. What are the norms for establishing urban VBD scheme?

The norms for establishing Urban VBD Scheme:
  a. The towns should have a minimum population of 40,000
  b. The annual parasitic index should be 2 or above
  c. The towns should promulgate and strictly implement the civic by-laws to prevent/eliminate domestic and peri-domestic breeding places

Q 37. Briefly describe other common fever in India.

Domain	Japanese Encephalitis	Chikungunya	Filariasis	Kala-azar or visceral leishmaniasis
Causative agent	Japanese encephalitis virus	Chikungunya virus	*Wuchereria bancrofti* (most cases)	*Leishmania donovani*
Vector	*Culex vishnui Culex tritaeniorhynchus*	*Aedes aegypti* (mostly in India), *Aedes albopictus*	*Culex quinquifasciatus*	Phlebotomine sandflies
Clinical features	Fever, neurological symptoms ranging from headache, convulsion, disorientation and loss of co-ordination	Fever, joint pain which predominantly affects small joints of hand, feet, ankle and wrist, and macular-papular rash	Despite most patients being asymptomatic, mostly lymphatic system (lymphoedema, elephantiasis, hydrocele) and kidney are affected.	Fever, grayish discolouration of hand, feet, abdomen and face Hepatospleno-megaly
Treatment	No specific antiviral treatment. Ensure airway is patent and management of fluid and electrolyte balance	No specific antiviral treatment. Non-pharmacological measures. Tepid water for sponging. Cold compresses for painful joints.	Co-administer single dose of diethylcar-bamazine (DEC) and albendazole (Alb) (i) 2 to 5 years: 100 mg DEC and 400 mg (Alb) (ii) 6 to 14 years: 200 mg DEC and 400 mg (Alb) (iii) 15 years and above: 300 mg DEC and 400 mg (Alb)	First line of treatment. Single intramuscular injection of sodium stibogluconate (20 mg/kg body weight)

ANTENATAL AND POSTNATAL

D Surendra Babu

Q 1. What is the duration of a normal pregnancy?
Duration of normal pregnancy is 40 weeks (37 to 42 weeks).

Q 2. What is the first trimester of pregnancy?
It is the first 12 weeks of gestation.

Q 3. What are the common symptoms in the first trimester of pregnancy?
The common symptoms in the first trimester of pregnancy are amenorrhea, morning sickness, increased frequency of micturition, breast discomfort, fatigue, Braxton Hicks contraction and others.

Q 4. What are the common signs in the first trimester of pregnancy?
The common signs in the first trimester of pregnancy are breast changes, Chadwick's sign, cervical sign, Goodell's sign, soft cervix, Hegar signs, and others.

Q 5. What is the pregnancy hormone?
Human chorionic gonadotropin is pregnancy hormone. Its t½ is 24 hours. It is detected by 8–9 days after fertilization. Doubling time is every 48 hours. It is maximum (100–200 IU/ml) at 60–70 days of gestation. It is increased in hydatidiform mole and it disappears 2 weeks after delivery.

Q 6. What are the findings in abdominal ultrasound in the first trimester of pregnancy?
    a. Gestational sac at 5 weeks
    b. Foetal pole at 6 weeks
    c. Cardiac activity at 6 weeks
    d. Foetal movements at 7 weeks

Q 7. What is the second trimester of pregnancy?
The second trimester of pregnancy is 13 to 28 weeks of gestation.

Q 8. What is quickening?
It is the perception of foetal movements. It starts in the second trimester of pregnancy. In nullipara at approximately 20 weeks and in multipara 16 weeks quickening is felt.

Q 9. What is the third trimester of pregnancy?
The third trimester of pregnancy is 29 to 40 weeks of gestation.

Q 10. What is engagement and lightening?
Engagement is the descent of foetus into the pelvic cavity. It starts in the late third trimester of pregnancy. Lightening is a sense of relief of the pressure due to engagement.

Q 11. What do you mean by early registration in the antenatal mother?
Early registration means registering every pregnancy within 12 weeks of gestation.

Q 12. How many minimum and ideal number of antenatal visits should a pregnant woman do?
Minimum number of ANC visits recommended:
    a. 1st visit: Within 12 weeks—preferably as soon as pregnancy is suspected
    b. 2nd visit: Between 14 and 26 weeks
    c. 3rd visit: Between 28 and 34 weeks
    d. 4th visit: Between 36 weeks and term

Ideal number of ANC visits recommended:
    a. 0 to 7 months: Once every month
    b. 8th month: Twice a month
    c. 9th month onwards: Once a week

On an average total maximum visits are 11–13 (14)

Q 13. What is obstetric care under RMNCH+A?

Essential obstetric care	Basic emergency obstetric care	Comprehensive emergency obstetric care
Early registration	Essential obstetric care plus	Basic emergency obstetric care plus
Examination	Manual removal of placenta	Blood transfusion
Iron folic acid	Remove retained products (e.g. dilatation and curettage)	Perform surgery (e.g. caesarean section)
Tetanus toxoid	Perform assisted vaginal delivery (ventouse/forceps)	
	Administer parental antibiotics	
	Administer parental oxytocin	
	Administer parental anticonvulsants for pre-eclampsia and eclampsia (i.e. magnesium sulphate)	

Q 14. What are the different methods to calculate the expected date of delivery?
a. Naegele's formula: EDD = Date of LMP + 9 months + 7 days
b. Parikh's formula: EDD = Date of LMP + 9 months – 21 days + duration of previous menstrual cycles in days.
c. Ultrasound dating is most accurate if undertaken in the first trimester
d. Date of quickening: Begins at around 18–22 weeks of pregnancy

Q 15. What is the normal weight gain during pregnancy?
A pregnant woman's weight should be recorded at each ANC visit. The weight taken during the first visit/registration is the baseline weight.

Normally, a woman should gain 9–11 kg during her pregnancy (in India average is 6.5 kg).

Usually, after the first trimester, a pregnant woman gains around 2 kg every month. Weight gain by trimester:
1st trimester   1 kg
2nd trimester   5 kg
3rd trimester   5 kg

Pre-pregnancy weight	BMI (kg/m²)	Total weight gain range (kg)
Normal weight	18.5 to 24.9	11.5 to 16
Underweight	<18.5	12.5 to 18
Overweight	25 to 29.9	7 to 11.5
Obese	≥30	5 to 9

Of the total weight gain, reproductive weight gain is ≈6 kg [foetus, placenta, liquor, uterus, and breast] and net maternal weight gain ≈6 kg [blood volume, extracellular fluid and fat].

Q 16. What is rapid weight gain in an antenatal woman?
In an antenatal woman rapid weight gain is when >0.5 kg (1 lb) in a week or >2 kg (5 lb) in a month. The common causes are pre-eclampsia, multiple pregnancies, or diabetes. Take the woman's blood pressure and test her urine for proteinuria or sugar.

Q 17. What is Dawn's rule of ten for antenatal mothers?
Dr CS Dawn's rule of ten for pregnant mothers is a care calendar to grow 10 kg mother's weight and 3 kg baby.

Ten times pregnancy check-ups for high-risk pregnancy and minimum 5 check-ups for normal pregnancy starting from 10 weeks of gestation.

a. Ten kg mother's weight gain during pregnancy.

b. Ten hours rest and sleep (2 hours afternoon rest, 8 hours sleep at night) to grow the baby.

c. Ten gram percent blood haemoglobin is tested raised to 11 gm.

d. By ten months, tetanus vaccine

e. Ten to twelve hours normal labour management in first pregnancy, 5–6 hours in second pregnancy

f. Ten Apgar score for baby

g. By ten weeks, contraceptive in the postnatal period.

h. Ten months breastfeeding.

i. By ten months, infant immunization is completed.

Q 18. What is precocious pregnancy?
Precocious pregnancy is the occurrence of gestation at an unusually early age. The development of ripe Graafian follicles takes place long before puberty, and it is not uncommon to find one, or even a second pregnancy occurring before the onset of menstruation.

Q 19. What investigation will you prefer to do as a medical officer in PHC if an antenatal mother visit for the first time?
Physical examination: Blood pressure measurement, Weight in kg, height

Laboratory investigation: Haemoglobin, CBC, HIV status, blood group with RH typing, blood sugar, urine proteins, and others.

Q 20. What investigation will you do as a medical officer in CHC/DH if an antenatal mother visit for the first time?
Physical examination: Blood pressure measurement, weight in kg, height

Laboratory investigation: Haemoglobin, HIV status, blood group with RH typing, blood sugar, IgG rubella, VDRL, anti-HCV, Hbs antigen, lipid profile, thyroid hormone, urine proteins, and others.

Q 21. How do you measure the fundal height?

Fundal height measures the progress of the pregnancy and foetal growth. The uterus is an abdominal organ after 12 weeks of gestation. To measure the fundal height, the woman's legs should be kept straight and not flexed.

Number of weeks	Able to palpate
12	Just palpable above the symphysis pubis
16	At lower one-third of the distance between the symphysis pubis and umbilicus
20	At two-thirds of the distance between the umbilicus and xiphisternum
24	At the level of umbilicus
28	At lower one-third of the distance between the umbilicus and xiphisternum
36	At the level of xiphisternum
40	Sinks back to the level of the 32 weeks, but the flanks are full unlike that in the 32 weeks

After 24 weeks fundal height measured in cm corresponds to number of weeks up to 36 weeks (± 2 cm)

Q 22. What are the causes for fundal height more than gestational age?
a. Wrong date of LMP
b. Full bladder
c. Multiple pregnancy/large baby
d. Polyhydramnios
e. Hydrocephalus
f. Hydatidiform mole

Q 23. What are the causes for fundal height less than gestational age?
a. Wrong date of LMP
b. IUGR
c. Missed abortion
d. Intrauterine death (IUD)
e. Transverse lie

Q 24. How do you palpate to determine the foetal lie and presentation?
Fundal palpation/fundal grip: To determine the lie and presentation of the foetus
    Lateral palpation/lateral grip: To determine the foetal back
    a. Back—smooth resistant feel
    b. Limbs—knob-like structures

First pelvic grip/superficial pelvic grip: To determine whether the head or the breech is present at the pelvic brim. If the head cannot be moved, it indicates that the head is engaged. In case of a transverse lie the third grip will be empty.

Second pelvic grip/deep pelvic grip: To determine the degree of flexion of the head

Q 25. What is the normal foetal heart sound and foetal heart rate?

If the foetal heart rate (FHR) is between 110 and 150 beats per minute with base line variability 5 to 25 beats per minute. The FHS cannot be heard through the abdomen with the help of a stethoscope or foetoscope before 24 weeks of pregnancy. FHS is below umbilicus in cephalic presentation and above umbilicus in breech.

Q 26. How to count foetal movements?

Ask the woman to lie down in the left lateral position for an hour, three times a day after meals. Count the number of foetal movements in each hour. Normally the total number of movements in all three periods is more than 10.

Q 27. What do you mean by at-risk approach? Who are at-risk mothers?

At-risk approach: It is an approach to identify high-risk antenatal cases (as early as possible) to provide appropriate care.

At-risk mothers:
  a. Anaemia
  b. Antepartum haemorrhage, threatened abortion
  c. Elderly grand multipara (≥4 parity)
  d. Elderly primi (>30 years)
  e. History of previous CS or instrumental delivery
  f. Malpresentations (breech, transverse lie, etc.)
  g. Pre-eclampsia, eclampsia
  h. Pregnancy with comorbidities (diabetes, TB, etc.)
  i. Previous stillbirth, IUD, manual removal of placenta
  j. Prolonged pregnancy
  k. Short statured primi (<140 cm)
  l. Twins, hydramnios
  m. Body weight <45 kg

Q 28. What are the high-risk pregnancies?
  a. Malpresentation
  b. Multiple pregnancy
  c. Any bleeding P/V during pregnancy
  d. Preclampsia, eclampsia
  e. Severe anaemia
  f. Premature rupture of membranes before 37 weeks

Q 29. What are the warning signs in pregnancy requiring immediate health facility visit?
  a. Fever>38.5°C/for more than 24 hours
  b. Headache, blurring of vision
  c. Generalized swelling of the body and puffiness of face
  d. Breathlessness at rest
  e. Pain in abdomen
  f. Vaginal bleeding
  g. Reduced foetal movements

Q 30. What is true labour?
True labour is characterized by onset of regular uterine contractions (1–2 contractions in 10 minutes) associated with progressive cervical dilatation.

Q 31. What are the stages of labour?
a. First stage is onset of true labour pains until full dilatation of cervix (active labour: cervix ≥4 cm).
b. Second stage is full dilatation of cervix until delivery of the baby.
c. Third stage is delivery of baby until the delivery of placenta.
d. Fourth stage is for one hour after delivery.

Q 32. What is normal and prolong labour?
Prolonged labour is when 1st and 2nd stage of labour is more than 18 hours arbitrary.

Phase of labour	Primipara normal labour	Multipara
Latent phase	8 hours	4 hours
First stage	12 hours	6 hours
Second stage	2 hours	½ hour
Prolong labour		
Latent phase	>20 hours	>14 hours
First stage	>12 hours	>12 hours
Second stage	>2 hours	>1 hour
Cervical dilation	<1 cm/hr	<1.5 cm/hr
Descent of head	<1 cm/hr	<2 cm/hr

Q 33. What is the active management of the third stage of labour?
AMTSL is done to facilitate the delivery of placenta by increasing uterine contraction and retraction by using parenteral oxytocin and uterine massage (if oxytocin is not available, misoprostol can be given orally).

Q 34. What is postpartum haemorrhage?
Postpartum haemorrhage is blood loss of 500 ml or more from the genital tract after childbirth leading to deterioration of maternal condition.

Q 35. What is protraction of descent?
It is the failure of head to descent within 1 hour of full dilation.

Q 36. What is preterm labour?
When labour starts before 37th completed weeks (<259 days).

Q 37. What is involution of uterus?
Non-gravid uterus is 60 gm in weight and 7.5 cm in length. A term gravid uterus is 900–1000 gm in weight and 35 cm in length.

Immediately after delivery uterus measures 20 × 12 × 7.5 (length × breadth × thickness)

Immediately after delivery, fundal height is 13.5 cm above symphysis. Fundal height decreases by 1.25 cm per 24 hours postpartum. By 2 weeks uterus is a pelvic organ and by 6 weeks uterus is of normal pregnancy size.

Q 38. What are the salient features of placenta?
a. Diameter: 15–20 cm
b. Thickness: 2.5 cm
c. Weight: 500 gm
d. Lobes: 15–20
e. Uterine artery: 2
f. Vein: 1

Q 39. What is lochia?
Lochia is vaginal discharge, which occurs in the first fortnight during puerperium. It is of three types:
a. Rubra (1–4 days) contains blood, decidua, vernix
b. Serosa (5–9 days) contains RBCs, more leucocytes, mucus
c. Alba (10–15 days) contains decidual cells, leucocytes, mucus

The amount of lochia in first 5–6 days is 250 ml. If less or more amount of lochia is present, suspect infection. If colour red continues in lochia, suspect subinvolution or bits of conceptus. If the duration is more than 15 days, suspect local genital lesion.

Q 40. What is the short umbilical cord?
The short cord is umbilical cord less than 20 cm or 8 inches.

Q 41. What are oligohydramnios and polyhydramnios?
Normal amniotic fluid at 12 weeks of gestation is 50 ml, 36–38 weeks of gestation is 1000 ml and at term is 600–800 ml.

Oligohydramnios is amniotic fluid ≥2000 ml/single pool >8 cm/amniotic fluid index >25 cm

Polyhydramnios is amniotic fluid ≥200 ml/single pool >5 cm/amniotic fluid index >5 cm

Q 42. What is antepartum haemorrhage?
It is bleeding from or into genital tract after 28 weeks of gestation but before birth of baby.

Q 43. What is pre-eclampsia?
Pre-eclampsia is after 20 weeks of gestation, blood pressure more than 140/90 plus proteinuria in previously normotensive and nonproteinuric patient.

Q 44. What is pregnancy-induced hypertension?
Pregnancy-induced hypertension is systolic BP >30 mm Hg, diastolic >10 mm over previous known BP. There is oedema after rest. The weight gain >2 kg in 1 month. It is of three types:
a. Gestational hypertension
b. Pre-eclampsia
c. Eclampsia

Q 45. What is cut-off of clinically significant proteinuria?
When total proteinuria in 24 hours is >0.3 gm/l, i.e 2 + [trace is 0.1 gm/l, 1 + is 0.3 gm/l, 2 + is 1 gm/l, 3 + is 3 gm/l, 4 + is 10 gm/l]

Q 46. What are the risk factors for pre-eclampsia?
The risk factors for pre-eclampsia is primipara, family history, mole, placenta abnormality.

Q 47. What is the management of pre-eclampsia?
a. The drugs like methyldopa, labetalol, nifedipine, hydralazine and others.

b. Blood pressure monitoring

c. Rest

d. Monitoring liver and kidney function

e. No salt restriction

f. Adequate protein

g. Assessment of foetal well-being

Q 48. What are the complications of eclampsia?
The complications of eclampsia are injuries, acute left heart failure, pulmonary oedema, cerebral haemorrhage, renal failure, hepatic failure, shock, and others.

Q 49. What is the drug of choice for eclampsia?
The drug of choice for eclampsia is magnesium sulphate intramuscular (pritchard regimen) or intravenous (zuspan regimen).

Q 50. What is morning sickness in pregnancy?
Morning sickness is simple vomiting in pregnancy. It has no impairment of health and disappears by 1st trimester. It is managed by taking dry toast or biscuit in morning and avoiding spicy of fatty food.

Q 51. What is hyperemesis gravidarum?
It is vomiting in pregnancy with the deleterious effect on health. It impairs day-to-day activity. Its management is IV fluids and drug promethazine 25 mg BD or TDS.

Q 52. What is Hellin's rule of twins (1895)?
Chances of:
a. Twins 1 in 80 pregnancy

b. Triplet 1 in 800 pregnancy

c. Quadruplet 1 in 8000 pregnancy

Q 53. What is the pathognomic sign of twin pregnancy in ultrasound?
Twin peak sign

Q 54. What are the complications of twin pregnancy?
The complications of twin pregnancy are nausea and vomiting, antepartum haemorrhage, malpresentation, preterm and others. During puerperium, there are chances of lactation failure and subinvolution of uterus. There can be a miscarriage, foetal anomaly, or intrauterine death also.

Q 55. What are the complications of Rh negative pregnancy?

The complications of Rh negative pregnancy to foetus are hydrops fetalis, icterus gravis neonatorum, anaemia and others. The complications of Rh negative pregnancy to mother are pre-eclampsia, big size baby, polyhydramnios, postpartum haemorrhage and others.

Q 56. What is the management of Rh negative pregnancy?

To a Rh negative mother at 28 weeks of gestation intramuscular anti-D gamma globulin, 300 µg is given as prophylaxis to avoid foetal complications. Liley's chart is used to predict the severity of disease. After delivery, if the baby is Rh positive intramuscular anti-D gamma globulin 300 µg is given within the 72 hours of delivery but if the baby is Rh negative, nothing is done.

Q 57. What is the treatment given to a pregnant woman with no complication in the first trimester?

  a. Tab folic acid 500 µg once daily
  b. Injection tetanus toxoid as early as possible

Q 58. What is the treatment giving to a pregnant woman with no complication in second and the third trimester?

  a. Tab iron folic acid twice daily for 6 months
  b. Tab calcium twice daily for second and the third trimester
  c. Injection tetanus toxoid as per the previous immunization status

Q 59. What is the protocol for calcium supplementation during pregnancy?

All pregnant and lactating women should be counseled calcium rich foods like
  a. Milk and milk products such as cheese and curd
  b. Green leafy vegetables such as spinach and fenugreek
  c. Sweets made of sesame seeds and ragi.
  d. Oral calcium tablets to be taken twice a day from 14 weeks of pregnancy up to six months postpartum.
  e. Calcium tablets should not be taken empty stomach since it causes gastritis.
  f. Calcium and iron folic acid (IFA) tablets should not be taken together
  g. Calcium tablet should contain 500 mg elemental calcium and 250 IU vitamin D_3.

Q 60. What is the deworming during pregnancy?

Nearly half of iron deficiency anaemia in pregnant women is attributed to hookworm infestation. Albendazole 400 mg is recommended drug of choice for deworming of pregnant women, preferably during the second trimester. In first trimester albendazole is contraindicated, therefore the drug of choice is mebendazole.

Q 61. What is gestational diabetes mellitus?

Gestational diabetes mellitus (GDM) is impaired glucose tolerance with first recognition during pregnancy.

Q 62. What are the consequences of GDM?

The consequences of GDM are:
  a. Maternal: Polyhydramnios, pre-eclampsia, prolonged labour and others
  b. Foetal: Macrosomia, hypoglycaemia, hypocalcaemia, spontaneous abortion, intrauterine death and others

Q 63. How will you manage a case GDM?

a. The pregnant woman who is diagnosed with GDM (2 hours postprandial glucose >140 mg/dl) for the first time should be started on medical nutrition therapy for 2 weeks.

b. After 2 weeks, postprandial glucose is retested.

c. If 2 hours postprandial glucose<120 mg/dl, repeat test every fortnight in the second trimester and every week in the third trimester

d. If 2 hours PPPG ≥120 mg/dl insulin, therapy is to be started

e. Postpartum evaluation by a 75 g oral glucose tolerance test at 6 weeks.

Q 64. What is primary maternal hypothyroidism?

Primary maternal hypothyroidism is the presence of elevated thyroid stimulating hormone levels during pregnancy. Pregnancy-specific and trimester-specific reference levels for TSH are as follows:

First trimester	0.1–2.5 mIU/l
Second trimester	0.2–3 mIU/l
Third trimester	0.3–3 mIU/l

Q 65. What are the consequences of untreated hypothyroidism?

Untreated hypothyroidism in pregnancy is associated with adverse maternal effects like miscarriages, anaemia, pre-eclampsia and others.

Q 66. When do you screen for hypothyroidism in pregnancy?

Indian Thyroid Society recommends screening of TSH levels in all PW at the time of their first visit, ideally during pre-pregnancy evaluation or as soon as pregnancy is confirmed.

Q 67. What is the drug of choice for treatment of hypothyroidism in pregnancy?

The drug of choice for treatment of hypothyroidism in pregnancy is levothyroxine (25, 50, 100 g).

Q 68. What is partograph/prasavgraph?

The partograph is a graphic recording of the progress of labour and the condition of the mother and foetus. It helps to identify the need for action and recognises referral at the appropriate time. It records the following:

a. Identification data—name, age, parity, date, time of admission, registration number, and time of rupture of the membranes.

b. Foetal/maternal condition: FHR, cervical dilatation condition of the membranes, the colour of the amniotic fluid, number of uterine contractions, maternal pulse, blood pressure, temperature and drug administered during labour

Q 69. What is Janani Suraksha Yojana (JSY)?

Janani Suraksha Yojana is an initiative to reduce maternal mortality ratio and infant mortality rate, by increasing institutional deliveries from below poverty line families. India is the first country to declare National Safe Motherhood Day on 11th April.

Q 70. What is the eligibility for cash assistance under JSY?

Category	All pregnant women or accredited private institutions	Limitation of cash assistance
LPS states	BPL pregnant women, aged 19 years and above	All births
HPS states	All SC and ST women delivering in a government health centre accredited private institutions	Up to 2 live births

Q 71. What is the scale of cash assistance for institutional deliveries?

Category	Rural area		Total	Urban area		Total
	Mother's package	ASHA package	Rs.	Mother's package	ASHA package	Rs.
LPS	1400	600	2000	1000	200	1200
HPS	700	200	900	600	200	800

Q 72. What is Pregnancy Aid Yojana Scheme?
Expansion of cash benefit to INR 6000 for 1st delivery.

Global Strategy for Women's, Children's and Adolescent's Health (2016–30)
Vision: By 2030, a world in which every woman, child and adolescent in every setting realize their rights to physical and mental health and well being, has social and economic opportunities, and is able to participate fully in shaping prosperous and sustainable societies.
   Objectives and targets aligned with SDGs:
   a. Survive: End preventable deaths
   b. Thrive: Ensure health and well-being
   c. Transform: Expand enabling environments

Q 73. What is Pradhan Mantri Surakshit Matritva Abhiyan?
It was launched on 9th June 2016. In it on the 9th of every month, free health check-ups for pregnant women in 14 states will be done. If any poor pregnant women come to private practitioners, then they should give her free treatment.
   Colour coded:
   a. Red: High-risk pregnancy
   b. Blue: Pregnancy-induced hypertension
   c. Yellow: Pregnancy with comorbidities (DM; STIs; Hypothyroid)
   d. Green: No risk factor

Q 74. When to start contraceptive use in a postpartum women?
Contraceptive use in nonlactating women is started after 3 weeks postpartum and in lactating women it is started after 3 months postpartum.

Q 75. What is the drug to improve lactation?
Metoclopramide (10 mg TDS)

Q 76. What is the drug to stop lactation?

Bromocriptine 2.5 mg OD for 14 days

Q 77. What advises will you give in normal puerperium?

    a. Balance diet + extra calories and proteins

    b. Care of bladder

    c. Care of bowel

    d. Care of breast

    e. Care of vulva of episiotomy wound

    f. Hygiene

    g. Immunization

    h. Rest and ambulance

    i. Rooming in

    j. Sleep

Q 78. What are three delay models in health?

The three types of delays are:

    a. Delay 1: Delay in recognizing the problem (lack of awareness of danger signs) and deciding to seek care (due to inaccessible health facility, lack of resources to pay for services/supplies and medicines)

    b. Delay 2: Delay in reaching the health facility (due to unavailability of transport, lack of awareness of appropriate referral facility)

    c. Delay 3: Delay in receiving treatment once a woman has arrived at the health facility (due to inadequately equipped health facility, lack of trained personnel, emergency medicines, blood, etc.)

Q 79. What is Janani Shishu Suraksha Karyakram (JSSK)?

JSSK is an initiative to assure free services to all pregnant women and sick neonates accessing public health institutions launched in 2011.

    a. Beneficiaries are all pregnant women; entitlements provided till 3 days in normal vaginal delivery and 7 days for caesarean section) and infant (1 year).

    b. Facilities for mother: Free diagnostics, free diet, free delivery services, free drugs, free transport and free blood

    c. Facilities for child: NRCs, IMNCI, FIMNCI, NBCC, NBSU, SNCU

Q 80. What are the activities of ASHA to provide home-based postnatal care [HBPNC]? [Annexure 17]

The ASHA must undertake 6 home visits per newborn:

Day 1 of birth

Day 2–3 after birth

Day 5–7 after birth

Day 14–17 after birth

Day 23–28 after birth

Day 42–45 after birth

Q 81. What are the activities of ANM/block health supervisor to provide home-based postnatal care?
1. Identify facilities and/or medical personnel for referrals.
2. Support ASHA/AWW in developing the referral system in the village
3. Random validation of home visits
4. Ensure availability of referral funds with the ASHAs

Q 82. What is lactational amenorrhoea method (LAM)?
It is a method of contraception with three prerequisites:
   a. The mother's monthly bleeding has not returned
   b. The baby is exclusively breastfed
   c. The baby is less than 6 months old, can become pregnant after 6 months of childbirth

Q 83. What are the different types of contraceptive methods for postpartum period?
Timing of method use in the postpartum period

Intrauterine device	Postplacental insertion Immediate postpartum <48 hours of delivery Postpartum >6 weeks for an interval insertion	
Tubectomy	Within 7 days, otherwise wait 6 weeks	
Male or female condom	Immediately or when sex is resumed	
Combined oral contraceptives	6 months after childbirth	3 weeks after childbirth if not breastfeeding
Progestin only methods (pills/injectables)	6 weeks after childbirth	Immediately if not breastfeeding
Vasectomy	Immediately or during wife's pregnancy	

Q 84. What is Dakshata?
Dakshata is a package of training to empower providers for improved maternal and neonatal health during institution deliveries.

ADULT

Human Immunodeficiency Virus (HIV)
Acquired Immuno Deficiency Syndrome (AIDS)

Puja Dudeja

Introduction

Q 1. What is the size of HIV virus?
The size of HIV virus is 1/10000 of a millimeter.

Q 2. HIV replicates in which cell?
HIV replicates in actively dividing T4 lymphocytes.

Q 3. Can HIV cross blood–brain barrier?
HIV can cross blood–brain barrier.

Q 4. Mention the types of HIV.
The types of HIV are: HIV-1 and HIV

Q 5. AIDS is also known as————?
Slim disease

Burden

Q 6. What is the global prevalence of HIV?
The global prevalence of HIV is 36.7 million.

Q 7. What is the global incidence of HIV?
The global incidence of HIV is 2.1 million.

Q 8. What is burden of HIV/AIDS in India?
India: 3rd largest population living with HIV in the world

 People living with AIDS (prevalence): 21.17 lakhs

 New infections/year (incidence): 86,000

 AIDS related deaths: 1.48 lakhs

 Manipur: State with maximum adult HIV prevalence

 Adult HIV prevalence = 0.26%

Q 9. Prevalence of HIV in which age group is considered a proxy for incidence/new cases in the general population?
Prevalence of HIV in the pregnant woman in the age group of 15–24 years is considered a proxy for incidence/new cases in the general population.

Q 10. What is the target related to HIV under SDGs?
To end AIDS epidemic by 2030.

Q 11. What is HIV 90-90-90 target of WHO?
By 2020:
 – 90% of all people living with HIV will have been diagnosed
 – 90% of all people with diagnosed HIV infection will receive antiretroviral therapy
 – 90% of all people on antiretroviral therapy will have viral suppression

Q 12. What is the WHO/UNAIDS classification of HIV epidemic?
The WHO/UNAIDS classification of HIV epidemic is:
 a. Lower level HIV epidemic
 b. Concentrated HIV epidemic
 c. Generalized HIV epidemic

Q 13. How do you define low level HIV epidemic?
Low level HIV epidemic is HIV prevalence <5% in any defined subpopulation.

Q 14. What is concentrated HIV epidemic?
Concentrated HIV epidemic is HIV prevalence >5% in at least one subpopulation but below 1% in pregnant woman in urban areas.

Q 15. How do you define generalized HIV epidemic?
Generalized HIV epidemic is when HIV prevalence is consistently over 1% in the pregnant woman.

Q 16. Describe HIV epidemic in India.
HIV epidemic in India shifted from highest risk groups (commercial sex workers, homosexual men, drug users) to bridge population and then to general population. The shift occurs when the prevalence in the first group reaches 5%. There is a time lag of 2–3 years between the shifts from one group to another.

Q 17. Name the six states with highest HIV prevalence.
The six states with highest HIV prevalence are:
   a. Maharashtra
   b. Andhra Pradesh
   c. Tamil Nadu
   d. Karnataka
   e. Manipur
   f. Nagaland

Risk Factor

Q 18. Mention the high risk group for HIV.
The high risk groups for HIV are:
   a. Male homosexual and bisexual
   b. Heterosexual partners (including prostitutes)
   c. Injection drug users
   d. Transfusion recipients of blood and blood products
   e. Haemophilics
   f. Clients of STD

Q 19. List the bridge population.
The bridge population are:
   a. Clients of sex workers
   b. STD patient
   c. Migrant population
   d. Population in conflict areas
   e. Partners of drug users

Q 20. List the common routes of transmission of HIV.
The common modes of transmission of HIV are:
   a. Heterosexual (88.2%)
   b. Parent to child (5%)
   c. Injecting drug users (1.7%)
   d. Homosexual (1.5%)
   e. Blood and blood products (1%)
   f. Unknown (2.7%)

Q 21. Who are the reservoirs of HIV infection?
The reservoirs of HIV infection are cases and carriers.

Q 22. What are the sources of HIV infection?
The sources of HIV infection are blood, urine, semen, cervical and vaginal secretions, cerebrospinal fluid, brain tissue, tears, lymph node, saliva, bone marrow, breast milk, and skin.

Q 23. In which age group is HIV more common?
HIV is more common in 20–49 years.

Q 24. What are the factors that increase the risk of HIV?
The factors that increase the risk of HIV are:
   a. Presence of STD
   b. Sex and age of uninfected partner
   c. Type of sexual act
   d. Stage of illness of the infected partner
   e. Virulence of HIV strain involved

Q 25. What are the chances of transmission of HIV from male to female as compared to female to male?
The chances of transmission of HIV from male to female as compared to female to male is twice more.

Q 26. What are the reasons for women being more vulnerable to HIV?
The reasons for women being more vulnerable to HIV are:
   a. The large surface of exposure
   b. Semen contains higher concentration of HIV than vaginal or cervical fluids

Q 27. Why anal intercourse carries a higher risk of transmission than vaginal intercourse?
Anal intercourse carries a higher risk of transmission than vaginal intercourse because it is more likely to injure tissues of the receptive partner.

Q 28. Why are adolescent girls more prone to HIV?
Adolescent girls are more prone to HIV because the cervix is less efficient barrier for HIV in adolescents.

Q 29. Why are women over 45 years of age more prone to HIV?
Women over 45 years of age are more prone to HIV because of thinning of mucosa at menopause and lack of cervical mucous.

Q 30. By how many times do the chances of acquiring HIV increases in the presence of STD?
HIV increases in the presence of STD by 8–10 times.

Q 31. What is the reason for increased chances of acquiring HIV in presence of STD?
The reason for increased chances of acquiring HIV in presence of STD is presence of STD causes inflammation and accumulation of T-cells and monocytes/macrophages in the genital area, which facilitates infection.

Q 32. Transfusion of which contaminated blood products may cause HIV?
Transfusion blood products that may cause HIV are:
   a. Whole blood cells
   b. Platelets
   c. Factors VIII and IX

Q 33. Transfusion of which blood products is not known to transmit HIV?
Transfusion blood products that do not cause HIV are:
   a. Albumin
   b. Immunoglobulin

Q 34. What is the risk of contracting HIV after transfusion of a unit of infected blood?
The risk of contracting HIV after transfusion of a unit of infected blood is 95%.

Q 35. What are the modes of transmission of HIV from mother to child?
The modes of transmission of HIV from mother to child are:
   a. Through placenta
   b. During delivery
   c. By breastfeeding

Q 36. In the absence of any intervention, what is the rate of transmission of HIV from mother to child?
The rate of transmission of HIV from mother to child is 20–25%.

Q 37. What are the leading causes of HIV-related morbidity in Sub-Saharan Africa?
The leading causes of HIV-related morbidity in Sub-Saharan Africa are:
   a. Tuberculosis
   b. Bacterial infection
   c. Malaria

Q 38. What are the risk factors in infants influencing PPTCT?
The risk factors in infants influencing PPTCT are:
   a. Premature birth
   b. Low birth weight (<2500 gm)
   c. First infant of multiple birth
   d. Altered skin integrity
   e. Immature GI tract.

Clinical Features

Q 39. What is window period?
The window period is period between acquiring of HIV infection and appearance of antibodies.

Q 40. What is the importance of window period?
The importance of window period is although the person is infectious, because of high concentration of virus in blood, he will test negative on standard antibody blood test.

Q 41. What is the incubation period of HIV?
The incubation period of HIV is a few months to 10 years.

Q 42. What are the major signs of HIV?
The major signs of HIV are:

  a. Weight loss of ≥10% of body weight
  b. Chronic diarrhoea for >1 month
  c. Prolonged fever for >1 month

Q 43. What are the minor signs of HIV?
The minor signs of HIV are:

  a. Persistent cough for >1 month
  b. Generalised pruritic dermatitis
  c. History of herpes zoster
  d. Oropharyngeal candidiasis
  e. Chronic progressive or disseminated herpes simplex
  f. Generalised lymphadenopathy

   The presence of either generalized Kaposi sarcoma or Cryptococcal meningitis is sufficient for the diagnosis of AIDS (for surveillance).

Q 44. What are the stages of HIV?
The stages of HIV are:

  a. Initial infection with virus and development of antibodies
  b. Asymptomatic carrier state
  c. AIDS related complex
  d. AIDS

Q 45. What are the symptoms of initial infection of HIV?
The symptoms of initial infection of HIV are fever, sore throat and rash.

Q 46. After how many weeks do the antibodies usually appear in the bloodstream?
The antibodies usually appear in the bloodstream in 2 to 12 weeks.

Q 47. Name the clinical features seen in asymptomatic carrier state.
The clinical features seen in asymptomatic carrier state is persistent generalised lymphadenopathy.

Q 48. What are the clinical signs seen in AIDS related complex?
The clinical signs seen in AIDS related complex are:

  a. Unexplained diarrhoea lasting for more than 1 month
  b. Fatigue, malaise
  c. Loss of >10% body weight
  d. Fever, night sweats
  e. Oral thrush
  f. Generalised lymphadenopathy
  g. Enlarged spleen

Q 49. What are the opportunistic infections seen when CD4 count is between <500 cumm?

The opportunistic infections seen when CD4 count is between <500/cumm are:
- a. Bacterial infections
- b. Tuberculosis
- c. Herpes simplex
- d. Herpes zoster
- e. Vaginal candidiasis
- f. Hairy leukoplakia
- g. Kaposi's sarcoma

Q 50. What are the opportunistic infections seen when CD4 count is between 50 and 200/cumm?

The opportunistic infections seen when CD4 count is between 50 and 200/cumm are:
- a. Pneumocytosis
- b. Toxoplasmosis
- c. Cryptococcosis
- d. Coccidioidomycosis
- e. Cryptosporidiosis

Q 51. What are the opportunistic infections seen when the CD4 count is <50 cells/cumm?

The opportunistic infections seen when the CD4 count is <50 cells/cumm are:
- a. Disseminated *Mycobacterium avium* complex
- b. Histoplasmosis
- c. CMV retinitis
- d. CNS lymphoma

Q 52. What is the manifestation of CNS involvement by HIV?

CNS involvement by HIV manifests as AIDS encephalopathy or AIDS dementia

Q 53. By how many times does HIV infection increase the chances of developing TB?

HIV infection increases the chances of developing TB by 30–50 times.

Q 54. Define persistent generalised lymphadenopathy.

Persistent generalised lymphadenopathy is lymph node >1 cm in diameter in two or more sites other than the groin area for a period of at least 3 months.

Q 55. Describe the features of Kaposi sarcoma.

The features of Kaposi sarcoma are reddish brown or purplish plaques or nodules on the skin or mucosa.

Q 56. What are the symptoms of *Pneumocystis carinii* pneumonia?

The symptoms of *Pneumocystis carinii* pneumonia are dry nonproductive cough, inability to take a full breadth, occasional pain on breathing, weight loss, and fever.

Q 57. Describe hairy leukoplakia.

Hairy leukoplakia is white patches on the sides of the tongue in vertical folds resembling corrugations.

Q 58. What is the WHO case definition for AIDS in children?

The WHO case definition for AIDS in children is 2 major signs and 2 minor signs, if there is no other known cause of immunosuppression.

Q 59. What are the major signs of HIV in children?
The major signs of HIV in children are:
   a. Weight loss or abnormally slow growth
   b. Chronic diarrhoea >1 month
   c. Prolonged fever for >1 month

Q 60. What are the minor signs of HIV in children?
The minor signs of HIV in children are:
   a. Generalised lymph node enlargement
   b. Oropharyngeal candidiasis
   c. Recurrent common infections
   d. Persistent cough
   e. Generalised rash
   f. Confirmed HIV infection in mother

Q 61. What is HIV wasting syndrome?
HIV wasting syndrome is weight loss >10% of body weight, with unexplained diarrhoea for >1 month or chronic weakness and unexplained fever for >1 month.

Q 62. Define HIV encephalopathy.
HIV encephalopathy has clinical features of disabling mental or motor dysfunction, interfering with activities of daily living progressing over weeks and months in the absence of a concurrent illness or condition other than HIV infection, which could explain the findings.

Q 63. What is WHO clinical stage 2 for children?
The WHO clinical stage 2 for children is:
   a. Unexplained chronic diarrhoea
   b. Severe persistent or recurrent candidiasis
   c. Weight loss or failure to thrive
   d. Persistent fever
   e. Recurrent reverse bacterial infection

Q 64. What is WHO clinical stage 3 for children?
The WHO clinical stage 3 for children is:
   a. AIDS defining opportunistic infection
   b. Severe failure to thrive
   c. Progressive encephalopathy
   d. Malignancy
   e. Recurrent septicemia or meningitis

Management

Q 65. What are the 5 Cs principles of WHO for testing of HIV?
   a. Consent   b. Confidentiality
   c. Counseling   d. Correct test results
   e. Connection to care and treatment

Q 66. Which cells are depleted in HIV infection?
Specialised group of WBC called T-helper or T4 cells are depleted in HIV infection.

Q 67. What are the cells other than T-helper cells that are infected by HIV?
â-cells, macrophages, nerve cells other than T-helper cells that are infected by HIV.

Q 68. What happens to helper cell: Suppressor cell ratio in HIV?
Helper cell: suppressor cell ratio in HIV is reversed.

Q 69. What makes an individual more susceptible to neoplasm and opportunistic infections in HIV?
Alteration in T-cell function makes an individual more susceptible to neoplasm and opportunistic infections in HIV.

Q 70. What is the screening test for HIV?
The screening test for HIV is ELISA.

Q 71. What is the confirmatory test for HIV?
The confirmatory test for HIV is Western blot.

Q 72. Western blot test is based on which antibody?
Western blot test is based on antibodies to viral core protein P24 and envelop glycoprotein gp41.

Q 73. What is the indicator of active HIV replication?
p24 antigen.

Q 74. What is the method to isolate HIV?
The method to isolate HIV is by cultured lymphocytes.

Q 75. What is the prognostic marker in HIV?
The prognostic marker in HIV is CD4 lymphocytes.

Q 76. What is the normal CD4 count?
The normal CD4 count is >950 CD4 cells/cumm of blood.

Q 77. How often should CD4 count assessment be done in a patient with CD4 >500 cells/cumm?
The CD4 count assessment is done in a patient with CD4 >500 cells/cumm once every 3 months.

Q 78. When should you start prophylactic therapy for *P. carinii*?
The prophylactic therapy for *P. carinii* is started when CD4 count <200/cumm.

Q 79. What percent of CD4 count, the risk of progression to AIDS is high?
The risk of progression to AIDS is high with <14% of the CD4 count.

Q 80. What is the sensitivity of ELISA test in HIV?
The sensitivity of ELISA test in HIV is 99.9%.

Q 81. How do you reduce the transmission of HIV to haemophiliacs?
The transmission of HIV to haemophiliacs is reduced by heat treatment of factors VII and IX.

Q 82. Classify ART drugs.

ART drugs are classified as:

a. Nucleoside reverse transcriptase inhibitors, e.g. abacavir, didanosine, emtricitabine, lamivudine, stavudine, zidovudine.

b. Nucleotide reverse transcriptase inhibitors, e.g. tenofovir

c. Non-nucleotide reverse transcriptase inhibitors, e.g. Efaviren and etravirive and nevirapine

d. Protease inhibitors, e.g. atazanavir, ritonavir

e. INSTI, e.g. raltegravir

Q 83. What is the preferred first line ART for adults?

The preferred first line ART for adults is 2 NRTI + 1 NNRTI/INSTI [tenofovir + lamivudine + efavirenz].

Q 84. Which drug is given as the first line ART in children <3 years?

The first line ART in children <3 years is lopinavir-based regimen.

Q 85. What is the first line ART regimen for children <3 years who develop TB?

The first line ART regimen for children <3 years who develop TB is abacavir + lamivudine + zidovudine.

Q 86. What is the preferred NNRTI for children <3 years?

Efavirenz is the preferred NNRTI for children<3 years.

Q 87. What are the preferred drugs for second line ART in adults?

2 NRTI + Ritonavir boosted PI are preferred drugs for second line ART in adults.

Q 88. What are the preferred drugs for second line ART in children?

2 NRTI + EFV in children older than 3 years is the preferred drugs for second line ART
In children <3 years, the preferred regime is RAL-based regime

Q 89. Exposure to which body fluids require PEP.

The body fluids which require PEP are parental or mucous membrane exposure to blood, blood stained saliva, breast milk, genital secretions, CSF, amniotic fluid, rectal, peritoneal, synovial, pericardial, or pleural fluid.

Q 90. Exposure to which body fluids does not require PEP.

The body fluids which do not require PEP are:

a. When the exposed individual is already HIV positive

b. When the source is established to be HIV negative

c. Exposure to body fluids like tears, no blood stained saliva, urine, and sweat.

Q 91. When should PEP be started?

PEP should be started as early as possible or within 72 hours.

Q 92. What is the preferred AR regimen for adults PEP?

The preferred AR regimen for adults PEP is tenofovir + lamivudine + LPV/r.

Q 93. What is the preferred AR regimen for children PEP?

The preferred AR regimen for children PEP is zidovudine + lamivudine.

Q 94. Postexposure prophylaxis should be given for how many days?
Postexposure prophylaxis is given for 28 days.

Q 95. When is co-trimoxazole prophylaxis started in adults?
The co-trimoxazole prophylaxis started in adults who are WHO stage 3 or 4 or CD4 count <350 cells/cumm

Q 96. When is co-trimoxazole prophylaxis started in children?
The co-trimoxazole prophylaxis started in children irrespective of clinical or immune conditions.

Q 97. When is co-trimoxazole prophylaxis started in infants who are HIV exposed?
The co-trimoxazole prophylaxis started in infants who are HIV exposed from 4 to 6 weeks of age.

Q 98. What is the revised treatment guideline recommended by WHO in 2016?
The revised treatment guideline recommended by WHO in 2016, an initiation of ART of all adults irrespective of WHO clinical stage and CD4 count. As a priority ART is to be given to all adults with severe or advanced clinical disease (WHO clinical stage 3 or 4) and adults with a CD4 count <350 cells/mm^3.

Q 99. Which drug is contraindicated in HIV?
The drug contraindicated in HIV is thioacetazone.

Q 100. What is drug of choice for prophylaxis against *Mycobacterium avium* complex?
The drug of choice for prophylaxis against *Mycobacterium avium* complex is rifabutin.

Q 101. What are the problems with the treatment of paediatric HIV?
The problems with treatment of paediatric HIV are:
  a. Lack of adherence
  b. Life long treatment required
  c. Malnutrition
  d. Growing brain and encephalopathy

Q 102. Which is the gold standard test to measure CD4 cells?
The gold standard test to measure CD4 cells is immunofluorescence assays by flow cytometry.

Q 103. How much is the CD4 cell count drop in a typical progression?
The CD4 cell count drop in a typical progression is 35–50 cells/year.

Q 104. How much is the CD4 cell count drop in a rapid progress?
The CD4 cell count drop in a rapid progression is 50 cells/month.

Q 105. What is the side effect of zidovudine?
The side effects of zidovudine are lactic acidosis, bone marrow suppression.

Q 106. What is the side effects of lamivudine?
The side effects of lamivudine are lactic acidosis, pancreatitis in children.

Q 107. What are the side effects of nevirapine?
The side effects of nevirapine are hepatitis, Stevens-Johnson syndrome.

Q 108. Rifampicin can be given with which NNRTI?
Rifampicin can be given with efavirenz.

Q 109. ART decreases the effectiveness of which two groups of drugs?
ART decreases the effectiveness of anticonvulsants and OCPs.

Q 110. What is immunological failure with respect to treatment with ART?
The immunological failure with ART when patients with persistent CD4 cell count less than 50 cells/cumm after 12 months on ART.

Q 111. What is the prevalence of HIV and HCV co-infection?
The prevalence of HIV and HCV co-infection is 30–40%.

Q 112. For how long can a hepatitis B virus survive in dried blood?
Hepatitis B virus can survive in dried blood for 7 days.

Q 113. Who is labelled as loss to follow-up in ART?
Patients who do not return for 3 or more continuous months or miss 4th drug packet in a row is labelled as a loss to follow-up in ART.

Q 114. What is the drug of choice for cryptosporidia?
Nitazoxanide 500 mg orally twice daily is the drug of choice for cryptosporidia.

Q 115. What is the drug of choice for giardiasis?
Metronidazole 250 mg orally 3 times daily for 5 to 10 days is the drug of choice for giardiasis.

Q 116. What is the case fatality rate among HIV infected TB cases?
The case fatality rate among HIV infected TB cases is 13–14%.

Q 117. Is HIV testing in all TB cases mandatory?
HIV testing in all TB cases is not mandatory. It is voluntary.

Q 118. What are the ART eligibility criteria for HIV infected TB patient?
The ART eligibility criteria for HIV infected TB patient are:
   a. All patients with extrapulmonary TB
   b. All those with pulmonary TB unless CD4 count <350 cells/mm^3

Q 119. When should a person tested positive for HIV be referred to ART centre?
A person tested positive for HIV should be immediately referred to ART centre.

Q 120. When should a person with pulmonary TB and HIV be referred to ART centre?
A person with pulmonary TB and HIV should be referred to ART centre after at least 2 weeks of anti-TB treatment.

Prevention

Q 121. What are the mechanisms by which HIV can be inactivated?
The mechanisms by which HIV can be inactivated are heat, ether, acetone, ethanol (20%), β-propiolactone (1:400 dilution).

Q 122. What are the mechanisms by which HIV cannot be inactivated?
The mechanisms by which HIV cannot be inactivated are ionizing radiation and UV light.

Q 123. How can you prevent transmission of HIV from mother to child?
The transmission of HIV from mother to child is prevented by:
   a. ART prophylaxis
   b. Elective caesarean section before the onset of labour or rupture of membranes
   c. Refraining from breastfeeding

Q 124. Define universal precautions.
Universal precautions are a set of precautions to protect health care workers from occupational exposure to bloodborne pathogens.

Q 125. What is the prophylaxis given to infants of mothers who are receiving ART and are breastfeeding?
The prophylaxis given to infants of mothers who are receiving ART and are breastfeeding is nevirapine for minimum 6 weeks daily.

Q 126. NACO is under which ministry?
NACO is under Ministry of Health and Family Welfare.

Q 127. Who conducts community-based HIV screening?
ANM conducts community-based HIV screening.

Q 128. As per NACO guidelines, what are included by ART centre staffing pattern?
ART centre staffing pattern includes:
   a. Doctor
   b. Counsellor
   c. Lab Technician
   d. Data manager
   e. Pharmacist (when number >500)
   f. Nurse
   g. Case co-ordinator

Q 129. What is the minimum space required for an ART centre?
The minimum space required for an ART centre is 800 sqft for a centre housing an average of 500 patients.

Q 130. What are the different type of surveillance in HIV?
The different types of surveillance in HIV are:
   a. HIV sentinel Surveillance
   b. HIV sero surveillance
   c. AIDS case surveillance
   d. STD surveillance
   e. Behavioural surveillance

Q 131. What are the objectives of HIV sentinel surveillance?
The objectives of HIV sentinel surveillance are:
   a. To determine the level of HIV infection among general population
   b. To understand the trends of HIV epidemic
   c. To understand the geographical spread of HIV infection and to identify emerging pockets
   d. To estimate HIV prevalence and HIV burden in the country

Q 132. What is the WHO case definition for AIDS surveillance?

The WHO case definition for AIDS surveillance is an adult or adolescent is considered to have AIDS if at least two of the major signs are present in combination with at least one of the minor signs and if these signs are not due to a condition unrelated to HIV infection.

Q 133. What is the expanded WHO case definition for AIDS surveillance?

The expanded WHO case definition for AIDS surveillance is adult or adolescent is positive for HIV antibody and one or more are present.

    a. More than 10% body weight loss with diarrhoea or fever for at least one month

    b. Cryptococcal meningitis

    c. Pulmonary/extrapulmonary TB

    d. Kaposi sarcoma

    e. Neurological impairment

    f. Recurrent pneumonia

    g. Candidiasis

    h. Invasive cervical cancer

Q 134. Where are the sentinel surveillance done for HIV?

The sentinel surveillance for HIV is done at:

    a. Antenatal clinics

    b. Suraksha clinics

    c. IV drugs

    d. Female sex workers

    e. Men having sex with men

Q 135. What are the services provided by ICTC?

The services provided by ICTC are:

    a. VCTC—voluntary confidential counselling and testing

    b. PMTCT—prevention of mother to child transmission

    c. ART—counselling, which includes access to the following services through linkages; IEC/BCC, condom promotion, STI treatment linkages, prophylaxis and early management of opportunistic infections, DOTS for TB, and ART services.

Q 136. What is care, support, treatment services through ART centres?

    a. Psychological support

    b. Prevention of treatment of opportunistic infections and tuberculosis

    c. Free antiretroviral therapy

    d. Facilitating home-based care and impact mitigation

Q 137. What is the name of the approach which is used to manage STDs?

Syndromic approach is used to manage STDs.

Q 138. Under what name NACO has branded the STI/RTI services?

Suraksha Clinic is NACO brand for the STI/RTI services.

Q 139. What is the link worker scheme?

The link worker scheme is a case-based outreach strategy to address HIV prevention and care needs of HRG and vulnerable population in the rural area.

LEPROSY

Introduction

Q 1. What is the type of organism *Mycobacterium leprae*?
Mycobacterium leprae is intra-cellular obligate parasite.

Q 2. What is the division time for *Mycobacterium leprae* bacillus?
The division time for *Mycobacterium leprae* bacillus is 12–14 days.

Q 3. What is the source of infection?
The source of infection is untreated human being (multibacillary case).

Q 4. What is the portal of exit from the patient?
The portal of exit from the patient is respiratory tract especially the nose, nasal mucosa apart from skin ulcers.

Q 5. Name the nonhuman reservoir of leprosy?
The nonhuman reservoirs of leprosy are armadillos, mangabey monkeys, and chimpanzees.

Q 6. What are the various types of classification of leprosy?
  a. Ridley Jopling (clinical and immune histological scale): Tuberculoid (TT), borderline tuberculoid (BT), borderline borderline (BB), borderline lepromatous (BL) and lepromatous (LL)
  b. Indian: Indeterminate (I), tuberculoid, borderline, lepromatous and pure neuritic
  c. Madrid: Indeterminate, tuberculoid, borderline, lepromatous
  d. WHO Classification: Paucibacillary (1–5 skin lesions), multibacillary (6 or more skin lesions)

Burden

Q 7. What is the contribution of India in total worldwide incident case?
The contribution of India in total worldwide incident case is 60% (2016 WER update—data of 2015)

Q 8. When was the goal of elimination achieved?
The goal of elimination was achieved in 2005.

Q 9. How many states/UTs have achieved the goal of elimination?
34 states/UTs have achieved the goal of elimination.

Q 10. Which states/UTs have not yet achieved the goal?
Chandigarh, Dadra and Nagar Haveli, Lakshadweep, Chattisgarh, Odisha, and Delhi have not achieved the goal of elimination.

Q 11. What is the prevalence rate of leprosy presently in India?
The prevalence rate of leprosy presently in India is 0.69/10000 population.

Q 12. What is the child case rate of leprosy in India?
The child case rate of leprosy in India is 0.88 per 1,00,000.

Q 13. What is the minimum compliance rate under NLEP?
The minimum compliance rate under NLEP is 95%.

Q 14. In how many countries have leprosy been eliminated?
Leprosy is eliminated in 119 countries.

Q 15. What is the percent of relapses?
The percent of relapses is 0.88%.

Q 16. What is the contribution of SEAR in the global prevalence of leprosy?
The contribution of SEAR in the global prevalence of leprosy is 67.28%.

Q 17. What is the annual new case detection rate?
The annual new case detection rate is 9.98 per lakh population.

Q 18. What is the attack rate of lepromatous cases?
The attack rate of lepromatous cases is 4.4 to 12% among household contacts.

Q 19. What is the most sensitive index of transmission of leprosy?
The most sensitive index of transmission of leprosy is incidence.

Risk Factor

Q 20. What age group affected more quickly by leprosy?
10–20 years more quickly affected by leprosy.

Q 21. Which gender is affected more by leprosy?
Males are more quickly affected by leprosy.

Q 22. Which climate favours leprosy?
Tropical and sub-tropical climates favour leprosy.

Q 23. What are the modes of transmission?
The modes of transmission are droplet infection (commonest), less common are contact transmission through direct skin to skin contact or indirect with contaminated soil or fomites, breast milk, insect vectors, and by tattooing needles.

Q 24. What is the incubation period of leprosy?
The incubation period of leprosy is a few weeks to 20 years. Average is 5–7 years.

Clinical Features

Q 25. What is a case of leprosy?
The case of leprosy is a person with the cardinal sign of leprosy and yet to complete a full course of MDT.

Q 26. What are the cardinal signs of leprosy?
The cardinal signs of leprosy are:
   a. Hypopigmented patches
   b. Partial or total loss of cutaneous sensation in the affected area (the earliest sensation to be affected is usually light touch)
   c. Presence of thickened nerves
   d. Presence of acid-fast bacilli in the skin or nasal smears

Q 27. Which peripheral nerves are most commonly affected in leprosy?
Ulnar, lateral popliteal, common peroneal, and posterior tibial nerves are most commonly affected in leprosy.

Q 28. What is the feature of involvement of ulnar nerve?
The feature of involvement of ulnar nerve is clawing of 4th–5th fingers.

Q 29. What is the feature of involvement of radial nerve?
The feature of involvement of radial nerve is wrist drop.

Q 30. What is the feature of involvement of lateral popliteal nerve?
The feature of involvement of lateral popliteal nerve is foot drop.

Q 31. What is the feature of involvement of posterior tibial nerve?
The feature of involvement of posterior tibial nerve is claw toes.

Q 32. What is the feature of involvement of facial nerve?
The feature of involvement of facial nerve is lagophthalmos.

Q 33. What is the feature of involvement of trigeminal nerve?
The feature of involvement of trigeminal nerve is loss of sensation over cornea.

Q 34. How many lesions are present in paucibacillary leprosy?
1–5 many lesions are present in paucibacillary leprosy.

Q 35. What is a leprosy reaction?
Leprosy reaction is an altered immune response either following treatment (MDT) or due to improvement of immunological status, leading to the inflammation of skin or nerves and even other tissues

Q 36. What are the types of lepra reactions?
Type I and II are two types of lepra reactions.

Q 37. What is the other name of type I reaction?
The other name of type I reaction is reversal reaction.

Q 38. In which type of leprosy is type I reaction seen?
Leprosy type I reaction is seen both in paucibacillary (PB) and multibacillary (MB).

Q 39. What is the other name of type II reaction?
The other name of type II reaction is erythema nodosum leprosum (ENL)

Q 40. In which type of Leprosy is type II reaction is seen?
Leprosy type-II reaction is seen in MB leprosy.

Management

Q 41. How many sites are examined for skin smears?
A minimum of 7 sites (smears: 4 from skin lesions, from both ear lobes, and one nasal swab).

Q 42. What is the bacterial index?
The bacterial index is total number of (+) scored in all smears/no. of smears per microscopic field in oil immersion.

Q 43. What is the morphological index?
The morphological index is number of uniformly stained bacilli/total number of bacilli counted.

Q 44. Name some laboratory tests for diagnosing leprosy.
IgM antibodies to phenolic glycoprotein, glycolipid, PGL ELISA, FLAABS and PCR on skin sample is used for diagnosing leprosy.

Q 45. What is the lepromin test?
Lepromin test is done by injecting 1 ml of lepromin intradermally in the forearm. It is used to classify lesions. It is strongly positive in tuberculoid, negative in lepromatous and variable in borderline. It helps to assess the prognosis as a positive test indicates good prognosis. It can be used to assess the response of the patient to treatment and resistance of individual to leprosy.

Q 46. When and how are the readings of lepromin test taken?
The readings are taken at 48 hours and 21 days. At 48 hours induration of more than 10 mm at the site of inoculation indicates a positive test and this is a delayed hyper-sensitivity to a soluble antigen of lepra bacilli. The second reading is taken at 21 days and presence of a nodule >5 mm at the site of inoculation indicates a positive test. This gives the cell mediated immunity of patient. Early reaction is also called Fernandez reaction and late on Mitsuda reaction. Early reaction is superior to the late reaction.

Q 47. How does BCG vaccine inoculation interfere with readings of lepromin test?
BCG vaccine inoculation can convert the late reaction from negative to positive.

Q 48. Name certain tests which can be done to test cell mediated immunity in leprosy case.
Lepromin test, lymphocyte transformation test, lymphocyte migration inhibition test are used to test cell mediated immunity in leprosy case.

Q 49. Name certain tests which can be done to test humoral immunity in leprosy case.
Fluorescent leprosy antibody test, monoclonal antibody test, ELISA, radioim-munoassay are used to test humoral immunity in leprosy case.

Q 50. What is ROM strategy?
ROM strategy is given by WHO where a patient with single lesion paucibacillary leprosy can be treated with rifampicin, ofloxacin, and minocycline.

Q 51. In which type of leprosy corticosteroids can be used?
Corticosteroids can be used in pure neuritic leprosy.

Q 52. Which drugs are used in MDT of leprosy?
Cap rifampicin, tab dapsone, and cap clofazimine are used in MDT of leprosy.

Q 53. What are the doses of rifampicin, dapsone and clofazimine?
Rifampicin—10 mg/kg, dapsone—2 mg/kg, Clofazimine—6 mg/kg monthly and 1 mg/kg daily.

Q 54. What are the precautions taken before starting MDT?
The precautions taken before starting MDT are evaluate for jaundice, anaemia, tuberculosis, and allergy to sulpha drugs.

Q 55. Which drug can be given to patients allergic to sulpha drugs in place of dapsone?

Clofazimine can be given to patients allergic to sulpha drugs in place of dapsone.

Q 56. What is AMDT?

AMDT stands for accompanied MDT. This is a WHO recommended policy where patient is provided the entire supply of MDT drugs at the time of diagnosis (6 months for PB and 12 months for MB), and asking someone close to the patient to ensure complete full course of treatment.

Q 57. Who is a defaulter?

A defaulter is a patient who has not collected treatment for 12 consecutive months. Once a patient has been categorized as a defaulter this patient should be removed from the register. However, all efforts should be made to trace the individual.

Q 58. How much stock should be maintained at the district level?

Three months stock should be maintained at the district level.

Q 59. Who keeps the records of leprosy at district level?

District Leprosy Officer keeps the records of leprosy at district level.

Q 60. What is the drug of choice for type I lepra reaction?

The drug of choice for type I lepra reaction is prednisolone.

Q 61. What is the duration of corticosteroids therapy in severe type II reactions?

The duration of corticosteroids therapy in severe type II reactions is 2–3 weeks.

Q 62. What is a relapse?

Relapse is re-occurrence of a disease any time after the completion of a full course of treatment.

Q 63. What are the signs of relapse?

The signs of relapse are slow and insidious onset with erythema and infiltration in old lesions and involvement of single nerve and usually occurs when chemotherapy has been discontinued.

Q 64. How is relapse differentiated from reversal in PB leprosy?

Reversal occurs during chemotherapy or within 3 years of stopping treatment, whereas a relapse occurs after the chemotherapy has been discontinued after a period of three years.

Q 65. What is a BCP and who maintains it?

Blister calendar packs (BCPs) are medicines packed together for four weeks (28 days). There are 4 types of BCPs used in India:
   a. PB BCP for 15 years and above
   b. PB BCP for 10–14 years
   c. MB BCP for 15 years and above
   d. MB BCP for 10–14 years
   e. PB BCP contains 2 drugs.
   f. MB BCP contains 3 drugs.
   g. There are no BCPs for ages less than 10 years of age.

Q 66. What is EHF scoring?

EHF score is the sum of all the individual disability grades for the two eyes, two hands and two feet. Each organ is scored for disability from 0 to 2. Thus the EHF score ranges from 0 to 12. A score of 12 would indicate grade 2 disability of both eyes, both hands, and both feet.

Q 67. What are the dietary precautions to be taken before starting prednisolone?

The dietary precautions to be taken before starting prednisolone is restricted salt intake.

Q 68. What is ichthyosis?

Ichthyosis is a condition where the skin is dry and scaly like that of a fish.

Q 69. What is Lucio's phenomenon?

Lucio's phenomenon is seen in lepromatous leprosy when an untreated case develops recurrent crops of large sharply marginated, ulcerative lesions, especially on lower extremities.

Q 70. Name a few candidate vaccines for leprosy.

BCG, heat killed *Mycobacterium leprae* vaccine.

Q 71. When was the National Leprosy Control Programme launched by Government of India?

The National Leprosy Control Programme was launched in 1955.

Q 72. Can leprosy be eradicated?

Leprosy is not amenable to eradication because it has a long and variable incubation period, absence of effective vaccine, extra human reservoir, multiple modes of transmission, presence of subclinical cases, hiding of disease by cases due to stigma and broad spectrum of presentation.

Q 73. When did MDT come into wide use?

The MDT came into wide use from 1982, following the recommendation of the WHO Study Group, Geneva.

Q 74. When was the National Leprosy Eradication Programme (NLEP) introduced?

NLEP was introduced in 1983 with the objective to reduce the case load by turn of century to <1/10000.

Q 75. Who sponsors NLEP?

NLEP is sponsored by Central Government.

Q 76. Who supplies free drugs for leprosy?

WHO supplied free MDT only between 2001 and 2004 after that all budget components are under MOHFW-GOI and subsequently under NHM.

Q 77. Who is the head of Global Leprosy Programme?

The head of Global Leprosy Programme is Regional Director SEAR.

Q 78. Where is the office of Global Leprosy Programme?

The office of Global Leprosy Programme is in New Delhi.

Q 79. Where was the office of Global Leprosy Programme located earlier?

The office of Global Leprosy Programme was earlier located in Geneva.

Q 80. When was the office shifted from Geneva to New Delhi?

The office shifted from Geneva to New Delhi on July 1st 2005.

Q 81. What is the proposed global target of reducing the rate of new cases with grade II disabilities?

The proposed global target of reducing the rate of new cases with grade II disabilities is the reduction by at least 35% by the end of 2015 compared to the baseline at the end of 2010.

TUBERCULOSIS (TB)

Introduction

Q 1. Define a presumptive case of TB.

Presumptive case refers to a patient who presents with symptoms/signs suggestive of TB.

Q 2. Define monoresistance, polydrug resistance, multidrug resistance and extensive drug resistance.

   a. Monoresistance: Resistance to one first-line anti-TB drug
   b. Polydrug resistance: Resistance to more than one first line anti-TB drug (other than both INH and rifampicin)
   c. Multidrug resistance: Resistance to at least both INH and rifampicin
   d. Extensive drug resistance: Resistance to only fluoroquinolones and at least one of three second-line injectable drugs (capreomycin, kanamycin, amikacin), in addition to MDR.

Q 3. Define treatment relapse and treatment failure.

Relapse: Those who have been previously treated for TB, were declared cure or treatment completed at the end of their most recent course of treatment, and are now diagnosed with a recurrent recent episode of TB.

Failure: Those who have previously been treated for TB and whose treatment failed at the end of their most recent course of treatment.

Q 4. Define rifampicin resistance.

Resistance to rifampicin detected using phenotypic or genotypic methods, with or without resistance to other anti-TB drugs.

Q 5. Define HIV-positive TB patient.

Any bacteriologically confirmed or clinically diagnosed case of TB who has a positive result from HIV testing conducted at the time of TB diagnosis or other documented evidence of enrollment in HIV case.

Q 6. Define HIV-negative TB patient.

Any bacteriologically confirmed or clinically diagnosed case of TB who has a negative result from HIV testing conducted at the time of TB diagnosis.

Q 7. Define HIV status unknown TB patient.

Any bacteriologically confirmed or clinically diagnosed case of TB who has a no result of HIV testing and no other documented evidence of enrollment in HIV case.

Q 8. Which are the "seeds of future relapse" in TB?

The seeds of future relapse in TB are slow multipliers/persisted. Effective anti-microbial treatment reduces infectivity by 90% within 48 hours.

Q 9. What is the incubation period of TB?

The incubation period of TB varies from weeks/months/years. Time for receipt of infection to the development of a positive tuberculin test ranges from 3 to 6 weeks.

Q 10. Define mortality from TB.

A number of deaths caused by TB in HIV-negative people, according to the latest revision of ICD-10.

Q 11. What are the different classifications under which a bacteriological confirmed or clinically diagnosed case is classified?

The different classifications under which a bacteriological confirmed or clinically diagnosed case are:

    a. Anatomical site of disease

    b. History of previous treatment

    c. Drug resistance

    d. HIV status

Burden

Q 12. What is the burden of TB in India?

As per TB India 2017 Annual Report

    a. India has the highest burden of TB and MDR TB in world

    b. India has the second highest burden of HIV TB in world

    c. Incidence: 217 per lakh population (2015)

    d. Mortality: 36 per lakh population (2015)

Q 13. Define DOTS coverage.

DOTS coverage is percentage of the national population living in areas where health services have adopted DOTS.

Q 14. Define case notification rate of TB.

New recurrent episodes of TB notified to WHO for a given year, expressed per 1,00,000 population. It is an important estimate of TB incidence.

Q 15. Define tuberculin-conversion index.

Tuberculin-conversion index is the percent of the population under study who will be newly infected by *M. tuberculosis* among the non-infected of the preceding survey during the course of one year. It is also known as annual infection rate or incidence of infection.

Clinical Features

Q 16. What are the 4S symptoms in adults?

The 4S symptoms in adults are:

    a. Current cough   b. Fever

    c. Weight loss   d. Night sweats

Q 17. What are the 4S symptoms in children?
The 4S symptoms in children are:
   a. Cough   b. Fever
   c. Poor weight gain   d. Contact with TB case

Management

Q 18. What are the curative components and preventive components of TB control?
   a. Curative component: Case finding and treatment
   b. Preventive components: BCG vaccine

Q 19. How many sputum samples should be collected minimum TB for case finding?
Two sputum samples should be collected minimum for TB case finding.

Q 20. How many specimens should test positive to declare a patient smear positive TB?
One specimen should test positive to declare a patient smear positive TB.

Q 21. How many organisms need to be present for sputum smear microscopy for tubercle bacilli to be positive?
At least 10,000 organisms per ml of sputum are needed to be present for sputum smear microscopy for tubercle bacilli to be positive.

Q 22. Which is the stain used in fluorescent microscopy?
Auramine is the stain used in fluorescent microscopy.

Q 23. Which is the media used in micro colony detection in solid media?
Middle brook 7H11 agar medium is the media used in micro colony detection in solid media.

Q 24. Which system detects the presence of mycobacteria based on their metabolism?
Radiometric BACTEC-460 TB method detects the presence of mycobacteria based on their metabolism.

Q 25. Which is the most common target used in PCR?
1S6110 is the most common target used in PCR.

Q 26. MB/BaCT system is based on what?
MB/BaCT system is based on colorimetric detection of CO_2.

Q 27. Which is the current gold standard for TB diagnosis?
Cartridge-based nucleic acid amplification test is the current gold standard for TB diagnosis.

Q 28. Name the specific test for detecting rifampicin resistance.
GeneXpert MTB/RIF is the specific test for detecting rifampicin resistance.

Q 29. Who discovered the tuberculin test?
Von Piraquet, 1907, discovered the tuberculin test.

Q 30. Which is the only method of detecting the prevalence of TB in a population?
Tuberculin test is the only method of detecting the prevalence of TB in a population.

Q 31. Which are the tuberculins accepted by WHO?
Derivative-S (PPD-S) and PPD-RT 23 are the tuberculins accepted by WHO.

Q 32. Define standard 5 tuberculin unit dose of PPD-S.
Standard 5 tuberculin unit dose of PPD-S is delayed skin activity contained in a 0.1 µg/0.1 ml dose of PPD-S.

Q 33. Which is the PPD used in India?
PPD used in India is PPD-RT 23 with Tween 80.

Q 34. What is Tween 80?
Tween 80 is a detergent added to tuberculin to prevent their adsorption on glass or plastic surface.

Q 35. What is the strength of PPD used in India for the standard Mantoux test?
The strength of PPD used in India for the standard Mantoux test is 1 TU.

Q 36. When is the result of tuberculin test read? Where is the site for inoculation?
The tuberculin test read after 48–96 hours; 72 hours is ideal. The site for inoculation is intradermally, flexor surface of left forearm, mid-way between elbow and wrist.

Q 37. Who are the "strong reactors" of tuberculin test?
The "strong reactors" of tuberculin test are those showing induration 20 mm or more.

Q 38. Which is the only bacteriological drug effective against "persisters"?
The only bacteriological drug effective against "persisters" is rifampicin.

Q 39. Where in India is the Tuberculosis Chemotherapy Centre located?
Tuberculosis Chemotherapy Centre located in Chennai, India.

Q 40. What was the old DOTS regime followed by category 1 and category 2 patients?
Cat 1 (red box)—2 (HRZE) 3 + 4 (HR) 3
Cat 2 (blue box)—2 (HRZES) 3 + 1 (HRZE) 3 + 5 (HRE) 3

Q 41. When is daily self-administered non-DOTS regime followed?
Daily self-administered non-DOTS regime is followed:
  a. When there is an adverse reaction to drugs used in short-course chemotherapy.
  b. When the patient cannot comply with this regime.

Q 42. What is non-DOTS regime for new smear positive pulmonary seriously ill patients and extra pulmonary seriously ill patients (ND1) who interrupt treatment?
Non-DOTS regime for new smear positive pulmonary seriously ill patients and extra pulmonary seriously ill patients is 2 (SHE) + 10 (HE).

Q 43. What is non-DOTS regime for new smear negative pulmonary not seriously ill patients and extrapulmonary not seriously ill patients (ND2) who interrupt treatment?
Non-DOTS regime for new smear negative pulmonary not seriously ill patients and extrapulmonary not seriously ill patients is 12 (HE).

Q 44. Name the second line anti-TB drugs.

Fluoroquinolones, ethionamides, capreomycin, kanomycin, amikacin, cycloserine, thioacetazone, and macrolides.

Q 45. What is the treatment regimen for MDR-TB?

RNTCP regimen for MDR-TB—6 drugs—6(m) Km Lvx, Eto, Cs, Z, E/18 Lvx, Eto, Cs, E for 24 to 27 months depending upon the intensive phase duration, where

 a. Lvx: Levofloxacin   b. Eto: Ethionamide

 c. Cs: Cycloserine   d. Z: Pyrizineamide

 e. E: Ethambutol

Q 46. When should be a patient of MDR-TB be first reviewed?

A patient of MDR-TB is first reviewed after 6 months of treatment

If culture positive, extended by 1 month.

If 4th or 5th month culture result negative, switch over to CP phase.

Q 47. What is the treatment regimen for XDR-TB?

RNTCP regimen for XDR-TB 6–12 Cm, PAS, Mfx, high dose-H, Cfz, Lzd, Amx/Clv/18PAS, Mfx, high dose-H, Cfz, Lzd, Amx/Clv for 24 to 30 months, where

 a. Cm: Capreomycin   b. Mfx: Moxifloxacin

 c. H: INH   d. Cfz: Clofazamine

 e. Lzd: Linezolid

Q 48. How much induration is considered as positive for tuberculin test in paediatric age group?

Induration of 10 mm or more is considered as positive for tuberculin test in paediatric age group.

Q 49. What is the dose of isoniazid for TB preventive therapy?

The dose of isoniazid for TB preventive therapy is 10 mg/kg, administered daily for 6 months.

Q 50. Where is the BCG laboratory located in India?

BCG laboratory is located in Guindy, Chennai, India.

Q 51. Where is the International Reference Centre for BCG quality control located?

The International Reference Centre for BCG quality control is located in Copenhagen.

Q 52. Define primary or pre-treatment resistance.

Primary or pre-treatment resistance is resistance shown by bacteria in a patient who has not received the drug in question before.

Q 53. Define secondary or acquired resistance.

Secondary or acquired resistance is when bacteria were sensitive to the drug at the start of the treatment but became resistant to it during the course of the treatment.

Q 54. Which is the most peripheral lab under the RNTCP?

The most peripheral lab under the RNTCP is designated microscopic centre (DMC), serving a population of 1,00,000 (50,000 for tribal and hilly areas).

Q 55. What is the population ratio under one TB unit?
The population ratio under one TB is one per block, one per 1.5 to 2.5 lakh population.

Q 56. How many microbiologist and lab technician have been provided to each NRL under RNTCP?
Under RNTCP each NRL has three microbiologists and four lab technician.

Q 57. Is case finding under RNTCP active or passive?
Case finding under RNTCP is passive.

Q 58. How much incentive is a DOTS agent paid in RNTCP?
DOTS agent is paid Rs 150/- per patient completing the treatment.

Q 59. Name the newer drug (diarylquinoline antibiotic) being investigated as an adjunct to existing therapies for MDR-TB.
Bedaquiline.

Q 60. What is the basic requirement for the patient to be initiated on bedaquiline?
A case of pulmonary MDR-TB who is more than 18 years old.
The additional requirements for the patient to be initiated on bedaquiline are:
   a. Females should not be pregnant nor be using hormone-based birth control methods
   b. The patients should be willing to continue practice birth control methods
   c. The patient should be postmenopausal for 2 years
   d. Patient with controlled stable arrhythmia

Q 61. What are the 3 Is under TB-HIV co-ordination?
The 3 Is under TB-HIV co-ordination are:
   a. IPT: Isoniazid preventive therapy   b. AIC: Airborne infection control
   c. ICF: Intensive case finding

Q 62. What are the screening strategies under RNTCP 2016?
The screening strategies under RNTCP 2016 are:
   a. Community screening   b. Institutional screening

Q 63. What are the targets of DOTS programme?
The targets of DOTS programme are successful treatment or cure rate of 90% of new smear positive cases and detection of 90% of such cases (85% for drug sensitive previously treated).

Q 64. When did WHO launch the stop TB strategy?
The stop TB strategy was launched in 2006.

Q 65. When was the End TB strategy launched?
The End TB strategy was launched in 2015.

Q 66. What are the salient principles of the End TB strategy?
The salient principles of the End TB strategy are:
a. Integrated, patient centered care and prevention
b. Bold policies and supportive programme
c. Intensified research and innovation

Q 67. What are the targets of END TB strategy?

The targets of End TB strategy are:

a. 95% reduction in a number of TB deaths compared with 2015

b. 90% reduction in TB incidence rate compared with 2015

c. Zero TB affected families facing catastrophic expenditure

Q 68. What are the stop TB partnership targets?

By 2015: The global burden of TB will be reduced by 50% relative to 1990 levels.

By 2050: The global incidence of TB disease will be less than or equal to one case per million population per year.

Q 69. What are the objectives of the National Strategic Plan for Tuberculosis Elimination 2017–2025?

The objectives of the National Strategic Plan for Tuberculosis Elimination 2017–2025 are:

a. To achieve 90% notification rate for all cases

b. To achieve 90% success rate for all new and 85% for re-treatment cases

c. To significantly improve the successful outcomes of treatment of DR-TB cases

d. To achieve decreased morbidity and mortality of HIV-associated TB

e. To improve outcomes of TB care in the private sector

Q 70. What is 99 DOTS?

It is an ICT-based tool to improve drug adherence.

Q 71. How do 99 DOTS works?

Patients send a free call each time they take their medication so that providers can monitor adherence records. The calls are toll-free, so patients do not have any additional costs.

Q 72. What is 90-90-90 by 2035 in TB?

It is 90% reduction in incidence, mortality and catastrophic health expenditures due to TB by 2035.

ELDERLY

(A person aged more than 60 years)
HYPERTENSION

Swagata Mandal, Sahil Goyal, Arti Gupta

Introduction

Q 1. Define hypertension.

According to Joint National Committee on prevention, detection, evaluation, and treatment of high blood pressure (JNC 7), hypertension is defined as a systolic BP (SBP) of more than 139 mm of Hg and/or diastolic BP (DBP) of more than 89 mm of Hg in an adult aged 18 years or more, who is not taking antihypertensive drugs and not actually ill.

Q 2. Classify hypertension according to blood pressure level.

Blood pressure			Category	
Systolic (mm of Hg)		Diastolic (mm of Hg)	JNC7	2017 ACC/AHA
<120	And	<80	Normal	Normal
120–129	And	<80	Pre-hypertension	Elevated
130–139	Or	80–89	Pre-hypertension	Hypertension stage 1
140–159	Or	90–99	Hypertension stage 1	Hypertension stage 2
≥160	Or	≥100	Hypertension stage 2	Hypertension stage 2
≥180	Or	≥110	Hypertension stage 3	

When SBP and DBP fall in different classifications, the higher classification should be selected to classify the patient's BP. For example, a patient with BP of 160/94 should be classified as stage 2 hypertensive as per JNC 7.

Q 3. What is sustainable development goal 3: target 3.4?
By 2030 reduce by one-third pre-mature mortality from non-communicable diseases (NCDs) through prevention and treatment, and promote mental health and well-being.

Q 4. What is Framingham Heart Study?
The Framingham Heart Study is widely acknowledged as a premier longitudinal study. Framingham was the study site. This study elaborated detailed hypothesis representing multifactorial causes of cardiovascular diseases.

Q 5. When is World Hypertension Day?
May 17

Q 6. Hypertension was the theme of which World Health Day?
2013: Healthy heart beat, Healthy blood pressure

Q 7. What is primary or essential hypertension?
Hypertension which has no known cause.

Q 8. What is secondary hypertension?
Hypertension secondary to a systemic disease commonly renal.

Q 9. Define isolated systolic hypertension.
SBP of 140 mm of Hg or more and a DBP of less than 90 mm of Hg.

Q 10. What is malignant hypertension?
Hypertension with the following features:
- a. Blood pressure >200/140 mg Hg
- b. Encephalopathy
- c. Renal disease
- d. Fundus changes like papilledema

Q 11. What is hypertensive urgency?

Severe asymptomatic hypertension (systolic >180 mm, diastolic >120 mm)

Q 12. What is hypertensive emergency?

Severe hypertension accompanied by cardiac (e.g. acute left ventricular failure), neurological (e.g. hypertensive encephalopathy), or acute renal dysfunction.

Q 13. What is white coat hypertension?

It is increasing blood pressure in normal individual when BP is recorded by doctor or in hospital.

Q 14. What is pseudohypertension?

It is the false increase in blood pressure due to stiffening of vessels, commonly seen in old age group.

Q 15. What is paradoxical hypertension?

It is a paradoxical increase in blood pressure in patients even on antihypertensive medicines.

Q 16. What is accelerated hypertension?

It is the recent significant increase over baseline BP that is associated with target organ damage [like vascular damage on fundus examination].

Q 17. Explain "Rule of halves".

In the 1970s it was found evidence that in the most developed countries, only half of the hypertensive subjects were aware of the condition, among them only half with the problem was being treated, and only half among treated were considered adequately treated.

Q 18. What is "tracking" of blood pressure?

If we follow-up BP levels of individuals over a period of years starting from early childhood to adult life, then those individuals whose BP were initially high in the distribution, would probably continue on the same "track" as adults. For example, low BP levels tend to remain low, and high BP levels tend to become higher as the individual grows older. This phenomenon of persistence of rank order of blood pressure has been described as "tracking".

Implication: This knowledge can be applied to identify children and adolescents "at risk" of developing hypertension in the future.

Q 19. How to measure blood pressure?

Measurement of blood pressure

a. The diagnosis of hypertension should be based on multiple BP measurements taken on several separate occasions (preferably record at least 3 sets of readings on different occasions and minimum two)

b. Patients should be asked to refrain from smoking or drinking tea/coffee, exercise for at least 30 minutes before measuring the BP.

c. Blood pressure should be measured after the patient has emptied bladder and has been seated for five minutes with back supported and legs resting on the ground (not crossed).

d. The arm used for measurement should rest on a table, at heart-level.

e. Use a sphygmomanometer and stethoscope or automated electronic device.
f. Use a standard cuff with a bladder that is 12 cm × 35 cm. Use a large bladder for fat arms and a small bladder for children.
g. The bladder should encircle and cover two-thirds of the length of the arm.
h. For measurement, inflate the bladder quickly to a pressure 20 mm Hg higher than the point of disappearance of the radial pulse.
i. Deflate the bladder slowly by 2 mm Hg every second.
j. The pressure at which Korotkoff sound 1 is heard is taken to be systolic pressure. Though phase 4 sound (at which sounds first become muffled) can be taken, most settings use Korotkoff 5 sound to indicate diastolic pressure at which sounds disappear.

> * Consider checking standing readings after one and three minutes to screen for postural hypotension, especially in the elderly.

Burden

Q 20. What is the prevalence of hypertension in India?
The prevalence of hypertension is 22.2%.

Q 21. What is the prevalence of coronary vascular disease in India?
The prevalence of coronary vascular disease is 272 per lakh population.

Q 22. What are the three most common cause of mortality in India?
a. IHD = 15.7% of deaths
b. COPD = 10.0% of deaths
c. Stroke/cerebrovascular disease = 7.8% of deaths

Risk Factor

Q 23. What are the risk factors for hypertension?
They can be categorised as non-modifiable and modifiable risk factors. Non-modifiable risk factors include age, sex, genetic makeup of an individual and ethnicity. Black Americans and African origin people have been found to have higher blood pressure levels than white.

Modifiable risk factors include the presence of obesity, high salt intake, high intake of saturated fat, less intake of dietary fibre, less intake of alcohol consumption, high heart rate, low physical activity, socioeconomic status. The commonest secondary cause of hypertension these days is oral contraception (due to the estrogen component). Heart rate of hypertensives is higher than normotensives due to the resetting of sympathetic activity at a higher level.

Management

Q 24. Who should be treated with pharmacotherapy?
Recommendations according to JNC 8:
a. Patients <60 years of age: Start pharmacotherapy at 140/90 mm Hg.
b. Patients with diabetes: Start pharmacotherapy at 140/90 mm Hg.
c. Patients with CKD: Start pharmacotherapy at 140/90 mm Hg.
d. Patients 60 years of age and older: Start pharmacotherapy at 150/90 mm Hg.

> * Continue lifestyle changes in addition to pharmacotherapy.

Q 25. What is the goal blood pressure?
Recommendations according to JNC 8:

a. Patients <60 years of age: <140/90 mm Hg

b. Patients with diabetes: <140/90 mm Hg

c. Patients with CKD: <140/90 mm Hg

d. Patients 60 years of age and older: <150/90 mm Hg

e. In patients 60 years of age and older, no need to back off on tolerated treatment if lower systolic (e.g. <140 mm Hg) achieved.

f. Use clinical judgment; consider risk/benefit of treatment for each individual when setting goal.

g. Unproven clinical benefit of lower targets previously recommended for diabetes, CKD, and CAD.

Q 26. What pharmacotherapy is recommended?
Recommendations according to JNC 8:

a. Nonblack, including those with diabetes: Thiazide, calcium channel blockers (CCB), angiotensin converting enzyme inhibitor (ACEI), or angiotensin receptor blockers (ARB).

b. African American, including those with diabetes: Thiazide or CCB

c. CKD: Regimen should include an ACEI or ARB (including African Americans)

d. Can initiate with two agents, especially if systolic >20 mm Hg above goal or diastolic >10 mm Hg above goal.

e. If goal not reached:
   - Stress adherence to medication and lifestyle
   - Increase the dose or add a second or third agent from one of the recommended classes.
   - Choose a drug outside of the classes recommended above only if these options have been exhausted. Consider specialist referral.

Indications	Treatment choice
Heart failure	ACEI/ARB + BB + diuretic + spironolactone
Post-MI/clinical CAD	ACEI/ARB and BB
CAD	ACEI, BB, diuretic, CCB
Diabetes	ACEI/ARB, CCB, diuretic
CKD	ACEI/ARB
Recurrent stroke prevention	ACEI, diuretic
Pregnancy	Labetolol (first line), nifedipine, methyldopa

Prevention

Q 27. What is the lifestyle modifications recommended for blood pressure control?

a. Weight reduction: Maintain normal BMI (18.5–24.9 kg/m²), SBP reduction by 5–20 mm Hg/10 kg weight loss.

b. DASH diet, SBP reduction by 8–14 mm Hg

c. Dietary sodium restriction: Reduce dietary sodium intake to no more than 100 mEq/d (less than 2.4 gm/day), SBP reduction by 2–8 mm Hg

d. Salt should not be more than 5 gm per day

e. Physical activity: Brisk walking at least 30 minutes per day, SBP reduction by 4–9 mm Hg

f. Stop tobacco use if any

g. Moderation of alcohol consumption, if any [Men ≤60 ml/day, Women ≤30 ml/day]

Q 28. What is World Health Organization PEN for non-communicable diseases?

It is package of essential noncommunicable (PEN) disease interventions for primary health care in low-resource settings.

- **Primary prevention of heart attacks and strokes:**

  a. Tobacco cessation (level 1)

  b. Regular physical activity 30 minutes a day (level 1)

  c. Reduced intake of salt <5 g per day (level 1)

  d. Fruits and vegetables at least 400 g per day (level 2)

  e. Aspirin, statins, and anti-hypertensives for people with 10-year cardiovascular risk >30% (level 1)

  f. Anti-hypertensives for people with blood pressure ≥160/100

  g. Anti-hypertensives for people with persistent blood pressure ≥140/90 and 10-year cardiovascular risk >20% unable to lower blood pressure through lifestyle measures (level 1)

- **Acute myocardial infarction:**

  Aspirin (level 1)

- **Secondary prevention (postmyocardial infarction):**

  a. Tobacco cessation (level 1), healthy diet and regular physical activity (level 2).

  b. Aspirin, angiotensin-converting enzyme inhibitor, beta-blocker, statin (level 1)

Q 29. What is World Health Organization STEPS in NCD?

It is the WHO STEPwise approach (STEPS) to surveillance of NCD risk factors.

The STEPS instrument has three different levels or 'steps' of risk factor assessment:

Step 1 (questionnaire)

Step 2 (physical measurements)

Step 3 (biochemical measurements)

The STEPS instrument contains:

a. Core items: The core items for each section have questions required to calculate basic variables. For example, current daily smokers, mean BMI, etc.

b. Expanded items: The expanded items for each section assess more detailed information. Examples include use of smokeless tobacco, sedentary behaviour, etc.

c. Optional items: The expanded items for each section assess other detailed information. Examples include mental health, skin fold thickness.

Q 30. What is World Health Organization/International Society of Hypertension (WHO/ISH) risk prediction charts? [Annexure 18, 19]

They are charts to estimate the 10-year cardiovascular risk of an individual using the following parameters:

a. Presence or absence of diabetes
b. Gender
c. Smoker or non-smoker
d. Age
e. Systolic blood pressure
f. Total blood cholesterol

Q 31. What are the nonpharmacological treatment of hypertension?

a. Reduce salt/sodium intake
b. Increase physical activity
c. Moderating alcohol consumption
d. DASH diet
e. Losing weight
f. Yoga
g. Medication

Q 32. What are the targets of the national monitoring framework for prevention and control of NCDs?

a. A 25% relative reduction in risk of premature mortality from NCDs.
b. At least 10% relative reduction in the harmful use of alcohol
c. A 10% relative reduction in the prevalence of insufficient physical activity
d. A 30% relative reduction in mean population intake of salt/sodium
e. A 30% relative reduction in the prevalence of current tobacco use in persons age 15 + years
f. A 25% relative reduction in the prevalence of raised blood pressure
g. Halt the rise in diabetes and obesity
h. At least 50% of eligible people receive drug therapy and counseling to prevent heart attacks and stroke
i. An 80% availability of the affordable basic technologies and essential medicines required to treat major NCDs in both public and private facilities
j. A 50% relative reduction in household use of solid fuels as a primary source of energy for cooking [this target is added by India].

Q 33. Enumerate national initiatives for prevention and control of NCDs.

a. National Programme for cancer, diabetes, cardiovascular diseases and stroke
b. National Tobacco Control Programme
c. National Mental Health Programme
d. National Programme for Health Care of the Elderly

e. National Palliative Care Programme
f. Addressing comorbidities:
   a. TB-diabetes
   b. TB-tobacco
g. National Iodine Disorders Control Programme
h. National Oral Health Programme
i. National Programme for Prevention and Control of Deafness
j. National Programme for Control of Blindness
k. National Programme for Prevention and Control of Fluorosis
l. National Programme for Prevention of Burn Injuries
m. National Programme for Trauma Care

DIABETES MELLITUS

Sahil Goyal

Introduction

Q 1. What is diabetes mellitus?
Diabetes mellitus is a chronic disease due to lack or ineffectiveness of insulin. It is a state of raised blood glucose *(hyperglycemia)* associated with premature mortality.

Q 2. What is hyperglycemia?
Hyperglycemia seriously damages many of the body's systems, especially the blood vessels and nerves.

Q 3. What is diabetes mellitus known in Hindi?
Diabetes mellitus is also known as *madhumeha.*

Q 4. Who coined the term diabetes mellitus?
The term "diabetes" or "to pass through" by the Greek Apollonius of Memphis.
The term "Mellitus" or "from honey" was added by Thomas Willis.

Q 5. Who classified diabetes as type 1 and type 2?
Type 1 and type 2 diabetes were identified as separate conditions by the Indian physicians Sushruta and Charaka.

Q 6. Who discovered insulin?
Frederick Banting and Charles Best isolated a substance from the pancreas of dogs, which they named isletin, now known as insulin.

Q 7. Classify diabetes mellitus as per WHO 1985.
   a. Insulin-dependent DM
   b. Noninsulin-dependent DM
   c. Malnutrition-related DM
   d. Gestational DM
   e. Others

Q 8. Classify diabetes mellitus as per WHO 1999 and ADA 1997.
  a. Type 1 DM
  b. Type 2 DM
  c. Pancreatic DM (including Fibrocalculous pancreatic diabetes)
  d. Gestational DM
  e. Others

Q 9. What is type 1 diabetes mellitus?
It is also called insulin-dependent diabetes mellitus (IDDM) or juvenile-onset diabetes. It develops when the body's immune system destroys pancreatic beta cells of the pancreas. It is usually diagnosed in children and young adults.

Q 10. What is type 2 diabetes mellitus?
It is also called noninsulin-dependent diabetes mellitus (NIDDM) or adult-onset diabetes. It accounts for about 90% to 95% disease burden. It usually begins with insulin resistance.

Q 11. What is gestational diabetes mellitus?
It is a form of glucose intolerance that is diagnosed in women during pregnancy.

Q 12. What is LADA?
LADA is latent autoimmune diabetes in adults. It is a form of autoimmune type 1 diabetes. It is also known as late-onset autoimmune diabetes of adulthood, slow onset type 1 diabetes, and type 1.5 diabetes.

Q 13. What is MODY?
MODY is maturity onset diabetes of the young due to mutations in enzyme glucokinase leading to insufficient insulin release from pancreatic β-cells.

Q 14. What is metabolic syndrome?
The metabolic syndrome is the clustering of central obesity, dyslipidemia, hypertension, impaired glucose or diabetes mellitus, insulin resistance and other cardiovascular disease risk factor.

Q 15. What is secondary diabetes mellitus?
Diabetes mellitus is due to secondary causes, for example, acromegaly, Cushing syndrome, thyrotoxicosis, pheochromocytoma, and others.

Q 16. What is impaired glucose tolerance and impaired fasting glucose?
Impaired glucose tolerance (IGT) and impaired fasting glucose (IFG) is metabolic state intermediate between normal glucose homeostasis and diabetes. It is also known as pre-diabetes.

Burden

Q 17. What is the burden of diabetes mellitus globally?
In 2015 globally 415 million people had diabetes and 5 million died from diabetes mellitus.

Q 18. What is the magnitude of diabetes mellitus in India?
The prevalence of diabetes in adults (20–79 years) is 8.7%. The prevalence of DM type 2 is 20.3%.

Risk Factors

Q 19. What are the causes of type 1 DM?

Insulin deficiency is absolute in type 1 DM. This may be due to:

a. Auto-immunity

b. Decreased number of insulin receptors

c. Defects in the formation of insulin

d. Destruction of beta cells by viral infections or chemical agents

e. Genetic defects like mutation of insulin gene

f. Pancreatic disorders like inflammatory or neoplastic

Q 20. What are the causes of type 2 DM?

The causes of type 2 DM are:

a. Elderly age

b. Region/race: South-East Asia.

c. Overweight/Obesity

d. Sedentary lifestyle

e. Unhealthy eating

f. Stress

g. Unhealthy habits like alcoholism

h. Physical inactivity

i. Others

Clinical Features

Q 21. What are the clinical features in a patient of diabetes mellitus?

Hyperglycemic (osmotic) symptoms:

a. Polyuria and nocturia

b. Polyphagia

c. Polydipsia

d. Weight loss

Non-specific symptoms:

a. Tiredness

b. Weakness

c. Blurred vision

d. Giddiness

Q 22. What are the short-term complications of diabetes mellitus?

a. Hyperosmolar hyperglycemic nonketotic syndrome—ketoacidosis leading to coma and even death.

b. Recurrent or persistent infections like tuberculosis.

c. Skin complications like styes, boils, folliculitis, carbuncles and others.

Q 23. What are the long-term complications of diabetes mellitus?

The long-term complications of diabetes mellitus are classified as follows:

Macrovascular complications affect the larger blood vessels, such as those supplying blood to the heart, brain, and legs.

    a. Coronary artery disease (heart attack)

    b. Stroke

Microvascular complications affect the small blood vessels, such as those supplying blood to the eyes and kidneys.

    a. Retinopathy

    b. Nephropathy

    c. Peripheral neuropathy

Q 24. What is meant by acanthosis nigricans?

Acanthosis nigricans is a velvety, papillomatous overgrowth of the epidermis. The common sites are the axilla, neck, abdomen, and phalanges.

Management

Q 25. What are the criteria for the diagnosis of diabetes mellitus?

Sample	Fasting glucose (mg/dl)	2-hour post-glucose load (mg/dl)
Plasma—venous	≥126	≥200
Whole blood—venous	≥110	≥180
Whole blood—capillary	≥110	≥200

Q 26. What are the criteria for the diagnosis of impaired glucose tolerance?

Sample	Fasting glucose (mg/dl)	2-hour post-glucose load (mg/dl)
Plasma—venous	<126	≥140 to <200
Whole blood—venous	<110	≥120 to <180
Whole blood—capillary	≥110	≥200

Q 27. What is the cutoff for the diagnosis of diabetes mellitus using HbA1c?

The cutoff value for the diagnosis of diabetes mellitus using HbA1c is >6.5%.

Q 28. What is the range for the diagnosis of pre-diabetes using HbA1c?

The range for the diagnosis of pre-diabetes using HbA1c is 5.7– 6.4%.

Q 29. What is HbA1c?

HbA1c is glycated hemoglobin that helps in identifying the three-month average plasma glucose concentration as the lifespan of red blood cells is three months.

Q 30. What are the eligibility criteria for diabetes screening in an asymptomatic adult?

The various eligibility criteria for diabetes screening in an asymptomatic adult are:

a. HbA1c >5.7%
b. First-degree relative with diabetes
c. Women who were diagnosed with gestational diabetes mellitus, polycystic ovary syndrome
d. History of cardiovascular disease, hypertension, obesity
e. Altered lipid profile

Q 31. What is opportunistic screening for undiagnosed diabetes?

Nearly half or more of type 2 diabetic patients are undiagnosed. Opportunistic screening during a healthcare visit for other reasons can identify undiagnosed diabetes.

Q 32. What is the recommendation of opportunistic screening under National Program for Prevention and Control of Cancer, Diabetes, Cardiovascular disease, and Stroke (NPCDCS)?

For early diagnosis of non-communicable diseases, opportunistic screening of persons above the age of 30 years had to do at all level of health care. It includes history like tobacco consumption, physical measurements like blood pressure, and investigations like blood glucose, etc.

Q 33. What is the physical examination will you do in a patient of diabetes mellitus?

Physical examination includes:

a. Weight, body mass index, waist-hip ratio
b. Blood pressure
c. Peripheral pulses
d. Foot examination
e. Fundoscopy
f. Peripheral nervous system
g. Skin like acanthosis nigricans

Q 34. What are the investigations will you do in a patient with diabetes mellitus?

Investigations	Frequency
Fasting/postprandial blood glucose	3 monthly
HbA1c	3 monthly
Renal function test	Annually
Lipid profile	Annually
Liver function test	Annually
Fundus examination	Annual if normal
Foot examination	Every visit

Q 35. What are the oral anti-diabetic drugs prescribed in diabetes mellitus?

a. Biguanides, e.g. metformin
b. Sulphonylureas, e.g. glimepiride
c. Thiazolidinediones, e.g. pioglitazone
d. α-Glucosidase inhibitors, e.g. acarbose
e. Meglitinide analogues, e.g. repaglinide

Q 36. What are the monotherapy recommendations in diabetes mellitus?

Metformin is the best first-line agent, especially in obese patients. Glimeprides and others are less used as first-line monotherapy. They are more used in non-obese patients. Gliptins are commonly used second or third line drugs.

Q 37. What are the indications for insulin therapy in type 2 diabetes mellitus?

Insulin is indicated in a diabetic patient who has a poor response to two or three oral anti-diabetic agents. For example, glimepiride or repaglinide/metformin/glitazone.

Q 38. Enumerate some insulin formulation available in market.

a. Rapid acting: Insulin lispro
b. Short acting: Regular (soluble) insulin, semilente insulin
c. Intermediate acting: Insulin zinc suspension or lente, neutral protamine hagedorn
d. Long acting: Protamine zinc insulin, ultralente insulin

Q 39. What are the goals of comprehensive control of diabetes mellitus?

a. HbA1c <7%
b. Fasting plasma glucose: 90–130 mg/dl
c. Postprandial plasma glucose: <180 mg/dl
d. Blood pressure <130/80 mm of Hg
e. Low density lipoproteins: <100 mg/dl
f. Triglycerides: <150 mg/dl

Prevention

Q 40. What is self-care in diabetes mellitus?

Self-care in diabetes mellitus includes:

a. Adherence to drug regimens
b. Blood glucose monitoring
c. Body weight monitoring
d. Foot-care
e. Healthy lifestyle/diet
f. Identify targets for control
g. Moderate-intensity physical activity
h. Personal hygiene
i. Regular eye examination
j. Self-administration of insulin

k. Abstinence from alcohol and tobacco

l. Recognition of symptoms associated with hypoglycemia

Q 41. What is the dietary advice to be given to a patient with diabetes mellitus?

a. The diet should be divided into small and frequent meals

b. Total fat <30% of energy consumed

c. Saturated fat <10% of energy consumed

d. Increase in fibre intake to 15 g/1000 kcal

e. Ingestion of whole grain products, vegetables, fruit, low-fat milk and meat products

f. Use vegetable oils rich in MUFA

Q 42. What are components of primary prevention in diabetes mellitus?

The primary prevention of diabetes mellitus includes:

a. Regular physical activity

b. Maintenance of normal body weight

c. Healthy nutritional habits like high fibre diet and avoidance of sweet foods

d. Control of blood pressure and elevated cholesterol/triglyceride levels

e. Avoidance of alcohol and tobacco use

f. Stress management and avoidance of irregular sleeping patterns

Q 43. What are the components of secondary prevention in diabetes mellitus?

The secondary prevention includes early diagnosis and prompt treatment using exercise, diet, drugs or combination of one or more of these intervention strategies.

Q 44. What are the components of tertiary prevention in diabetes mellitus?

Tertiary prevention includes the screening for diabetic retinopathy, nephropathy, cardiovascular, and peripheral vascular disease.

Q 45. What is meant by glycaemic index of foods?

The glycaemic index is an extent to which they raise blood sugar levels after eating. It ranges from 0 to 100. Foods with a high GI are those which are rapidly digested, absorbed and metabolized and result in marked increase in blood sugar levels like ice-creams, cornflakes, and others.

Q 46. When is World Diabetes Day is celebrated?

World Diabetes Day is celebrated every year on 14th November.

Q 47. What was the theme of World Health Day 2016?

World Health Day 2016 theme was beat diabetes

Q 48. What is Indian Diabetes Risk Score (IDRS)?

Indian Diabetes Risk Score is developed by Madras Diabetes Research Foundation, Chennai. It uses four simple parameters—age, abdominal obesity/waist circumference, physical activity, and family history of diabetes. Out of the total score of 100, subjects with an IDRS of <30 are categorized as low risk, 30–50 as medium risk and those with >60 as high risk for diabetes.

Q 49. What is mDiabetes?

It is mobile health initiative for the prevention and care of diabetes—mDiabetes. This contributes to increasing awareness about diabetes and promoting healthy active lifestyle along with early healthcare seeking, better adherence to drug or dietary control, self-care and prevention of complications.

CHRONIC OBSTRUCTIVE PULMONARY DISEASE

Arti Gupta

Introduction

Q 1. What is chronic obstructive pulmonary disease (COPD)?

Chronic obstructive pulmonary disease is characterized by airflow limitation that is usually progressive and associated with an enhanced chronic inflammatory response in the airways and the lung to noxious particles or gases.

Burden

Q 2. What is burden of COPD?

The WHO estimated 2.74 million deaths globally from COPD in year 2000. It is the fourth leading cause of death in the United States.

Risk Factor

Q 3. What are the risk factors for COPD?

The risk factors for COPD are tobacco smoke, biomass fuel smoke, occupational exposure, alpha-1 antitrypsin deficiency, outdoor air pollution, pulmonary tuberculosis, poorly treated asthma, intrauterine growth retardation, malnutrition, low socioeconomic status and others.

Clinical Features

Q 4. What are the clinical features of COPD case?

The clinical features of COPD cases are:
    a. Patient is usually a smoker
    b. Common in fifth decade of life
    c. Productive cough
    d. Dyspnea
    e. Others

Management

Q 5. How is COPD diagnosed in a patient?

COPD is diagnosed
    a. Based on symptoms: Cough, sputum, dyspnea
    b. Exposure to risk factors
    c. Spirometry

Q 6. How is spirometry curve in COPD patient?

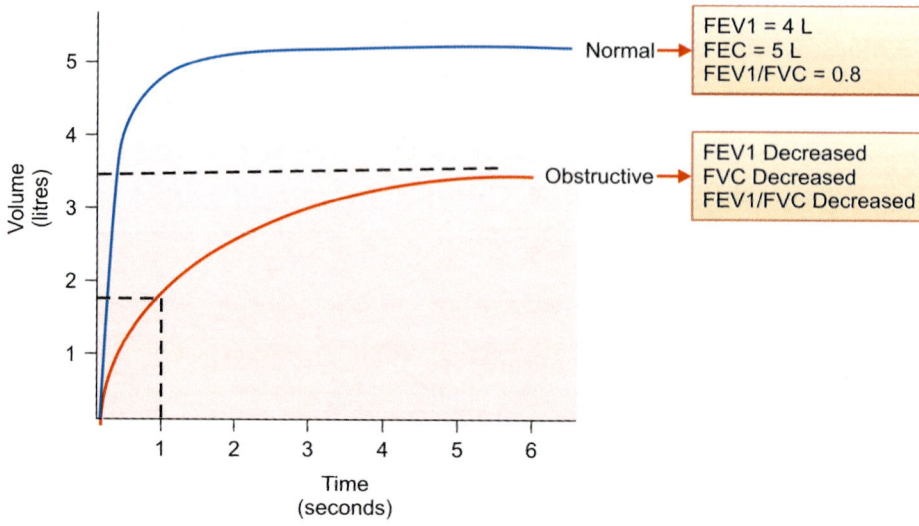

Q 7. What is GOLD classification of severity of airflow limitation in COPD?

In patients with FEV1/FVC <0.70:

a. GOLD 1: Mild COPD   FEV1>80% predicted

b. GOLD 2: Moderate COPD   50% <FEV1<80% predicted

c. GOLD 3: Severe COPD   30% <FEV1<50% predicted

d. GOLD 4: Very severe COPD   FEV1<30% predicted

Q 8. What is combined assessment of COPD in patient?

The combined assessment of COPD is based on symptoms, the degree of airflow limitation using spirometry, a risk of exacerbations and presence of comorbidities.

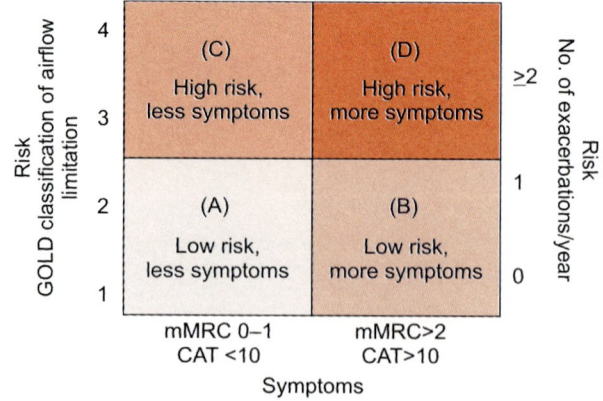

Note: mMRC is modified Medical Research Council questionnaire, CAT is COPD Assessment Test

Source: Global Initiative for Chronic Obstructive Lung Disease (GOLD) 2011 (www.goldcopd.org/)

Q 9. What is the treatment of choice for a COPD patient?

The treatment of choice for a COPD patient is as per the category.

Category A (low risk, less symptoms): Short acting beta agonists or short acting muscarinic antagonist

Category B (low risk, more symptoms): Long acting beta agonists or long acting muscarinic antagonist

Category C (high risk, less symptoms): Inhaled corticosteroids and long acting beta agonists or long acting muscarinic antagonist

Category D (high risk, more symptoms): Inhaled corticosteroids plus long acting beta agonists and/or long acting muscarinic antagonist

Q 10. When is oxygen therapy used in COPD patient?
   a. Very severe COPD (Stage IV)
   b. $PaO_2 < 55$ mm Hg or $SaO_2 < 88\%$
   c. PaO_2 55–60 mm Hg, if associated with cardiac failure

Prevention

Q 11. What is the non-pharmacologic treatment for a COPD patient?

The non-pharmacologic treatment for a COPD patient is smoking cessation, physical activity, vaccination, for example, flu vaccination, pulmonary rehabilitation and others.

Annexures

Annexure 1

Weight-for-age girls

Birth to 5 years (z-scores)

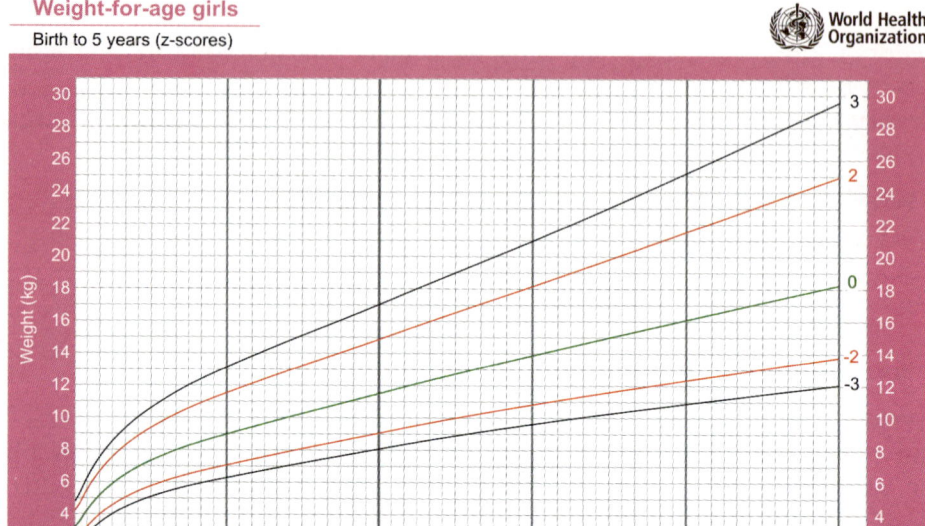

WHO Child Growth Standards

Annexure 2

Length/height-for-age girls

Birth to 5 years (z-scores)

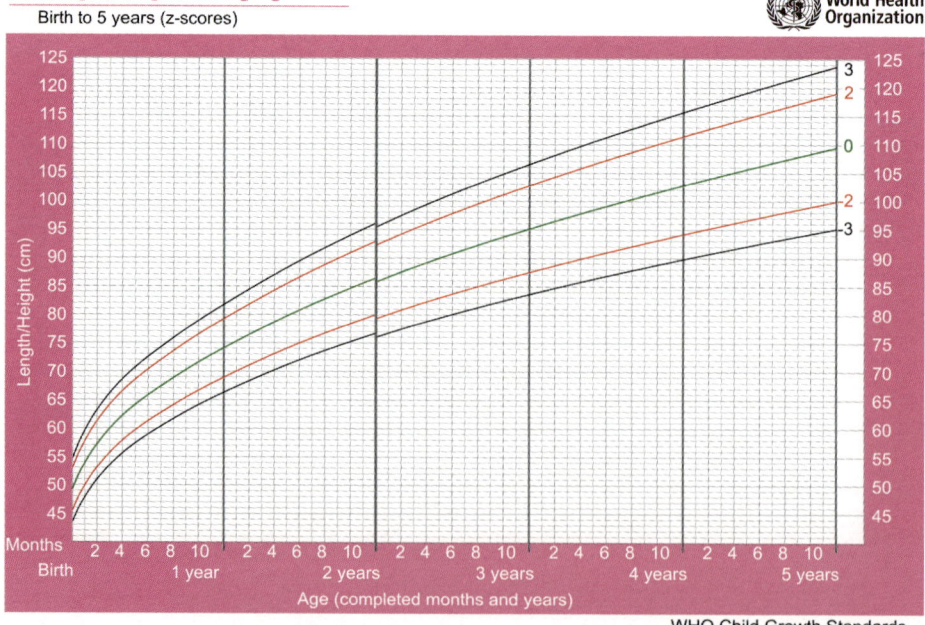

WHO Child Growth Standards

Annexure 3

Weight-for-length/height girls

Birth to 5 years (z-scores)

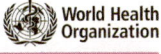

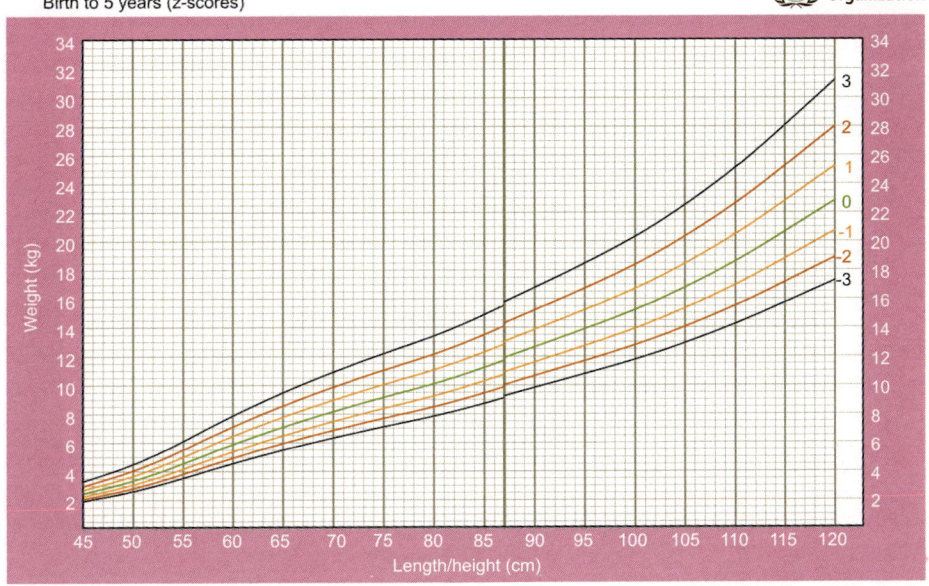

WHO Child Growth Standards

Annexure 4

Weight-for-age boys

Birth to 5 years (z-scores)

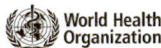

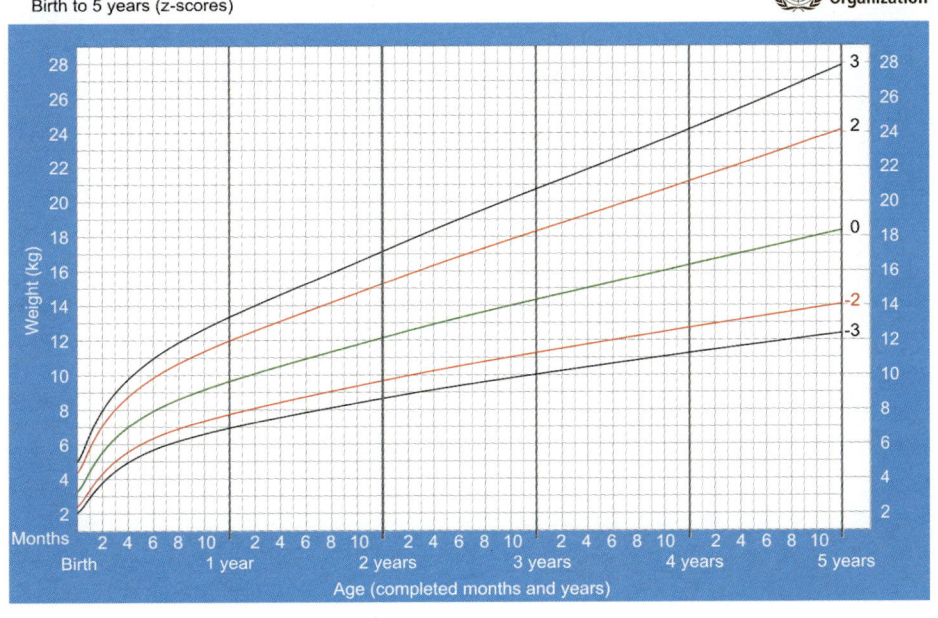

Annexure 5

Length/height-for-age boys

Birth to 5 years (z-scores)

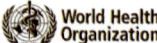

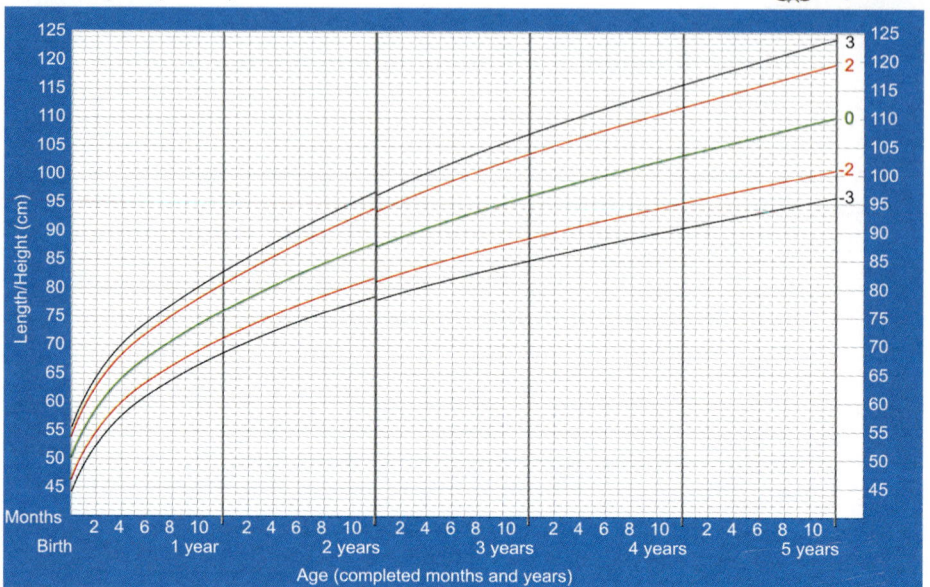

WHO Child Growth Standards

Annexure 6

Weight-for-length/height boys

Birth to 5 years (z-scores)

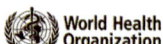

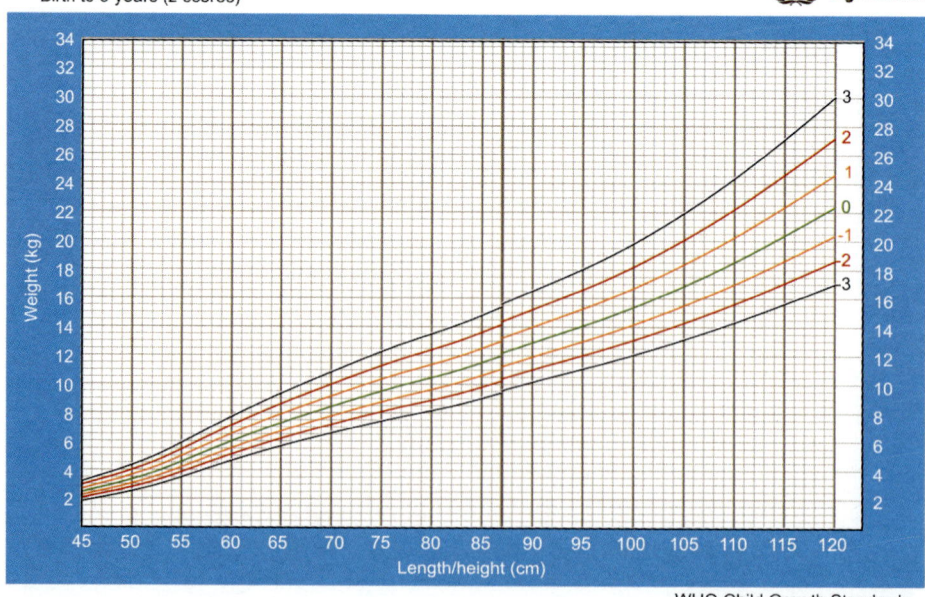

WHO Child Growth Standards

Annexure 7

Weight-for-age girls
5 to 10 years (z-scores)

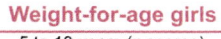
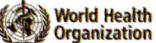

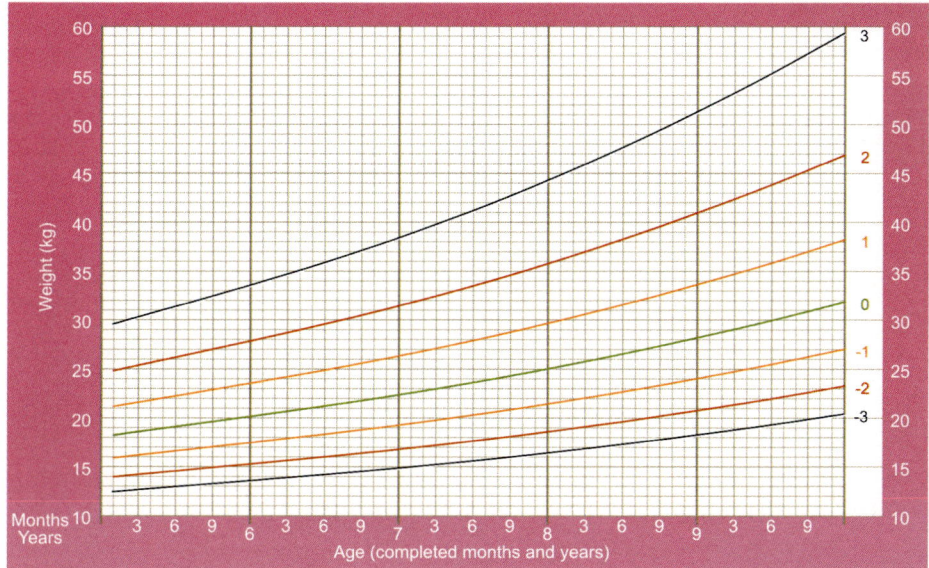

2007 WHO Reference

Annexure 8

Height-for-age girls
5 to 19 years (z-scores)

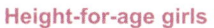
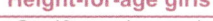
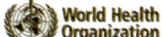

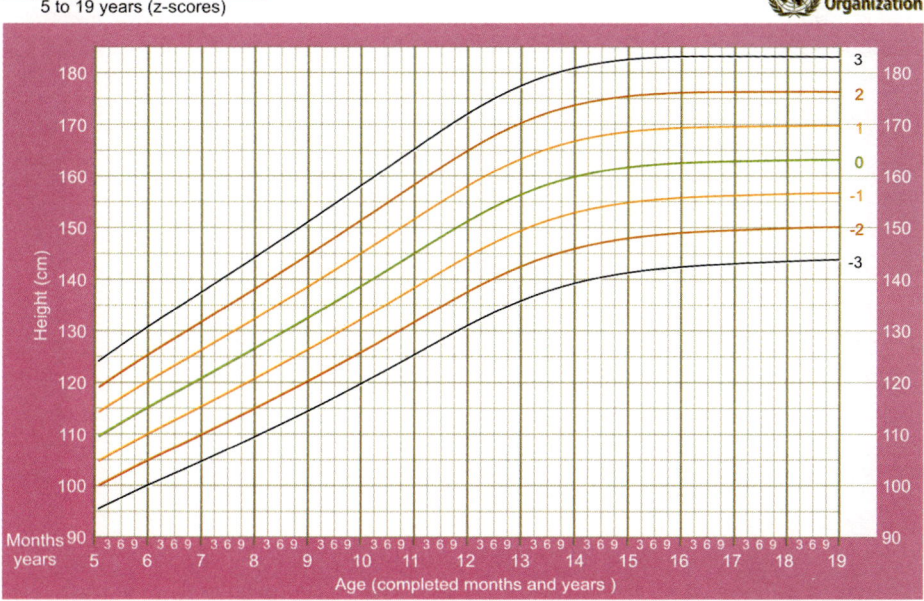

2007 WHO Reference

Annexure 9

BMI-for-age girls

5 to 19 years (z-scores)

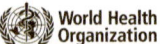

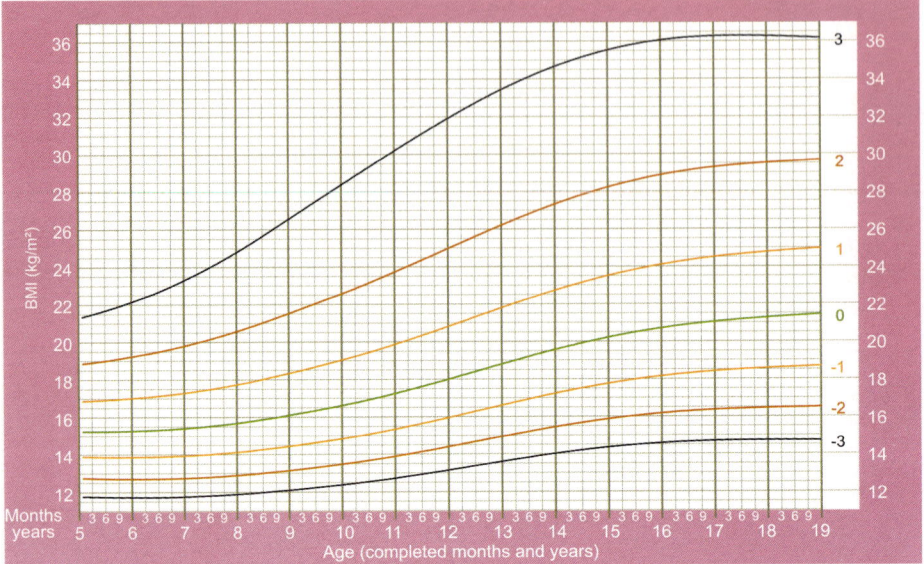

2007 WHO Reference

Annexure 10

Weight-for-age boys

5 to 10 years (z-scores)

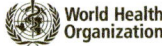

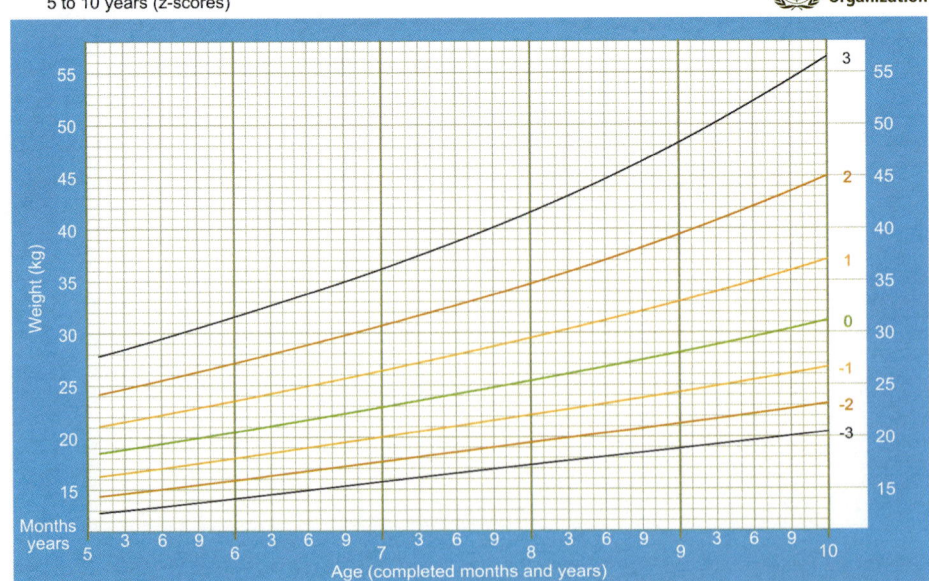

2007 WHO Reference

Annexure 11

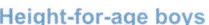

Height-for-age boys
5 to 19 years (z-scores)

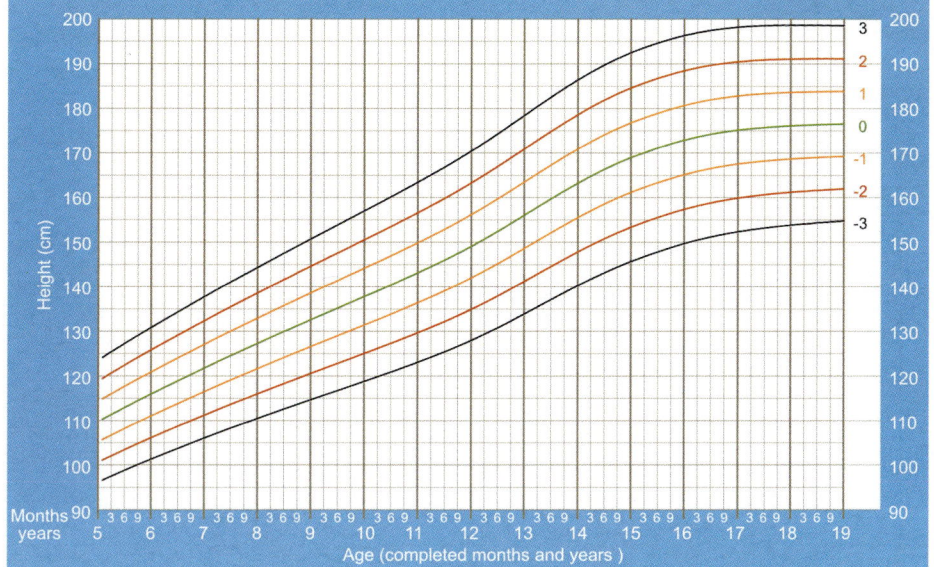

2007 WHO Reference

Annexure 12

BMI-for-age boys
5 to 19 years (z-scores)

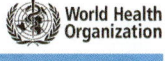

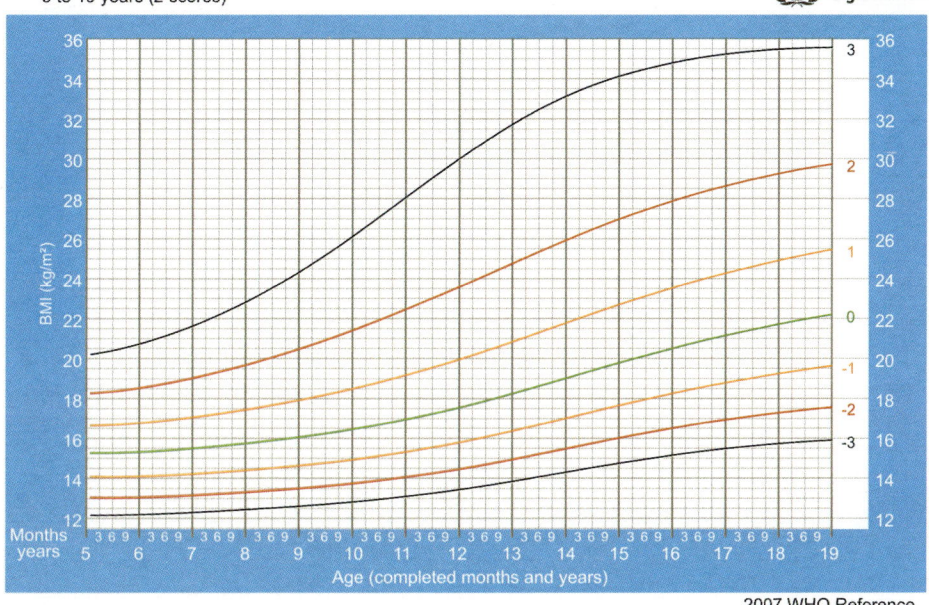

2007 WHO Reference

Annexure 13

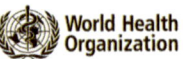

Windows of achievement for six gross motor milestones

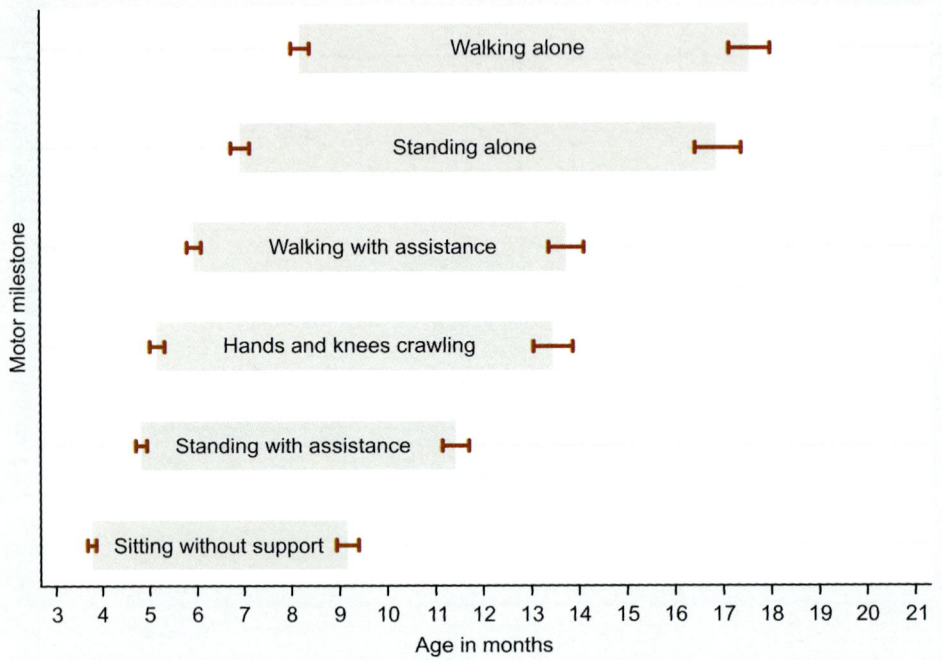

Reference: WHO Multicentre Growth Reference Study Group. WHO Motor Development Study: windows of achievement for six gross motor development milestones. Acta Paediatrica Supplement 2006;450:86–95.

Annexure 14

FORM P
(Weekly Reporting Format –IDSP)

Name of Reporting Institution:		I.D. No.:
State:	District:	Block/Town/City:
Officer-in-Charge	Name:	Signature:
IDSP Reporting Week:-	Start Date:-	End Date:-	Date of Reporting:-
	___/___/_____	___/___/_____	___/___/_____

S.no	Diseases/Syndromes	No. of cases
1	Acute Diarrhoeal Disease (including acute gastroenteritis)	
2	Bacillary Dysentery	
3	Viral Hepatitis	
4	Enteric Fever	
5	Malaria	
6	Dengue / DHF / DSS	
7	Chikungunya	
8	Acute Encephalitis Syndrome	
9	Meningitis	
10	Measles	
11	Diphtheria	
12	Pertussis	
13	Chickenpox	
14	Fever of Unknown Origin (PUO)	
15	Acute Respiratory Infection (ARI) / Influenza Like Illness (ILI)	
16	Pneumonia	
17	Leptospirosis	
18	Acute Flaccid Paralysis < 15 Years of Age	
19	Dog bite	
20	Snake bite	
21	Any other State Specific Disease (Specify)	
22	Unusual Syndromes NOT Captured Above (Specify clinical diagnosis)	
	Total New OPD attendance (Not to be filled up when data collected for indoor cases)	
	Action taken in brief if unusual increase noticed in cases/deaths for any of the above diseases	

Annexure 15

FORM L
(Weekly Reporting Format – IDSP)

Name of the Laboratory:		**Institution:**	
State:	**District:**	**Block/Town/City:**	
Officer-in-Charge:	**Name:**	**Signature:**	
IDSP Reporting Week:-	**Start Date:-**	**End Date:-**	**Date of Reporting:-**
	___/___/_____	___/___/_____	___/___/_____

Diseases	No. Samples Tested	No. found Positive	
Dengue / DHF / DSS			
Chikungunya			
JE			
Meningococcal Meningitis			
Typhoid Fever			
Diphtheria			
Cholera			
Shigella Dysentery			
Viral Hepatitis A			
Viral Hepatitis E			
Leptospirosis			
Malaria		PV:	PF:
Other (Specify)			
Other (Specify)			

Line List of Positive Cases (Except Malaria cases):

Name	Age (Yrs)	Sex (M/F)	Address: Village/Town	Name of Test Done	Diagnosis (Lab confirmed)

Annexure 16

Form S
Reporting Format for Syndromic Surveillance
(To be filled by Health Worker, Village Volunteer, Non-formal Practitioners)

State_____ District_____ Block_____ Year_____

Name of the Health Worker/Volunteer/Practitioner	Name of the Supervisor	Name of the Reporting Unit

| ID No./Unique Identifier (To be filled by DSU) | Reporting week | From | | dd | mm | yy |
| | | To | | | | |

	a	b	c	d	e	f	g	h	i	j	k	l	m	n
	Cases						Total	Deaths						Total
	Male		Total	Female		Total		Male		Total	Female		Total	
	< 5 yr	≥ 5 yr	Total	< 5 yr	≥ 5 yr	Total		< 5 yr	≥ 5 yr	Total	< 5 yr	≥ 5 yr	Total	
1. Fever														
Fever < 7 days														
1 Only Fever														
2 With Rash														
3 With Bleeding														
4 With Daze/Semiconsciousness/ Unconsciousness														
Fever > 7 days														
2. Cough with or without fever														
< 3 weeks														
> 3 weeks														
3. Loose Watery Stools of Less Than 2 Weeks Duration														
With Some/Much Dehydration														
With no Dehydration														
With Blood in Stool														
4. Jaundice cases of Less Than 4 Weeks Duration														
Cases of acute Jaundice														
5. Acute Flacid Paralysis Cases in Less Than 15 Years of Age														
Cases of Acute Flacid Paralysis														
6. Unusual Symptoms Leading to Death or Hospitalization that do not fit into the above.														

Date:

Signature

Annexure 17

S. No.	Tasks	Home-based postnatal care					
		Visit 1 Day 1 of birth	Visit 2 Day 2–3 after birth	Visit 3 Day 5–7 after birth	Visit 4 Day 14–17 after birth	Visit 5 Day 23–28 after birth	Visit 6 Day 42–45 after birth
1.	Examine the baby for Alertness Activity Breathing Color Temperature	√	√	√	√	√	√
2.	Malformations	√					
3.	Record weight	√	√	√	√	√	√
4.	Enquire about initiation of breast feeding within an hour after birth	√					
5.	Assess breast feeding positioning and attachment and demonstrate to the mother if needed	√	√	√	√	√	√
6.	Enquire about exclusive breast feeding	√	√	√	√	√	√
7.	In the baby Look for jaundice		√	√			
8.	In the baby look for Cord Skin pustules	√	√	√	√	√	√
9.	Ask for baby's passage of urine and stool		√				
10.	Check for birth registration	√	√	√	√	√	√
11.	Counsel the mother for birth spacing				√	√	√
12.	Counsel the mother Immunization of baby Breast feeding Keeping Baby Warm Hygiene Danger signs	√ √	√ √	√ √	√ √	√ √	√ √
13.	Examine mother Heavy vaginal bleeding Fever Pain Problems with urination Breast problem	√	√	√	√	√	√
14.	Look for dangers signs and decide on referral	√	√	√	√	√	√

Annexure 18

WHO/ISH Risk prediction chart
for 14 WHO epidemiological sub-regions

WHO/ISH risk prediction chart for SEAR D. 10-year risk of a fatal or non-fatal cardiovascular event by gender, age, systolic blood pressure, total blood cholesterol, smoking status and presence or absence of diabetes mellitus.

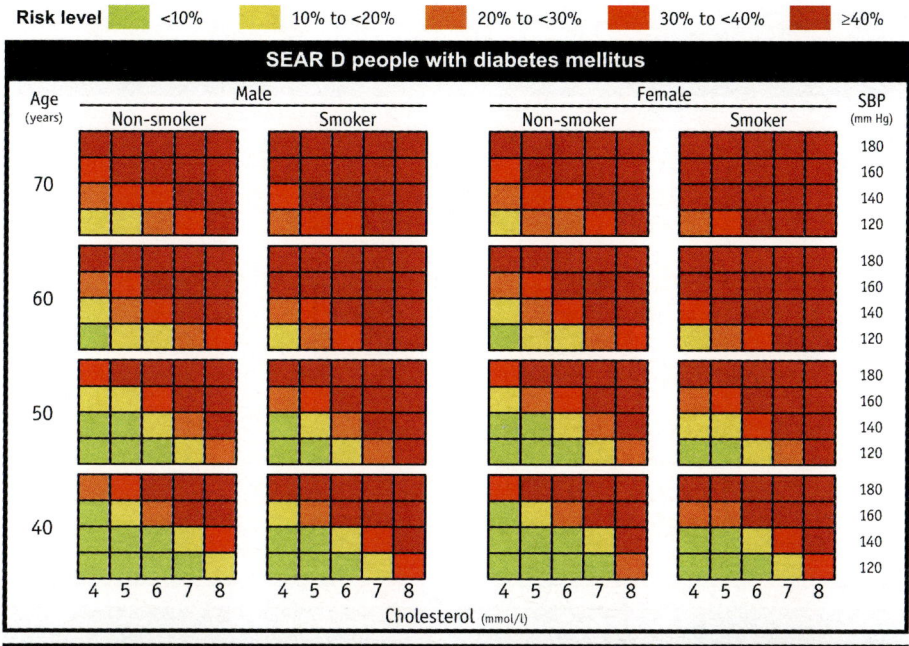

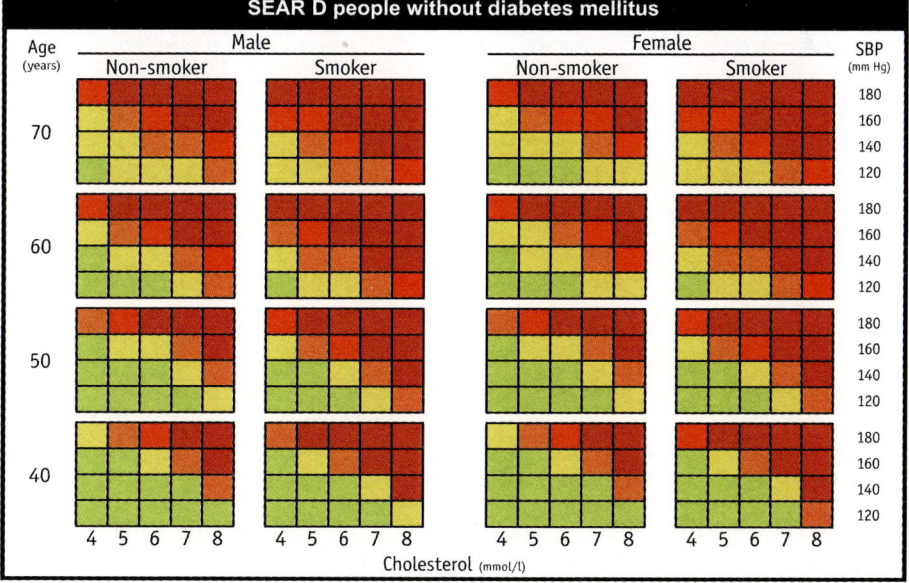

This chart can only be used for countries of the WHO region of South-East Asia, sub-region D, in settings where blood cholesterol can be measured.

WHO/ISH Risk prediction chart
for 14 WHO epidemiological sub-regions

WHO/ISH risk prediction chart for SEAR D. 10-year risk of a fatal or non-fatal cardiovascular event by gender, age, systolic blood pressure, smoking status and presence or absence of diabetes mellitus.

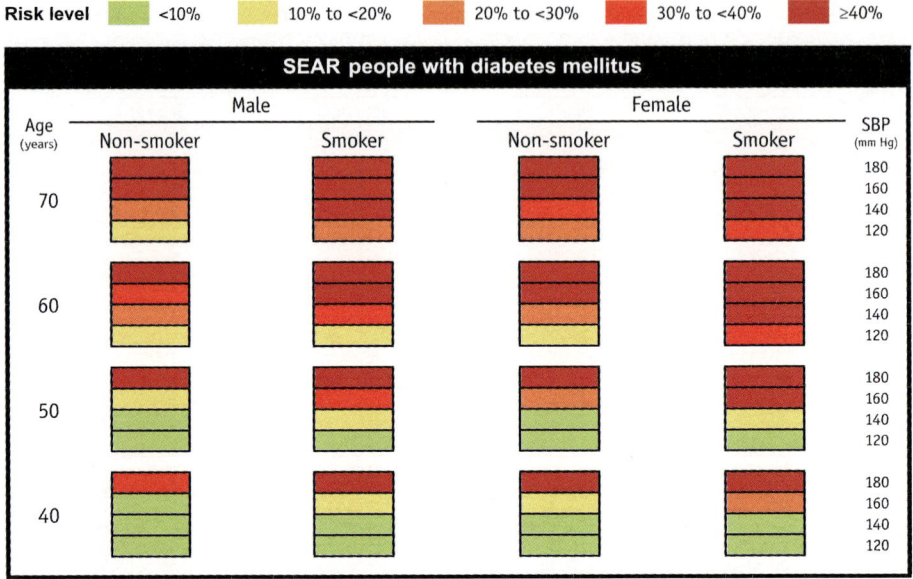

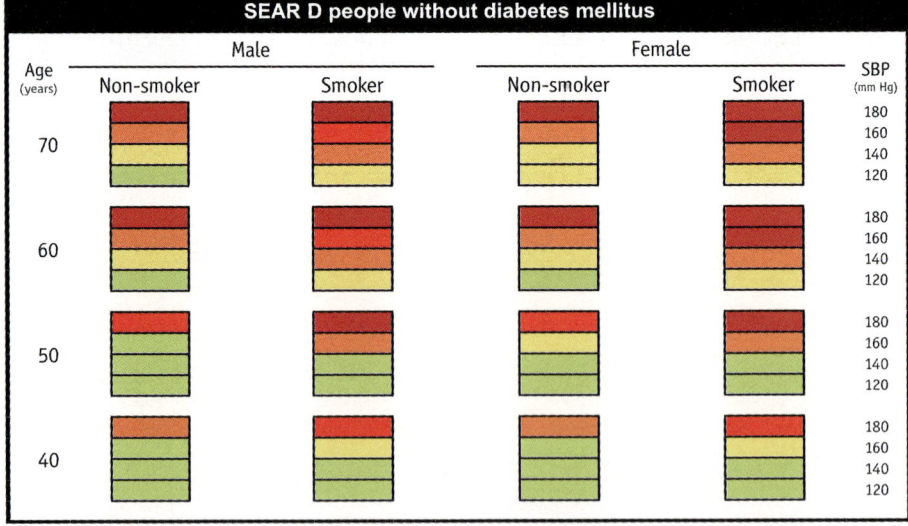

This chart can only be used for countries of the WHO region of South-East Asia, sub-region D, in settings where blood cholesterol CANNOT be measured.

Evolution and Critical Appraisal of National Health Programs

Arti Gupta

SWOT Analysis

SWOT "Strength Weakness Opportunity and Threat", is a planning tool. It detects the internal and external factors, which are advantageous as well as hostile to attain definite objective.

SWOT can be divided into two main categories:

Strength and weakness are always internal to the organization/programme.

Opportunities and threat are external to the organization/programme.

REVISED NATIONAL TUBERCULOSIS CONTROL PROGRAMME (RNTCP)

Evolution of TB in India

1906	First open-air sanatorium founded in Tilounia in Ajmer
1939	Establishment of the TB Association of India
1940	Start of domiciliary treatment
1946	Health Survey and Development Committee, outlined a conventional phased scheme for the management of TB for the first time
1947	TB Division established within in the Directorate General of Health Services
1948	The BCG campaign was introduced on a small scale in Madanapalli
1956	TB Chemotherapy Centre (TCC)/TB Research Centre (TRC) was established in Chennai
1959	National TB Institute (NTI) established in Bangalore
1961	NTP pilot-tested in Anantapur district of Andhra Pradesh
1962	National TB Programme (NTP) started
1983	TRC, Chennai pilot tested the SCC (short course chemotherapy) regimen
1986	Introduction of SCC and coverage scaled up to cover 252 districts
1992	Programme review of NTP [only 30% of patients diagnosed, of these, only 30% treated successfully]
1993	RNTCP (DOTS component) pilot began

(Contd.)

1997	Launch of RNTCP as National programme
1998	RNTCP scale-up
1999–2001	First national survey to estimate the Annual Risk of Tuberculosis Infection (ARTI)
2001–2003	Second national survey to estimate the Annual Risk of Tuberculosis Infection (ARTI)
2001	450 million population covered by RNTCP
2004	>80% of the country coveredby RNTCP
2006	Entire country covered by RNTCP, India adopted Stop TB Strategy, Phase II of RNTCP was started
2007	National framework of joint TB/HIV collaborative activities
2010	Introduction of DOTS plus guidelines
2012	TB declared a notifiable disease, ban on serological tests for the diagnosis of TB
2012–17	National Strategic Plan with the vision of TB free India
2012	Case-based Web-based TB notification system NIKSHAY was established
2013	Complete geographical coverage for diagnostic and treatment services for multi-drug resistant TB
2014	Government of India adopted the End TB strategy
2014	Development of the Standards for TB care in India
2014	The launch of first nationwide anti-TB drug resistance survey of India
2016	Introduction of new treatment guidelines, fixed drug combination, daily regimen was started
2017–25	National Strategic Plan for Tuberculosis Elimination highlighting four strategic pillars of "Detect – Treat –Prevent – Build" (DTPB)
2018	TB free India campaign
2018	The clinical establishments. Pharmacy, chemist and druggist not notify a tuberculosis patient to the nodal officer may attract the provision of Indian Penal Code.

Critical Appraisal- RNTCP

Strengths	Weaknesses
1. Strong political and administrative commitment	1. TB epidemiology in India is varied
2. Secured medium to long term financing	2. Unorganized private sector
3. Country wide network of TU and DMC	3. Noncompliance to treatment guidelines
4. Easily accessible DOTS Centre	4. Interrupted drug supply
5. Reaching targeted cure rate and case detection rate	5. Ignorance about TB
6. Availability of valid national treatment guidelines	6. Weak general health system
	7. Shortage of managerial staff
7. Effective anti-tubercular drugs	8. Rising burden of MDR
8. Evaluation and monitoring system incorporated in the program	9. Lack of diagnostic facility for MDR/XDR TB at all levels
	10. Criteria used for MDR classification only rifampicin resistance

(Contd.)

(Contd.)

9. Nationwide PMDT coverage
10. Management of HIV-TB co-infection
11. International standards of TB care
12. Involvement of NGOs, cooperate and professional bodies
13. Nikshay portal
14. Using CB NAAT for MDR-TB diagnosis
15. Training
16. Dedicated staff for TB
17. Use of IEC media

11. Long duration of treatment so adherence is difficult
12. Rifampicin main anti-tubercular drug since 1963
13. Lack of research on anti-tubercular drugs
14. Lack of interest of pharma companies
15. BCG vaccine ineffective
16. Effectiveness of alternate day anti-tubercular treatment is doubtful

Opportunities

1. Universal access
2. Fixed Drug Daily Regimen
3. Decrease human suffering and socioeconomic impact
4. Innovative operational research
5. Reducing stigma
6. Implementation of Airborne infection control guidelines
7. LED microscopy at all health care levels
8. Scale up of bedaquilline use
9. Introduction of Delamanid

Threats

1. Co-infection with HIV
2. Irrational use of drugs
3. Increasing urbanization
4. Challenges of integration with other program
5. Comorbidities like diabetes, hypertension, and tobacco use.

Disclaimer: This critical appraisal is a perspective and actual facts may be different. The primary purpose of this is to provide an insight to students on how to critically appraise a programme.

POLIO
Evolution of polio eradication in India

1988	Global Polio Eradication Initiative
1994	America certified Polio free, Pilot polio immunization campaign in Delhi
1995	Pulse polio immunization in India for children less than 3 years
1996	Pulse polio immunization in India for children less than 5 years
1997	National Polio Surveillance Project
1999	The India Expert Advisory Group (IEAG) for polio was constituted, type 2 polio virus eradicated from India (last case seen in Aligarh, UP), House to house strategy began, IPPI in India
2000	Western Pacific region certified polio free, modified IPPI in India
2001	Social mobilization network by UNICEF in India

(Contd.)

(Contd.)

2002	European region certified polio free
2003	Under served strategy introduced in Uttar Pradesh, India
2004	Six countries were endemic for polio (India, Pakistan, Afghanistan, Nigeria, Niger and Egypt), in India Transit Vaccination strategy introduced
2005	mOPV introduced
2006	Four countries were endemic for polio (India, Pakistan, Afghanistan, Nigeria)
2007	Migrant strategy was started
2008	Kosi river plan in Bihar, India
2009	107 Block plan in UP and Bihar, India
2010	Last confirmed WPV3 case in Jharkhand, bOPV introduced
2011	Large scale mop up in Howrah, last case seen in West Bengal
2013	Polio endgame strategic plan
2014	WHO South East Asia Region certified polio free
2015	IPV introduced in national immunization program
2016	Nationwide trivalent OPV to bivalent OPV switch and fractional dose of IPV introduced in eight states
2017	Nationwide scale up of fractional dose of IPV

Critical appraisal: Polio eradication

Strengths
1. Political commitment
2. International commitment and support
3. No financial constraints
4. WHO SEARO region certified polio free
5. Routine immunization bOPV, and IPV
6. National immunization day, Sub-National Immunization Days, immunization week
7. Good quality surveillance
8. Ability to detect, report and respond to importation
9. Social mobilization network
10. Special strategies for high risk area
11. Large number of staff working
12. Participation of NGOs, civil society, private sector
13. Legacy planning
14. Vaccination at international borders

Weaknesses
1. Many serotypes of polio virus
2. Subclinical cases
3. cVDPV, VAPP, iVDPV, aVDPV present
4. Environmental persistence of wild polio virus
5. Poor sanitation, drinking water quality
6. Less immunization coverage
7. Less exclusive breastfeeding
8. High incidence of diarrhoea
9. False beliefs
10. Vast diversity
11. Lack of mOPV stockpile
12. Lack of laboratory services at all levels

(Contd.)

(Contd.)

Opportunities	Threats
1. IPV introduction	1. Importation
2. Bio-containment	2. Retransmission establishment
	3. cVDPV outbreak
	4. Outbreak from research facility and laboratory
	5. Bioterrorism
	6. Increasing urbanization
	7. Population mobility

Disclaimer: This critical appraisal is a perspective and actual facts may be different. The primary purpose of this is to provide an insight to students on how to critically appraise a programme.

National AIDS Control Programme (NACP)

Evolution of AIDS Control Programme in India

1986	Ten out of 102 female sex workers were found HIV positive in Tamil Nadu, India
1986	AIDS task force was set up and National AIDS committee was formulated
1987	National AIDS control programme (screening of high risk groups and educational activity)
1992–1997	National AIDS Control Programme-I (It was up to 1997 but extended till 1999) Strategies in NACP I were mass IEC, national blood transfusion policy, condom promotion, annual sentinel surveillance, control of STDs, some elementary treatment facility
1999–2007	National AIDS Control Programme II Strategies in NACP II were targeted intervention, mass education campaigns, blood safety, ICTC, annual sentinel surveillance, opportunistic infection, treatment, antiretroviral therapy (ART) programme
2007–2012	National AIDS Control Programme III Strategies in NACP III were targeted intervention, condom promotion, blood safety, ICTC, prophylactic treatment, continue support and treatment, collaboration, mainstreaming, surveillance and strategic information management System (SIMS)
2013	Onwards National AIDS Control Programme IV Strategies in NACP IV are prevention, care support treatment, SIMS, IEC, and capacity building
2017–24	National Strategic plan for HIV/AIDS and STI

Critical Appraisal: National AIDS Control Programme

Strengths

1. Vertical programme
2. Meeting the targets
3. Condom use promotion by social marketing
4. Emphasis on safe blood transfusion
5. Integrated counseling and testing centre services provided
6. High cost ART given free
7. Colour coded kits for STI/RTI
8. Care Support and Treatment
9. Strategic Information Management System
10. Regular sentinel and behavioural surveillance
11. Unlinked anonymous testing in HSS
12. Community liaison
13. Opioid substitution therapy for injecting drug users
14. Targeted intervention for high risk group
15. Providing enabling environment
16. Three Ones principles
17. IEC activities
18. Guidelines for post-exposure prophylaxis
19. Prevention of Parent to Child Transmission (PPTCT)
20. International partners
21. Special strategies like red ribbon express, link worker scheme
22. Integrated Biological and Behavioural Surveillance (IBBS)

Weaknesses

1. Political commitment raised slowly
2. Funding raised slowly
3. No numerical targets set in NACP III
4. ART initiated late
5. Low coverage of ART- not available at all health care levels
6. Inadequate laboratory services
7. Poor coverage of ICTC services in rural areas
8. Drop outs from ART, and STD therapy
9. Low awareness in the community regarding ICTC, CCC
10. Issues with Availability of blood
11. Shortage of blood for transfusion
12. Private sector involvement is still inadequate
13. Infrastructure needs to be strengthened
14. Outreach services of ICTC are low in general population
15. Poor post-exposure prophylaxis implementation

Opportunities

1. Involvement of medical colleges
2. Evidence-based research on ART, HIV vaccine
3. Operational research

Threats

1. Stigma and discrimination
2. Increasing urbanization
3. Unnatural sex

Disclaimer: This critical appraisal is a perspective and actual facts may be different. The primary purpose of this is to provide an insight to students on how to critically appraise a programme.

National Vector Borne Disease Control Programme (NVBDCP)

Evolution of malaria control in India

1946	A countrywide comprehensive programme to control malaria was recommended by the Bhore committee
1953	National Malaria Control Programme (NMCP) was started
1958	NMCP transformed to National Malaria Eradication Programme
1965	Malaria cases reduced
1970–75	Resurgence of malaria
1977	Modified plan of operations implemented
1997	Enhanced Malaria Control Project (EMCP) launched
1999	Programme renamed as National Anti-Malaria Programme
2002	National Vector Borne Disease Control Programme was launched by merging National Anti-Malaria Programme, National Filaria Control Programme and Kala Azar Control Programmes. Japanese B encephalitis and dengue/DHF
2004–5	Rapid Diagnostic test (RDT) kit introduced for *P. falciparum*
2006	Artemisinin-based Combination Therapy (ACT) introduced in areas showing chloroquine resistance
2009	Introduction of long lasting insecticidal nets (LLINs)
2012–17	Strategic plan for malaria control in India
2013	Bivalent rapid diagnostic test kit introduced for *P. falciparum* and *P. vivax*, coloured coded kit for malaria treatment, National Drug Policy for malaria cases introduced with ACT-AL in north-eastern states
2017	National strategic plan for malaria elimination in India 2017–22 introduced
2018	Prohibited use of RDT for routine diagnosis of malaria

Critical Appraisal: National Vector Borne Disease Control Programme

Strengths	Weaknesses
1. Political commitment	1. Targets not achieved
2. LLINs	2. Antigen-based RDT not available
3. Indoor residual spraying	3. Delay in conducting microscopy
4. Surveillance (IDSP)	4. Stock out of RDT and primaquine
5. Microscopy	5. Poor coverage, quality and community acceptance of IRS
6. Involvement of private sector, NGOs, civil society	6. Poor coverage, and community acceptance of LLINs
7. Micro stratification	7. Underestimation of burden
8. ACT, colour coded treatment	8. No notifying mechanism
9. Research	9. Lack of supervised treatment
10. India is one of the leading producer of malaria diagnostics, drugs, and insecticides.	10. JE vaccination needs strengthening
11. Involving ASHA	11. Lack of intersectoral coordination
12. BCC, IEC	12. Weak laboratory testing for other VBDs
13. Social mobilization	13. Weak surveillance for other VBDs
14. Legislation	14. Non-availability of drugs in private sector for other VBDs
15. Monitoring and evaluation	15. Irrational use of DDT
16. Capacity building	16. Irrational use of chloroquine
17. Environment codes of practice	
18. Training	

Opportunities	Threats
1. Vaccine	1. Emergence of resistance to ACT
2. Developing capacity at the medical colleges (diagnostic virology network laboratory)	2. Emergence of resistance to insecticide
3. Operational research	3. Overloading of ASHA
4. Funds availability	4. Increasing urbanization
	5. Global warming
	6. International trade and travel
	7. Changing agricultural practices
	8. Social unrest
	9. Social and ecological constraints
	10. Resurgence

Disclaimer: This critical appraisal is a perspective and actual facts may be different. The primary purpose of this is to provide an insight to students on how to critically appraise a programme.

Public Health Update

Sidharth Sekhar Mishra

TUBERCULOSIS

Burden (TB India 2017 Annual Report)
- India has the highest burden of TB and MDR TB in the world
- 2nd highest burden of HIV *TB* in India
- Revised estimates**:
  - Incidence: 217 per lakh population (2015)
  - Mortality: 36 per lakh population (2015)

New Goals
- Cure
- Prevent resistance
- Break chain of transmission

Targets
- Detection: 90%
- Cure rate:
  - Drug sensitive new: 90%
  - Drug sensitive previously treated: 85%

90-90-90 by 2035
90% reduction in incidence, mortality and catastrophic health expenditures due to TB.

DEPRESSION

Global Status of Depression
- Depression is the leading cause of disability worldwide and major contributor to overall global burden of disease
- India and China account for 50% of global burden
- Globally maximum number of cases of depression (prevalence 4.5%) are in India

- Globally maximum number of cases of anxiety (Prevalence: 3%)
- Globally maximum number of suicide
- YLD (years lived with disability) in India is 7.1% of total YLD, and anxiety disorders, its YLD was 2.5% of total YLD
- Not included into the primary health care yet

Health manpower status
- 4000 to 4500 trained psychiatrists (2 psychiatrists per 10 lakh population)
- Almost 500 seats of psychiatry in India ever year; no PhD courses
- Number of psychiatric beds in country is about 0.2 per 1 lakh population

Mental Health Bill, 2017: Rights-based Approach from Assurance-based Approach
- Rights of mentally ill
- Advance directive
- Mental health authorities
- Decriminalizing suicide, prohibiting ECT (without medication)

VACCINATION

National Operational Guidelines: Measles Rubella Vaccine (2017)
- India in September 2013, resolved to eliminate measles and control rubella/congenital rubella syndrome (CRS) by **2020.**
- **Accordingly, MOHFW is introducing rubella vaccine in its UIP as measles-rubella (MR) vaccine**
- The vaccine will be introduced as MR campaign, targeting children from **9 months up to 15 years**, in a phased manner over 2 to 3 years, followed by inclusion of the vaccine in routine immunization (RI)
- Campaign targets a large birth cohort of starting in 1st quarter of 2017
- Campaign will be conducted over a period of 3–4 weeks, where vaccination will first be conducted in schools and later in community through outreach
- Largest campaign of the world
- 1st time rubella vaccine introduced in India and will replace measles with MR vaccine

Pneumococcal vaccine
- NTAGI recommendation that within 1 year India will start
- 6th, 14th weeks and 9 months
- Introduction of the pneumococcal conjugate vaccine (PCV) under UIP to be implemented in five states, from 2017
- The states, where it will be introduced, include Bihar, Uttar Pradesh, Rajasthan and Madhya Pradesh (already introduced in Himachal Pradesh)

Dengvaxia
- Tetravalent (recombinant) live attenuated vaccine
- 9–45 years or 9–60 years
- 0/6/12 months, subcutaneous route
- Vaccine Efficacy: 66%
- Precautions: Do not co-administer with other LA vaccines

- Introduction (National/subnational level): Dengue sero prevalence 70% or higher
  - NOT recommended when < 50%
  - Philippines: 1st country to start it in national immunisation program

Open vial policy
- Reconstituted vaccines (BCG, measles, JE and rotavirus) cannot be reused
  - All vaccines which are not reconstituted can be reused for up to a maximum period of 4 weeks/28 days if
  - Provided that all of the following conditions are met:
    - The expiry date has not passed. The vaccines are stored under appropriate cold chain conditions
    - The VVM has not been submerged in water
    - Aseptic technique has been used to withdraw all doses
    - VVM, if attached, has not reached the discard point

STATISTICS: INDIA

(as on 1 July, 2016)

Demographic
- Population: 1328 million
- Sex ratio (at birth): 906;
  - Adult: 940 (census); 919 (NFHS 4)
- Density: 401 persons/km²

Maternal and child health
- ANC visits: At least once: 74%; at least 4: 45%
- Institutional deliveries: 79%
- Deliveries by trained personal: 52%
- LBW: 18.5% (2014)
- Services coverage:
  - BCG: 91%
  - DPT 3/OPV 3, Measles: 83%
  - HBV 3: 70%
  - Fully immunized: 77.3%

Sample registration system
- Population doubling time = 50.0 years
- Annual growth rate: 1.4%
- CBR = 20.4/1000 population
- CDR = 6.4/1000 population
- Population doubling time = 50.0 years
- IMR = 34/1000 live births (rural = 38; urban = 23; maximum = Madhya Pradesh—47; minimum = Goa—8)
- Maternal mortality ratio (2014–16): 130/lakh live births
- Maternal mortality rate (2014–16): 8.8/lakh of women aged 15–49

- NMR: 25/1000 live births
- ENMR: 20/1000 live births
- LNMR: 5/1000 live births
- Postneonatal mortality rate: 24/1000 live births
- Under 5 mortality rate: 43/1000 live births
- SBR: 22/1000 live births (INAP), 4/1000 live births (SRS): follow INAP
- TFR: 2.3
- GRR: 1.1
- GMFR: 107.7
- Total MFR: 3.9
- General fertility rate: 21.0
- Mean age of marriage: 22.3
- Life span (India): GBD 2015 data
  - Males = 65.2 years
  - Females = 69.5 years

Miscellaneous

- Doctor population ratio: 7 per 10000 population
- Bed population ratio: 9 beds per 10000 population

MATERNAL AND CHILD HEALTH

Maternity Bill
- Apply to: All establishments employing 10 or more persons
- Facilities:
  - 26 weeks of paid leave allowed for first 2 surviving children
- Can take 8 weeks before the due date and remaining after that
  - 12 weeks of paid leave for third child
- Can take 6 weeks before the due date and remaining after that
  - 12 weeks for those who adopt a child below age of 3 months and for commissioning mothers (in case of surrogacy)
  - All establishments > 50 employees to provide crèche (visit four times a day)
- Challenge: 90% of female labour force is unemployed in unorganized sector and this bill does not apply to it

ANMOL
- ANMOL: ANM Online, mobile tablet based application for ANMs
- Online tab which helps to record and save data by ANM
- Online yet offline

Juvenile Justice Act, 2015
- Effect from: 15th January, 2016
- Replaces existing Indian Juvenile Delinquency Law, Juvenile Justice Act (2000)
- Juveniles in conflict with law in age group of 16–18; involved in heinous offenses, can be tried as adults

FAMILY PLANNING

- ASHA: New brand of condoms under the national program
- Tag line: *Achi Aadat Hai* (It is a good habit)
- New punch line: *Plan Banate Hain* (Let's make a plan)
- Injectable contraceptives under national program: Pilot tested in Haryana (Program: Salamati, all PHCs, CHCs, SDH and DH will be provided free of cost)
- Maximum contraceptive usage in India: Sterilisation (2015)

NUTRITION

Healthy Diet: WHO Definition 2015 (Adults)

- Protect against malnutrition and NCDs
- Total fat intake should not exceed 30%
- Salt intake (iodised) <5 grams
- Limiting intake of free sugars to <10% equivalent to 50 gram or around 12 level teaspoons (5%: best)
- 400 gram (5 portions) of fruit and vegetables a day
  - Potatoes, sweet potatoes, cassava and other starchy roots are not classified as fruits or vegetables

Coronary heart disease

- Dietary modification: Principle preventive strategy
- WHO recommended changes
  - Cholesterol/HDL ratio <3.5
  - Reduction of fat intake to <20% of total energy intake
  - Saturated fat to <7% of total energy intake
  - **Dietary cholesterol < 200 mg per day**
  - **High sodium consumption (>2 grams/day, equivalent to 5 g salt/day) and insufficient potassium intake (less than 3.5 grams/day) contribute to high blood pressure and increase the risk of heart disease and stroke**
  - Sugar consumption < 30 grams/day

New Recommendations in Mid-day Meal Program

- Reduction of cereal intake from 100 grams to 90 grams for primary schoolchildren and 150 grams to 125 grams for upper primary schoolchildren
- Addition of additional items like milk, milk products, eggs, banana
- Increase in oil/fat intake from 5 grams to 10 grams for upper primary children
- The oil should be a mix of 3 combinations:
  - Palmolein/coconut oil/ghee
  - Sunflower or mustard/soya bean or linseed
- Use of double fortified salt with iodine and iron

Revised Baby Friendly Hospital Initiative (BFHI), 2018 guideline

The topic of each step is unchanged, but the wording of each one has been updated in line with the evidence-based guidelines and global public health policy.

The steps are subdivided into:
  i. The institutional procedures
  ii. Standards for individual care of mothers and infants

Miscellaneous

Global Reference List of Core Health Indicators

- 100 indicators
- Prioritized by global community to provide concise information on health situation at national and international levels so that comparison becomes easy.
- Health status
- Risk factors
- Health system
- Service coverage

ICF scale

- International classification of functioning, disability and health
- Provides details about definition, measurement, and classification of disability
- Will be used as a holistic approach to manage patients
- In India now we have 21 diseases in list of disabilities (acid attack and Parkinson's disease)
- Organizes information into 2 parts:
  - Part 1: Functioning and disability
  - Part 2: Contextual factors

SDG: Sustainable development goals

  - MDG was outdated in the year 2015
- SDG/P 15 A
  - 5 Ps: People, planet, prosperity, peace, partnership
  - Health related goal: 3
- MDGs dealt only with developing countries. In contrast, the SDGs deal with all countries and has a wider perspective

Targets in SDG

- By 2030
  - Global MMR < 70/1 lakh live births
  - NMR 12/1000 live births
  - U5MR 25/1000 live births
  - Reduce by 33% premature mortality from NCDs
  - 50% reduction in global deaths and injuries from RTAs

Swachh Bharat Abhiyan

- Clean India by 2 October, 2019
- Objective:
  - Eliminate open defecation by constructing toilets
  - Eradicate manual scavenging
  - Introduce modern and scientific solid waste management
  - Enable private sector participation
- Swachhate Pakhwada 2018
  - Tagline "Swachhata se siddhi"
  - Innovative approaches and sustenance swachhata

Categorization of Health Facilities (IPHS)

Subcentre	
Type A	**Type B**
All recommended facilities except the facilities of delivery	MCH subcentres, also provide delivery facilities
Essential staff: 1 ANM and 1 male health worker	Essential staff: 2 ANM and 1 male health worker.
Desirable: 2 ANM	Desirable: 1 staff nurse or ANM (if 20 or more deliveries in a month)
Primary Health Centre (PHC)	
<20 delivery/month is the load	≥ 20 deliveries per month

A new norm for subhealth centre based on time to care within 30 minutes by walk from a habitation for selected hilly and desert areas.

National Health Accounts
- Estimates of 2013-14 (updated after 10 years)
- 51%: Government spends on primary health care
- 64.2%: Out of pocket estimates
- 4.02%: Total health expenditure of GDP (INR 3638/capita)
- 1.15: Government
- 3.4%: Private health insurance
- Health Expenditure: 29.5% (OPD) and 20.2% (IPD)

Miscellaneous
- HDI: Rank—131; Value—0.624
- From 1 April, 2017 India will move BS IV fuels
- DLHS and NFHS have covered 4 rounds
- Yellow fever vaccine validity now life long
- 88.2% of India now has a 12 digit identity (aadhar card)
- NeHA: National e-health Authority
  - Digitisation of health information

Program Updates
Global Strategy for Women's, Children's and Adolescent's Health (2016–30)
- Vision: By 2030, a world in which every woman, child and adolescent in every setting realizes his/her rights to physical and mental health and well-being, has social and economic opportunities, and is able to participate fully in shaping prosperous and sustainable societies
- Objectives and targets aligned with SDGs
- Survive: End preventable deaths

- Thrive: Ensure health and well-being
- Transform: Expand enabling environments

Saathiya Salah Mobile App

Saathiya salah initiative was introduced for the adolescent peer educators (saathiyas) who act as a person for generating demand and imparting age appropriate knowledge on key adolescent health issues to their peer group.

INFECTIOUS DISEASE

Case Definitions of RNTCP (New)
- Microbiologically confirmed TB case: Refers to a presumptive TB patient with biological specimen positive for AFB, or positive for *Mycobacterium tuberculosis* on culture, or positive for TB through quality assured rapid diagnostic molecular test (earlier called sputum positive).
- Clinically diagnosed TB case: Refers to a presumptive TB patient who is not microbiologically confirmed, but has been diagnosed with active TB by a clinician on the basis of X-ray abnormalities, histopathology or clinical signs with a decision to treat the patient with a full course of anti-TB treatment (earlier called sputum negative).

Follow Up under RNTCP (New)

New and previously treated drug sensitive pulmonary TB.
- No need to extend IP
- Sputum microscopy at the end of IP and end of treatment
- Weight monthly, chest X-ray if required

Drug resistant TB
- Sputum smear monthly 3, 4, 5, 6, 7 months in IP and at 3 months interval in CP at 9, 12, 15 months
- Monitoring health status of TB treated patients (for recurrence of TB) for 24 months after treatment

Treatment (New)

- **Drug Sensitive TB**
  - IP: For new TB cases, the treatment in IP will consist of 8 weeks of HRZE in daily dosages
- There will be no need for extension of IP
  - During CP
- Only Z will be stopped
- Other HRE for another 16 weeks
- Daily dosages

Previously Treated TB
- IP: 12 weeks: S will be stopped after 8 weeks, HRZE for next 4 weeks as daily dose
- CP: HRE will be continued for another 20 weeks as daily dose
- CP in both new and previously treated cases may be extended by 12–24 weeks in certain forms of TB like CNS TB, skeletal TB, disseminated TB, etc.

Sputum Collection in RNTCP (NEW)

- 2 samples are collected within a day or 2 consecutive days. One sample is collected on spot under supervision and other is collected early in the morning
- Sputum should be at least 2 ml in quantity, muco-purulent
- Results of sputum tests should be reported within a day
  - Labelling of sputum containers:
    - o Early morning sample is labelled B
    - o 1st spot sample is labelled A
    - o Labelling done on the container and not on lid

Diagnosis of Drug Resistance (New)

- If rifampicin resistance is confirmed by CBNAAT or LPA, start standardized regimen for MDR-TB and perform liquid culture DST at baseline to levofloxacin, moxifloxacin, kanamycin, capreomycin, ethambutol, ethionamide, linezolid and pyrazinamide along with LPA for isoniazid on sample/culture isolate (results of which would be received after 6–8 weeks).
- If isoniazid resistance is detected by LPA, report of result must also mention Kat G or INH-A mutation.

Control of pneumonia under GAPPD		
Indicators	**Target**	**Target year**
Hib immunization coverage	90%	2025
Measles immunization coverage	90%	2025
DTP3 immunization coverage	90%	2025
PCV3 immunization coverage	90%	2025
Care seeking for pneumonia	90%	2025
Antibiotic treatment for suspected pneumonia	90%	2025

Control of diarrhoea under GAPPD		
Indicators	**Target**	**Target year**
Rotavirus immunization coverage	90%	2025
Exclusive breastfeeding of children aged 0–5 months	50%	2025
ORS treatment for diarrhoea	90%	2025
Access to improved drinking water at household	90%	2030
Access to hygienic sanitation facility at household	90%	2040
Access to handwashing facilities at household	90%	2030
Access to clean and safe fuel used for cooking in the household	90%	2030

Global Health Sector Strategy on Viral Hepatitis 2016–2021

Global targets
- Reduce new cases of chronic HBV and HCV infections by 90% by 2030
- Reduce deaths due to viral hepatitis by 65% by 2030
- Preventive interventions:
  - 3 dose HBV vaccine for infants
  - Prevention of PTCT of HBV
  - Blood safety and injection safety
  - Harm reduction for drug users
- Treatment interventions:
  - Diagnosis of HBV and HCV
  - Treatment of HBV and HCV
  - Global health sector strategy on viral hepatitis 2016–2021

India Infective Trachoma Free in December 2017: National Trachoma Survey Report (2014–17) found prevalence of trachoma in India is 0.7%.

Ayushman Bharat/National Health Protection Scheme: It will cover more than 10 crore poor and vulnerable families by providing coverage up to 5 lakh rupees per family per annum for secondary and tertiary care hospitalization. It will subsume the ongoing centrally sponsored schemes.

POSHAN Abhiyyan/National Nutrition Mission (NNM): Multi-sectoral program to address maternal and child under-nutrition. The strategy is based on intense monitoring and convergence of ongoing nutrition programs across the ministries.

Intensified National Iron Plus Initiative (I-NIPI): Under POSHAN abhiyyan (2018–2020), anaemia mukt Bharat: The strategy emphasizes on improving supply chain, targeted monitoring and continuous social mobilization using various channels of communication.

Miscellaneous

Manish Taywade, Sudip Bhattacharya, Pallavi Lohani, Arti Gupta

PUBLIC HEALTH LITERATURE

Public Health Pioneers

S No.	Name of Founder	Date of birth and place	Date of death and place	Contribution
1	Edward Jenner	17 May 1749 Gloucestershire	26 January 1823 Berkeley	Smallpox vaccination
2	John Snow	15 March 1813 City of York	16 June 1858	Cholera
3	James Lind	4 Oct 1716 Edinburg	13 July 1794 Gosport	Treatment of Scurvy
4	Robert Koch	11 December 1843	27 May 1910	Tubercle bacillus anthrax, cholera
5	Joseph Lister	1827	10 February 1912 Walmer Kent	Antiseptic
6	John Simon	10 October 1816 London	23 July 1904 London	Public sanitation and sanitation science
7	Lemuel Shattuck	1793 Ashby Massachusetts	1859 Boston	Sanitation and vital statistics
8	Edwin Chadwick	24 January 1800 Manchester	6 July 1890	Sanitation
9	Sir Ronald Ross	1857 Almora India	16 September1932	Malaria
10	William Farr	30 November 1807 Kenley Shrophire	14 April 1883	Father of Modern epidemiological surveillance
11	SrJoshep William Bhore	15 August 1878	15 August 1960	Bhore committee recommendation

Nobel Prize Winners in Physiology or Medicine in last few years

Year	Name of scientist	Discoveries
2015	William C Chambell and Santoshi Omura Youyou Tu	Novel therapy against infections caused by roundworm parasite Novel therapy against malaria
2014	John O' Keefe May-Brit Moser and Edvard I. Moser	Cells that constitute a positioning system in the brain
2013	James E. Rothman, Randy W. Schekman and Thomas C. Sudhof	Discoveries of machinery regulatory vesicle traffic, a major transport system in our cells
2012	Sir John B. Gurdon and Shinya Yamanaka	Matures cells can be reprogrammed to become pluripotent
2011	Bruce A. Beutler and Jules A. Hoffman	Activation of innate immunity
2010	Robert G. Edwards	*In-vitro* fertilization
2009	Elizabeth H. Blackburn, Carol W. Greider and Jack W Szostak	How chromosomes are protected by teromers and the enzyme telomerase
2008	Haraldzur Hausen Francoise Barre-Sinoussi and Luc Montagnier	Human papillomavirus causing cervical cancer Human deficiency virus
2007	Mario R Capecchi, Sir Martin J. Evans and Oliver Smithies	Principles for introducing specific gene modifications in mice by the use of embryonic stem cells
2006	Andrew Z. Fire and Craig C. Mello	RNA interference-gene silencing by double-standard RNA
2005	Barry J. Marshall and J. Robin Warren	Bacterium *Helicobacter pylori* and its role in gastritis and peptic ulcer diseases

Famous Institute of Public Health in India

S No.	Name of institute	Place
1.	JALMA: National Jalma Institute of Leprosy and other Mycobacterial Diseases	Agra, UP
2.	National Institute of Occupational Health (NIOH), Ahemdabad	Gujarat
3.	National Institute of Epidemiology	Chennai
4.	Indian Institute of Public Health	Delhi
5.	INClen: Indian Clinical Epidemiology Network	Delhi
6.	Public Health Foundation of India	Delhi

(Contd.)

(Contd.)

S No.	Name of institute	Place
7.	National Institute of Health and Family Welfare [NIHFW]	Delhi
8.	Indian Institute of Public Health, Gandhi Nagar	Gujarat
9.	All India Institute of Hygiene and Public Health	Kolkata
10.	National Institute for Research in Reproductive Health	Mumbai
11.	NEERI: National Environmental Engineering Research Institute	Nagpur
12.	National Institute of Virology	Pune, Maharashtra
13.	National Tuberculosis Institute	Bangalore
14.	National AIDS Research Institute	Pune
15.	International Institute for Population Sciences	Mumbai

MANAGEMENT

Sudip Bhattacharya

Q 1. What is planning? Write down the steps of planning.

Planning is organizing the processes or activities to accomplish a desired objective or goal.

Steps of planning:
 a. Laying down the scope
 b. Situational exploration
 c. Resource exploration
 d. Strength, weakness opportunity and threat analysis
 e. Assertion of the "public needs"
 f. Set the importance
 g. Recognize the "high risk" population
 h. Utter clearly the goal, aims, objectives, indicators and targets
 i. Pick a strategy
 j. Make an action plan
 k. Confirm public involvement
 l. Systematise the money, material and manpower
 m. Commence a "pilot run"
 n. Conduct and evaluate the programme

Q 2. What is an action plan?

It describes how objectives are to be achieved. In other words, we can say that to achieve certain objectives, we use action plans.

Some basic steps for action plan:
   a. Correct selection of strategies
   b. Fixing the duty
   c. Resource distribution
   d. Progressive programming of precise activities so that resource can be utilized optimally.

Problem: If you are the chief medical officer of a district, after discussion with your peers, you have recognized two of your important activities as "computerization" at all PHCs and printing of leaflets on "basic knowledge on computers" for the whole district. Make an action plan.

Solution:

Activities	Objectives	Action plans							
		Jan	Feb	Mar	Apr	May	Jun	Jul	Aug
Computerization in all PHCs	Free timings of rooms in PHC								
	Est. of LAN at all PHCs and making electrical points								
	Making of computer rooms at all PHCs and purchasing of computers and accessories								
	Training of staffs								
Printing of education material	Funds release								
	Designing the leaflets. Printing and supply of educational material to the health staff								
Planning is depicted by **blue colour**				Execution of activities is depicted by **green color**					

Q 3. What is Gantt chart?

It is a management tool, commonly used in projects. In this tool, activities are displayed against time.

   On the left of the chart is a list of the actions are mentioned. At the top a time frame is declared. The bar is a symbol of activity. The relative location and length of the bar reveal the start date, duration and end date of the action.

It is important because at a glance we can see:

a. The several actions   b. Starting and ending time of each action

c. Time taken for each action   d. Where actions are overlapping

e. The duration of the whole project

Gantt chart

Timeline of events

Time	Sep 2017	Oct 2017	Nov 2017	Dec 2017	Jan 2017	Feb 2017	March 2017	April 2017	May 2017	June 2017	July 2017
Ethical clearance, pretesting	██	██									
Data collection			██	██							
Data entry				██	██						
Data analysis							██	██			
Project writing										██	██

Q 4. Describe Johari Window.

It is a communication model. It improves our interpersonal relations. It has four-quadrant. The objective of this tool is to expand area which is open, without revealing the private facts.

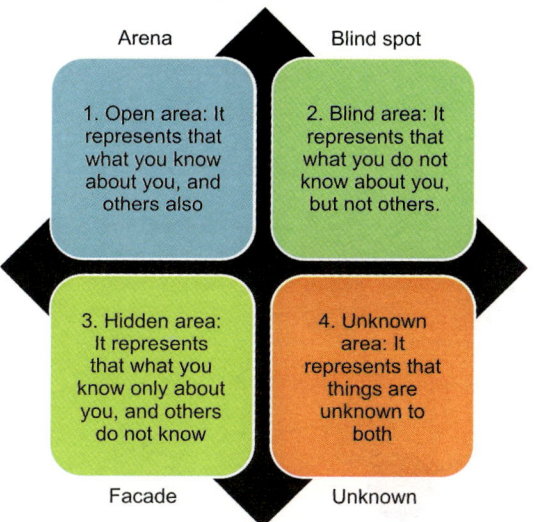

	Arena	Blind spot
	1. Open area: It represents that what you know about you, and others also	2. Blind area: It represents that what you do not know about you, but not others.
	3. Hidden area: It represents that what you know only about you, and others do not know	4. Unknown area: It represents that things are unknown to both
	Facade	Unknown

Q 5. What are network analysis, PERT, and CPM?

Network analysis is usually done for planning and controlling the processes of any activity.

In management critical path method, and project evaluation and review technique (PERT), are used to for completion of a project within time.

Critical Path Method (CPM): When time lengths of each action in a project are known accurately, we use CPM. In CPM we have to focus on critical path only, any delay in the critical path can delay the entire project.

Project Evaluation and Review Technique (PERT): In planning, monitoring and controlling of projects PERT is commonly used. The basic difference between PERT and CPM is the time required for each action in the project is not precisely known.

Problem: Make a PERT diagram regarding inauguration of a new hospital.

Activity	Description	Immediate predecessors
A	Organizational and health care staff selection	–
B	Selection and survey of site	–
C	Equipment selection	A
D	Making of master plans and layout	B
E	Bring services to the site	B
F	Recruitment hospital staffs	A
G	Purchase and delivery of instruments	C
H	Build the hospital	D
I	Develop the hospital information system	A
J	Instrument installation	E, G, H
K	Training of manpower	F, I, J

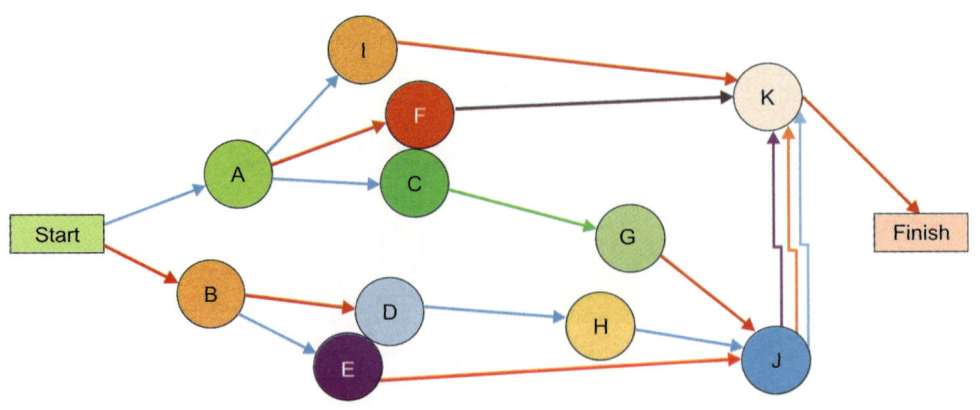

Paths —these are sequences of activities between a project's start and finish.	Time (weeks)
A-I-K	33
A-F-K	28
A-C-G-J-K	67
B-D-H-J-K	69
B-E-J-K	43

Q 6. What is an inventory?

An inventory is a detailed itemized list of assets held by an organization or institution.

Q 7. Classify various types of inventory management.

Abbreviation	Full form	Based on
ABC	Always better control	Annual consumption cost of items
VED	Vital, essential, desirable	Vital and critical items
FSN	Fast moving, slow moving and nonmoving	Issues from stores
SDE	Scare, difficult, easy	Availability of items
HML	High, medium and low	Unit price
XYZ		Value analysis
SOS	Season off season	Seasonal requirement

Q 8. What is ABC (Always Better Control) analysis?

Pareto's principle says that usually, a minor quantity of commodities incurs a large amount of cost and vice versa.

When we manage our items like medicines in our hospital, it is also categorized upon the cumulative annual cost of the different medicines.

a. 10% of the medicines would cost 70% of the total currency (Group-A commodities)

b. 20% of the medicines would cost around 20% of total currency (Group-B commodities)

c. 70% of medicines would cost only 10% of the total currency (Group-C commodities).

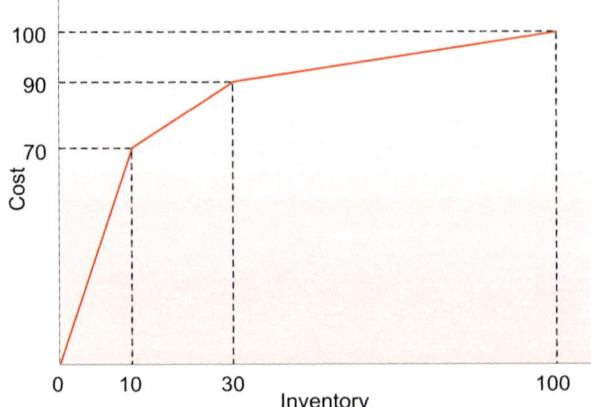

Q 9. What are the steps involved in ABC analysis in a hospital?

a. Firstly annual cost of each medicine is calculated.

b. Then the medicines are organized in detrimental value of total cost annually. That means the costliest will be at the top and the least costly being placed at the bottom.

c. The accumulative cost is then calculated and a table is prepared (Table given below).

d. From the table it is seen that about 10% of medicines would cost 70% of the total yearly cost. These are called group A commodities. The rest 20% items would cost nearly 20% of the total yearly cost. These are called group B commodities. The rest of 70% items account for only 10% of the total yearly cost. These are group C commodities.

		Table			
Sl No.	Name of the drug/item	Annual consumption costs (Rs)	Cumulative costs (Rs)	% of total costs	
1.	Inj Norfloxacin	9000	9000	9	
2.	Tab Norfloxacin	8500	17500	17.5	
3.	Inj Decadon	8300	25800	25.8	**Group A**
4.	Inj Amoxycillin	8000	33800	33.8	
—	—	—	—	—	
10.	Inj Alteplase	5000	70000	70	
—	—	—	—	—	**Group B**
30.	Oint Neosporin	1000	90000	90	
—	—	—	—	—	**Group C**
100.	Gauze	100	100000	100	

Q 10. What is VED (vital, essential, and desirable) analysis?

It is observed in hospitals that a medicine of low cost and low consumption but it is still live saving. We cannot ignore such drugs as per ABC analysis. As they fall in group 'C' category. For example, anti-rabies immunoglobulin may be used very rarely in a month. It has very low annual cost, but it is vital and life-saving. It should be available in every hospital round the clock.

For this reason, we used to do ABC–VED analysis.

ABC–VED analysis

	V items	E items	D items	
A Items	AV	AE	AD	Category 1 items
B Items	BV	BE	BD	Category 2 items
C Items	CV	CE	CD	Category 3 items

Q 11. What is zero-based Budgeting?

Under this approach of budgeting, in each budget cycle (i.e. the period for which budget is to be prepared), each program or project is put under scanner to justify the expenses to be incurred. Expenses items in the budget are justified if the benefits derived from them are more than the cost of it.

The focus in this approach is 'Why' the amount is to be spent rather than 'how much' to be spent.

As such, it is possible that a particular program or project, which has been in existence for past few years, will be discarded under approach if in current budget cycle the proposed budgeted expenses cannot be justified.

Zero-based budgeting provides competitive utilization of available funds and other resources among those programs and/or projects, which can be justified in each budget period.

Q 12. What is performance-based budgeting?

Performance-based budgeting is the allocation of funds based on programmatic results that contribute to organizational goals. Performance-based budgeting is not intended to punish or reward departments or agencies, but instead to focus on progress toward measurable goals during the budget process.

Performance-based budgeting is known by a variety of names: Outcome-based budgeting, results-based budgeting, or priority-based budgeting. All of these terms indicate a focus on increasing the use of data and evidence to improve the allocation of resources and achieve programmatically and community goals.

Performance-based budgeting allows strengthening the budgetary process in light of competing claims for resources by using objective criteria to:

a. Determine resource allocation;
b. Ensure accountability among those responsible for management;
c. Shift the budget focus to city priorities rather than department- or agency-specific goals;
d. Make the budget process more transparent; and
e. Engage the community in the budgeting process.

Q 13. Discuss the motivation theory of Maslow.

As per this theory, our basic needs are to be fulfilled first ONLY then our higher needs will be/can be fulfilled. For example, first our hunger, housing, and clothing etc. need to be provided. Only the creativity related aspects will get our attention. Our motivation works on these lines usually.

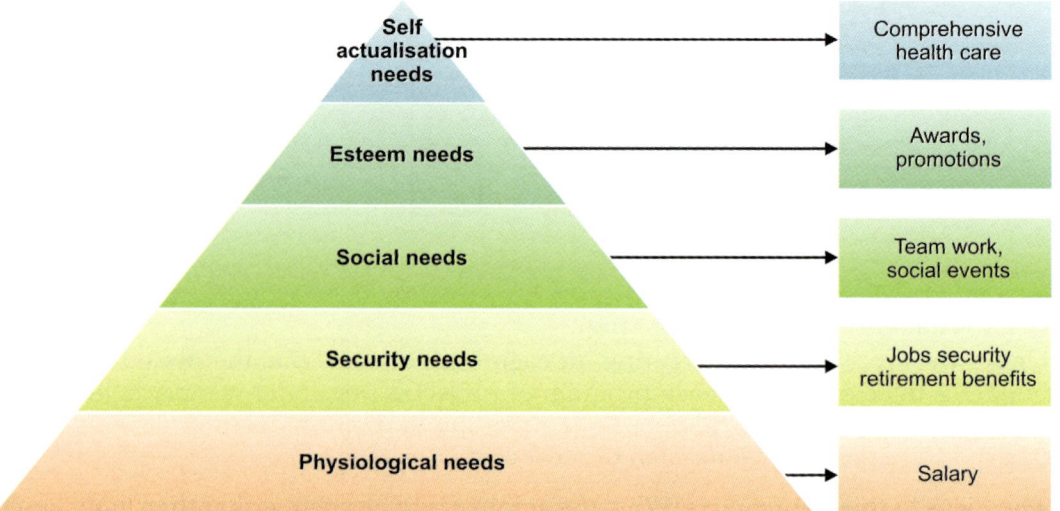

Q 14. What do you mean by audit in hospital and enumerate its important aspects?

Auditing is a financial authentication procedure grounded on past records, evaluated against a fixed rule, protocols, and principles.

It may be internal and may be external. Both have advantages and disadvantages.

Hospital audit is different from the usual audit. Because hospitals do not sell commodities and treatment, cost varies from person to person. The following things should be kept in mind during an audit in hospitals.

a. The policy of the hospitals (in every aspect) should be examined in details.
b. To detect internal discrepancies previous old documents should be examined.
c. Comparison of data must be cross checked by hospital records.
d. Every transaction must be recorded.
e. The procedure of taking grants or donations should be in place.
f. Competent authorities should verify discount to the poor free.

Q 15. Write down the steps of logistics and materials management activities.
  a. Tendering, procurement and inspection
  b. Storage, standardization, codification and classification
  c. Materials accounting and physical distribution
  d. Transportation
  e. Security of materials
  f. Condemnation and disposal of stores

Q 16 Enumerate various methods of total quality management.
  a. Acceptable quality level (AQL)
  b. Affinity diagrams
  c. Arrow diagram
  d. Bench marking
  e. Consensus reaching
  f. Contingency planning
  g. Cost-benefit analysis
  h. Deming Wheel or Plan, Do, Check and Act (PDCA) cycle
  i. Force analysis
  j. Gantt Chart
  k. Kaizen (change for the better)
  l. Pareto analysis
  m. Quality circles (QC)

Important Terminologies in Management

Auditing: Auditing is a financial authentication procedure grounded on past records, evaluated against a fixed rules, protocols and principles.

Break-even analysis: It is an economic tool to decide the level of manufacture where the total cost to manufacturer matches the total returns from transactions.

Break-even point (BEP): It is a point of 'no profit, no loss' status for the manufacturing company.

Budget: It is a statement of future expenditure plans defined in measurable and financial terms, for a definite period.

Fixed costs: The expenses that remain fixed and do not depend on the amount of output, e.g. making a hospital building.

Goals: These are time-bound, specific targets which are essential for the accomplishment of the objectives in the association.

Management: It is getting things done by and with the people.

Mission: It is described as the actual reason for the existence of any organization.

Motivation: It is the willingness of an individual to put extra effort into attaining goals.

Management by Objectives (MBO): Supervisors can improve their overall performance and effectiveness by a decision-making tool.

Objectives: Act direction of the mission.

Opportunity cost: It is the cost of foregoing an opportunity in favor of one alternative.

Out-of-Pocket cost: These are the cash expenditures, which would be saved, based on a decision.

Planning: It is the essential and initial process of any activity.

Policies: It gives us broad recommendations for whatever we wish to decide.

Quality: "The totality of features and characteristics of a product or service which have the ability to satisfy the clients felt or implied needs".

Rules: It delineates what should or should not be done.

Strategies: It may be any decision, plan or action which concerns the actions of opponents with the aim of accomplishing the objectives.

Social security: When a society protects individuals against the economic and social suffering is called social security. Like health insurance.

Step costs: Sometimes, the cost remains fixed for a certain considerable amount of output and then steps up to the next level of cost.

Variable costs: When costs vary with the output, it is called variable costs.

SOCIOLOGY

Pallavi Lohani

The social determinants of health according to Marmot review are:
 a. Give every child the best start in life
 b. Enable all children, young people and adults to maximise their capabilities and have control over their lives
 c. Create fair employment and good work for all
 d. Ensure healthy standard of living for all
 e. Create and develop healthy and sustainable places and communities
 f. Strengthen the role and impact of ill health prevention

Important terminologies in Sociology

Acculturation: When there is contact between two people with different types of culture, there is diffusion of culture both ways. For example, widespread use of tobacco

Achieved role: It is a role by virtue of age, sex, and birth status

Acquired role: It is by virtue of education or otherwise.

Anthropology: It deals with the social, physical, and cultural history of man.

Behavioral science comprises sociology, social psychology, and anthropology.

Below poverty line: It is defined in two ways
 a. The minimum level of income deemed adequate in a particular country C. Rangarajan committee (2012) recommended BPL when daily per capita expenditure to less than rupees 32 in rural and rupees 47 in urban areas.

b. The minimum amount of calories that a person take in rural and urban areas. K. Alagh committee (1977) measured poverty as starvation. The people consuming less than 2100 calories in urban and 2400 calories in rural areas are poor.

Community: A community is a social group determined by geographical boundaries with common values and interests interacting with each other.

Culture: It is a learned behavior that has been socially acquired, e.g. touching foot of our adults for blessings.

Custom: It is right ways of doing things, which are not written and is practise since long time by people, e.g. intercaste marriages are not allowed by some people.

Economics: It deals with human ownership of goods and services.

Emotion: An emotion is a mental and physiological state associated with a wide variety of feelings, thoughts, and behaviours. For example, fear, anger, anxiety, and love.

Gross Domestic Product (GDP): It is gross income generated within a country, i.e., it excludes net income received from abroad.

Gross National Income (GNI)/Gross National Product (GNP): Gross income within the country plus income received from abroad.

Habit: It is an accustomed way of doing things.

Human behaviour: It is the result of physical and mental factors interacting in complicated ways.

Leadership: It is the ability of a manager to influence and induce subordinates to work with confidence and zeal for the achievement of organizational goals.

The theories of leadership:
   a. Trait theory: Leaders are born, not made
   b. Behavioural theory: Leadership depends on behaviour of the leader
   c. Contingency theory: Leadership depends also on subordinates

The styles of leadership:
   a. Autocratic: Do as I say! It tends to humiliate people and make them irresponsible
   b. Anarchic: Do what you like
   c. Democratic: Let us agree on what we are to do—helps people grow, to become responsible and show initiative

Management makes decisions while administration carries out those decisions.

Medical sociology: The study of socio-cultural factors and their association with illness, the social principles in medical organization, and treatment.

Motivation: It is an inner force which makes a person to a certain action.

Net Domestic Product (NDP) is GDP minus the capital consumed due to depreciation, i.e. equipment, machinery, etc.

Net National Product (NNP): It is the market value of all final goods and services after subtracting capital consumed in the production process.

Operational research: It is a research providing results by advanced analysis in terms of quantitive basis for policy or programme change. For example, removal of category III from RNTCP.

Opinions: They are temporary judgement of people at a particular set of point. For example, mosquito bite more when one sleeps on floor.

Pedagogy: It is the science of teaching.

Political science: It is concerned with the study of laws and institutions that constitute government of whole societies.

Problem-based learning: It is a student based pedagogy. In it, students learn about a subject through the experience of solving an open-ended problem.

Psychology: It is a study of human behavior—of how people behave and why they behave in just the way, they do.

Purchasing power parity is the currency of a country required to buy the same amount of goods and services as one US dollar.

Social defence: It is a system developed to defend society against criminality by treating and defending the offended and creating conditions conducive for a healthy human life.

Social institution: It is an organized complex pattern of behaviour of persons in a group.

Social mobility: It is a change of socioeconomic status of a person over a time by virtue of literacy, occupation, and income.

Social problem: A social problem affects a large number of people. For example, dowry system, alcohol abuse and others

Social psychology: It is concerned with the psychology of individuals.

Social sciences: These are those disciplines which are committed to the scientific examination of human behaviour. These include:
   a. Economics
   b. Political Science
   c. Sociology
   d. Social Psychology
   e. Anthropology

Social security: Society provided security through an appropriate organization. For example, old age home.

Social structure: It is the pattern of the inter-relationships between persons.

Socialism: It is a system of production and distribution based on social ownership of goods and services for raising the living standards of the people.

Socialization: It is the process by which an individual gradually acquires culture and becomes a member of a social group. For example, children going to school.

Sociology: It is the study of individuals as well as groups in a society.

Urban Area: Urban areas are:
   1. All places with a municipality, corporation, cantonment board or notified town area committee, etc.
   2. All other places, which satisfied the following criteria, shall qualify to be called urban area:

a. A minimum population of 5,000;
b. At least 75 percent of the male main working population engaged in non-agricultural pursuits;
c. A density of population of at least 400 persons per sq. km.

Urban micro climate: Materials used in urban construction conduct more heat than vegetated areas. Buildings and vehicles release significant amounts of heat energy from burning of fossil fuels. Urbanization can, therefore, its own micro climate.

Wealth Index: The wealth index is a composite measure of a household's cumulative living assets, for example, televisions, bicycles and others.

K	**Knowledge:** It is information and skills acquired through experience or education, e.g. malaria is common in north India.
A	**Attitudes:** They are acquired characteristic of a person, which predisposes to act in a preferential manner in known/unknown situation. For example, Bednets are useless, as somehow mosquito will enter bednet.
B	**Belief:** It is an internal feeling that something is true, irrespective of facts. For example, I am 75 years old, malaria cannot occur to me.
P	**Practice:** It is real application of KAB. For example, I sleep on bed without bednets.

Alcohol and Tobacco

Q 1. What is the most common substance of abuse in India?
The most common substance of abuse in India is alcohol.

Q 2. How alcohol in beverages measured?
Alcohol in beverages is measured alcohol by volume, that is, how much pure alcohol is present in an alcoholic beverage.

Q 3. Which alcoholic beverage is commonly used in India?
The commonly used alcoholic beverage in India is country made liquor.

Q 4. What are the effects of alcoholism?
The effects of alcoholism are acute and chronic intoxication, cirrhosis of the liver, toxic psychosis, gastritis, pancreatitis, cardiomyopathy, peripheral neuropathy, cancer, suicide, accidents, violence, family disorganization, crime and loss of productivity.

Q 5. What is the safe limit of alcohol consumption?
According to Royal College of Physicians men/women can drink no more than 21/14 units of alcohol per week, no more than 4/3 units in any one day and have at least two alcohol-free days a week.

Q 6. Name the screening test used for problem drinking?
CAGE questionnaire is used for screening of alcoholism. It gives an indication that a person should be after investigated for alcohol dependence. It has four questions.

Q 7. What is the CAGE questionnaire?
It has four questions:
a. Have you ever felt you should **C**ut down on your drinking?
b. Have people **A**nnoyed you by criticizing your drinking?

c. Have you ever felt bad or **G**uilty about your drinking?

d. Have you ever had a drink first thing in the morning to steady your nerves or to get rid of a hangover (**E**ye opener)?

Q 8. Which device is used in the field by police to know the recent ingestion of alcohol?

Breath analyser

Q 9. What is alcohol abuse?

Alcohol abuse is when a person has at least one of the following occurring within 12 months:

a. Recurrent use of alcohol leading to a failure to perform the major role at work, school, or home

b. Recurrent alcohol use in physically hazardous situations

c. Recurrent alcohol leading to legal problems

d. Continued alcohol use despite having persistent or recurrent social or interpersonal problems

Q 10. What are the different forms of tobacco used?

a. Cigarette: Most common and most harmful

b. Bidi: Most popular

c. Tobacco chewing: 30% of total tobacco consumption

d. Sheesha Snuff: Moist and dry

Q 11. What is the composition of tobacco?

About 4000 toxic substances are present in cigarette smoke like nicotine, carbon monoxide, tar, toluene, ammonia, methanol, cadmium, stearic acid, and others.

Q 12. What are the detrimental effects of tobacco on health?

An important causative/risk factor for various diseases like lung cancer, chronic bronchitis, emphysema, ischaemic heart disease, stroke, obstructive peripheral vascular disease, cancer of lip, tongue, oesophagus, gastro-duodenal ulcers, stillbirths, abortions, pre-term birth, low birth weight, and others.

Q 13. What is Fagerstrom test?

Fagerstrom test is a standard instrument for assessing the physical dependence to nicotine and thus used by clinicians to decide whether to start medication for nicotine withdrawal. It provides an ordinal measure of nicotine dependence related to cigarette smoking. Evaluation of quantity of cigarette consumption, the compulsion to use and dependence can do through six items. The score ranges from 0 to 10; higher the count, more the dependence.

Q 14. What is the pharmacological treatment of smoking cessation?

Nicotine replacement therapy relieves cravings for nicotine and reduces withdrawal symptoms. It is presently available as patches, gums, nasal sprays, inhalers, e-cigarettes, and others.

Q 15. What are the 5A and 5R for tobacco cessation under RNTCP 2016?

5A	5R
a. Ask	Relevance
b. Advise	Risk
c. Assess	Reward
d. Assist	Road block
e. Arrange	Repetition

OTHER TOPICS

Arti Gupta

Important Personnel in Current Public Health in India

S. No.	Designation	Name
1.	Health Minister, India	Shri Jagat Prakash Nadda
2.	World Health Organization, Director General	Dr. Tedros Adhanom Ghebreyesus
3.	World Health Organization, Director South-East Asia Region office (SEARO)	Dr. Poonam Khetrapal
4.	Centers for Disease Control and Prevention	Dr. Brenda Fitzgerald
5.	Indian Public Health Association (IPHA), President	Dr. Prabir Kumar Das
6.	Indian Association of Preventive and Social Medicine (IAPSM), President	Dr. Ratan Srivastava
7.	Indian Council of Medical Research (ICMR), Director	Dr. Soumaya Swaminathan

Q 1. What are the various principles of ethics?
a. Essentiality
b. Voluntariness, informed consent, and community agreement
c. Nonexploitation
d. Risk minimization and precaution
e. Privacy and confidentiality
f. Transparency and accountability
g. Totality of responsibility
h. Professional competence
i. Institutional arrangement
j. Public interest and distributive justice
k. Public domain
l. Compliance

Q 2. What is impact factor?

The impact factor is a measure of the frequency with which the average article in a journal has been cited in a particular year.

Q 3. What is citation?

A citation is a reference to a published or unpublished source.

Q 4. What is the difference between referencing and bibliography in academic writing?

In referencing, references come at the end of a text. It mainly includes only those works that are cited within the text. Bibliography mainly includes works read as general background.

Q 5. What are bibliographic elements?

a. Authors (use et al. after 6 authors, if there are more than six authors, complete names should not be written. "et al." must be in italics)

b. Article title (should be exact as existing)

c. Journal name (should be in standard PubMed abbreviations)

d. Year

e. Volume

f. Page numbers

Q 6. What does "et al." means in academic writing?

It is a latin phrase, et al. meaning "and others."

Q 7. What are various styles of citation?

American Medical Association (AMA)
Modern Language Association (MLA)
American Psychological Association (APA)

For example:

AMA: Gupta A, Kalaivani M, Gupta SK, Rai SK, Nongkynrih B. The study on achievement of motor milestones and associated factors among children in rural North India. Journal of Family Medicine and Primary Care. 2016;5(2):378–382. doi:10.4103/2249–4863.192346.

MLA: Gupta, Arti, et al. "The Study on Achievement of Motor Milestones and Associated Factors among Children in Rural North India." Journal of Family Medicine and Primary Care 5.2 (2016): 378–382. PMC.Web. 23 June 2017.

APA: Gupta, A., Kalaivani, M., Gupta, S. K., Rai, S. K., and Nongkynrih, B. (2016). The study on achievement of motor milestones and associated factors among children in rural North India. Journal of Family Medicine and Primary Care, 5(2), 378–382. http://doi.org/10.4103/2249–4863.192346

Q 8. What is an annotated bibliography?

It is a list of citations to books, articles, and documents. Each citation is followed by a brief (usually about 150 words) descriptive and evaluative paragraph, the annotation. The purpose of the annotation is to inform the reader of the relevance, accuracy, and quality of the sources cited.

Q 9. What is an abstract?

They are the purely descriptive summaries often found at the beginning of scholarly journal articles or in periodical indexes. Annotations are descriptive and critical; they expose the author's point of view, clarity, and appropriateness of expression, and authority.

Q 10. What is referencing?

It is the process of citing or documenting the source that you have used in your writing.
   a. Harvard, we write number in text
   b. Vancouver, we write authors name in text.

Q 11. Enumerate some important critical appraisal tools of scientific research.

   a. CONSORT: Consolidated standards of reporting trials
   b. STROBE: Strengthening the reporting of observational studies in epidemiology
   c. PRISMA: Transparent reporting of systematic review and meta-analysis
   d. CASP: Critical appraisal skills programme
   e. MOOSE: Meta-analysis of epidemiological observation studies
   f. ARRIVE: For animal studies
   g. QUOROM: Systematic reviews and meta-analysis
   h. GRADE: Quality of evidence

Q 12. Enumerate some publications of World Health Organization.

   a. World Health Report
   b. World Health Statistics
   c. International Health regulation
   d. International Travel and Health

Q 13. Enumerate four journals of World Health Organization.

   a. Weekly Epidemiological record
   b. WHO Southeast Asia Journal of Public Health
   c. Pan American Journal of Public Health
   d. Eastern Mediterranean Health Journal

Q 14. What is PubMed?

It is a free electronic archive of biomedical and life sciences journal articles. PubMed is the interface.

Q 15. What is the difference between PubMed and PubMed central?

PubMed is a database of citations and abstracts, whereas **PubMed Central** is an electronic database of full-text journal articles.

Q 16. What is MEDLINE?

MEDLINE is journal citation database of the National Library of Medicine. PubMed is one of the ways to access MEDLINE.

Q 17. What is H index?

The H-index is an author-level metric that measures your research output and its citation impact. It is based on a set of your most cited work and the number of citations it received.

Q 18. Enumerate some database.
PubMed, EBSCO, ISI

Q 19. Enumerate some important public health journals.
   a. Indian Journal of Public Health
   b. Indian Journal of Preventive and Social Medicine
   c. Indian Journal of Community Medicine
   d. Indian Journal of Medical Research
   e. National Medical Journal of India
   f. Journal of Mahatma Gandhi Institute of Medical Sciences
   g. LANCET
   h. BMJ
   i. WHO bulletin

Q 20. What is multilateral organization?
Multilateral organizations are formed between three or more nations to work on issues that relate to all the countries in the organization. These are global, regional or international. For examples, SAARC (South Asian Association for Regional Cooperation).

Q 21. What is bilateral organization?
Bilateral organizations are governmental agencies in a single country which provide aid to developing countries. For example, the United States agency for International Development.

Q 22. What is intergovernmental organization?
Intergovernmental organization refers to modern international organizations that can be broken down into two main types: The public "variety" known as inter-governmental organizations, for example, the WHO; and the private variety, which are referred to as international non-governmental organizations, such as Amnesty International and the International Committee Red Cross, CARE, DFID.

Q 23. Enumerate some books on public health other than academics?
   a. House on fire: The Fight to Eradicate Smallpox by William Foege (Author).
   b. The Making of a Tropical Disease: A Short History of Malaria by Randall M. Packard (Author).
   c. The Ghost Map: The Story of London's Most Terrifying Epidemic—and How It Changed Science, Cities, and the Modern World by Steven Johnson.
   d. The Great Influenza: The Story of the Deadliest Pandemic by John M Barry.

Q 24. Enumerate some movies highlighting public health problems.
   a. Savdhaan on HIV
   b. Preg Rog: Widow remarriage
   c. Achhoot Kanya: Dalits
   d. Matrubhoomi: Female infanticide
   e. Vicky donor: Sperm donation
   f. Manthan: White revolution in India
   g. Toilet: Sanitation

Q 25. What is Pradhan Mantri Swasthya Suraksha Yojana [PMSSY]?

PMSSY was announced in 2003 with objectives of correcting regional imbalances in healthcare services and augmenting quality of medical education.

It approved in 2006 for building AIIMS like institutes [Patna, Jodhpur, Bhopal, Rishikesh, Bhubaneshwar, and Raipur] and 13 government medical colleges up-gradation.

Model Performa

Sidharth Sekhar Mishra

Name of HOH		Age	Sex	M/F
Type of the family (a) Nuclear, (b) Extended, (c) Single, (d) Joint				
H/o migration	**Original place of migration**	**Duration since migration**		

Demographic profile

No.	Name	Age	Sex	Relationship with HOH	Education	Occupation	Income

Chief complaints

Socioeconomic status

Family belongs to (a) APL, (b) BPL		
If family belongs to BPL, then does family have BPL/Ration card (a)Yes (b) No		
Availing any social security scheme	(a) Yes, (b) No, (c) NA	**If yes, then specify detail**

Obstetric H/o married females (18–49 years) in family						
Parity	Term	Sex	Place of delivery	Type of delivery	Birth weight	Present status/age
	a. Full term b. Preterm c. Abortion		a. Hospital b. Home	a. Vaginal b. LSCS		Live Dead

Eligible couple	(a) Present (b) Absent **Number of eligible couples**
Awareness of married woman regarding contraceptive methods	(a) Aware and using, (b) Aware but not using, (c) Not aware
Contraceptive methods used by eligible couple	(a) Not using any method, (b) Tubectomy, (c) Condoms Current (d) Oral Pills, (e) Cu T, (f) Vasectomy ——— (g) Injectables (h) Centchroman Ever used
Reason for not using any method	(a) Wish to have child, (b) Newly married, (c) Due to family pressure, (d) Scared of complication, (e) Other (specify)
Under five children	(a) Present **Number of under five children** (b) Absent

Anthropometry							Immunization status (for age) – (a) Complete
Number of children	Date of birth	Age months	Sex	Wt (kg)	Ht (cm)	MUAC	(b) Partial (c) Not immunized

Nutritional status of under five children

No (a) Normal (b) Wasted	**WHO Classification** (c) Stunted (d) Stunted and wasted

Is child attending/attended Anganwadi? (a) Yes (b) No	
Is child suffered from acute illnesses in last six months? (a) Yes (b) No	Diarrhoeal episode
	ARI
	Fever
Treatment history for illness	
If yes, did she know how to make ORS? (a)Yes, (b) No	
Does mother know how to make ORS at home? (a)Yes, (b) No	
Was the child given ORS for last diarrhoeal episode? (a)Yes, (b) No	
Development of child? (a) As per age (b) Delayed	
Time of start of breastfeeding after birth?	

Duration of breastfeeding	Duration of exclusive breastfeeding
Was the child given prelacteal feed	Age of complementary feeding (in months)

If there is a female who is pregnant or has delivered in the past one year then ask					
Gravida	Parity	Abortion	Live birth	Stillbirth	Lactating

Antenatal period

Registration (a) Booked, (b) Not booked
Number of antenatal care visits including all visits at all health facility
At least one dose of TT (a) Received, (b) Not received
IFA tablets (a) Consumed, (b) Not consumed
If consumed then how many tablets approx.

Any complications in pregnancy	(a) No complication, (b)HTN (c) DM (d) APH (e) Pre-eclampsia (f) Other obstetric complication (specify)

Postnatal period

Postnatal visits: Weeks of Postnatal visit	(a) No visits, (b) One visit, (c) ≥ Two visits
Postnatal complications	(a) No complication (b) Wound dehiscence (c) PPH (d) Infection (e) Other (Specify)

Is there any elderly (>60 years) in the family

Activities of daily living	Independent (a) Yes, (b) No
a. **Bathing**	
b. **Dressing** (wear clothes and dresses without any assistance except for tying shoes)	
c. **Toileting** (goes to toilet room, uses toilet, arranges clothes, and returns without any assistance (may use cane or walker for support and may use bedpan/urinal at night)	
d. **Continence:** Controls bowel and bladder completely by self (without occasional "accidents")	
e. **Feeding:** Feeds self without assistance	

H/o any chronic illness in elderly
(a) No illness, (b) Hypertension, (c) Diabetes mellitus (d) COPD, (e) Joint pain
(f) Other (specify)

Systolic BP	Diastolic BP

Joint examination			
a. Warmth	b. Stiffness	c. Tenderness	d. Redness

Eye examination		
Vision (with E- chart with available correction)	**Right eye**	**Left eye**

Cataract present (a)Yes, (b)No

Environmental history	
33. Type of house	(a) Own (b) Rented (a) Kutcha (b) pucca
Number of living rooms	**Overcrowding** (a) present (b) absent
Water hygiene	**Source:** (a) Public tap, (b) Private tap, (c) Hand pump
	Storage: (a) Covered utensils, (b) Uncovered utensils
Cooking done on (a) LPG, (b) Stove, (c) Chullah	
Ventilation (a) Adequate (b) Inadequate	
Toilet used (a) Sanitary latrine in house (b) Community latrine (c) Open	
Refuse disposal	(a) Through covered container (b) Through uncovered container (c) Dump outside
Is there any open drain near the house	

Nutritional history
Cooking oil used (a) Vanaspati, (b) Mustard oil (c) Refined oil, (d) Other
Average fat consumption per month
Average fat consumption per capita per month
Average sugar consumption per month
Average sugar consumption per capita per month
Salt used (a) Iodised, (b) Non-iodised, (c) Not known
Salt consumption per capita per day
H/o of addiction in family
Type of addiction (a) Smoke tobacco (b) Alcohol (c) Smokeless tobacco (d) Other
Duration of addiction

Requirement and Deficiency of protein:

Requirement and Deficiency of calories:

S. No.	Time of food intake	Food taken	Quantity	Raw materials	Method of Preparation	Energy in 100 gm	Protein in 100 gm	Energy intake by the index	Protein intake by the index

For references, assess the following link https://drive.google.com/file/d/1l6jJlfl3ZQRHPC3L3ZdxX1D2r0YOVFf0/view?usp=sharing

Index

A

5A for tobacco cessation 279
5A for tobacco cessation 279
5R for tobacco cessation 279
5R for tobacco cessation 279
99 DOTS 215
Abortion pills 82
Absolute risk 26
Abstract 281
Acanthosis nigricans 225
ACC/AHA 216
Acceptable quality level (AQL) 273
Accompanied MDT 207
Acculturation 274
Acquired role 274
Action plan 265
Adulteration 56–58
Age-specific fertility rate 44
Albendazole 103, 160, 185
Albert stain 68, 69
Alcohol/alcoholism 277
Alcohol thermometer 87
Almonds 96
Always Better Control 269
Angular stomatitis 157
ANMOL 256
Annapurna yojna 120
Anopheles 108
Antepartum haemorrhage 183
Anthropology 274
Anti-mosquito measures 106
Antiretroviral therapy 102
Antiseptics 104, 105
Antyodya Anna Yojna 120
Apgar score 149
Apple 97
Appraisal tools 281
Artemisinin 102

At-risk infants 147
At-risk mothers 181
Attack rate 17
Attributable risk 26
Auditing 272

B

Bacillus Calmette-Guérin vaccine 84
Basic emergency obstetric care plus 178
Beam balance 127
Bed bug 110
Behavioural science 274
Bengal gram 92
Bibliography 280
Biochemical oxygen demand 61
Biscuit 97
Bleaching powder 105
Blister calendar pack 207
Blood transfusion 158
Body mass index 52
Box and whisker plot 41
Bread 91
Brinjal 93
Broken family 114
Bromocriptine 188

C

CAGE questionnaire 277
Calcium 185
Case fatality rate 15
Cauliflower 93
Centchroman 83
Central tendency measures 1
Chadwick's sign 177
Chest circumference 128
Chi-square test 7
Chicken 95
Chikungunya 176

Chlorine tablets 105
Chloroquine 102
Chloroscope 63
Citation 280
Coefficient of variation 1
Colostrum 152
Communal family 115
Community 275
Continuous fever 169
Contraception 187
Contraceptive prevalence rate 43
Copper T 80
Cornflakes 91
Couple protection rate 43
Cow pea 92
Crude birth rate 43
Crude death rate 15
Culex 109
Culture 275
Curd 96
Custom 275

D

Dakshata 189
DASH diet 52
Dawn's rule 179
Day carrier 89
Deep freezer 88
Dehydration 140
Dengue 170–173
Dengvaxia 254
Depression 253
Deworming 185
Diabetic dietary guidelines 52
Diaphragm 79
Diarrhoea 138
Dietary assessment 49
Disinfectants 104, 105
Dispersion 1
Dog bite categories 122
Double toned milk 53
DPT vaccine 85
Drinking water standards 59

E

Early registration 177, 178
Eclampsia 178, 179, 181, 183, 184
Economics 275
Egg 95
EHF scoring 208
Eligible couple 42

Emergency contraceptive 82
Emotion 275
End TB strategy 214
Epidemic curve 13
Essential obstetric care 178
Extended family 113

F

F-100 132
F-75 132
Fagerstrom test 278
Family 113
Fast breathing 136
Female condom 78
Ferritin 158
Fever and rash 169
Field stain 71, 72
Filariasis 176
First trimester 176–178, 185, 186
Fish 95
Focal seizure 166
Food fortification 160
Forest plot 40
Framingham Heart Study 216
Full cream milk 53
Fundal height 180
Funnel plot 41
Fever of unknown origin 169

G

Gantt chart 266
GAPPD 138
General fertility rate 43
General marital fertility rate 44
Generalized seizure 167
Gerber method 54
Gestational diabetes mellitus 185, 186
Global health sector strategy on viral
    hepatitis 262
Global hunger index 124
Global Leprosy Programme 208
Global nutrition report 125
Global nutrition targets 125
Global strategy for women, children and
    adolescent health 259
Glycaemic index 228
GOLD classification 230
Goodells' sign 177
Gram's stain 67
Green gram 92

Grips 180
Gross domestic product 275
Gross national product 275
Gross reproduction rate 44
Growth chart 129
Grunting 136

H

H$_2$S strip test kit 63
Habit 275
Haemoglobinopathies 156
Hanging drop preparation 76, 77
Hard tick 111
Harpenden's caliper 128
HbA1c 225
HBPNC 188, 189
Head circumference 128
Health insurance 118, 119
Hegar's sign 177
Hellin's rule 184
Hepatitis B vaccine 85
High-risk pregnancy 181
Horrock's apparatus 66
Housefly 110
HUB cutter 89
Human chorionic gonadotropin (HCG) 177
Hydrometer 64
Hygrometer 64
Hyperemesis gravidarum 184
Hypertension 215
Hypothyroidism 186

I

ICDS 134
Ice pack 89
Ice-lined refrigerator 88
ICF scale 258
IDSP 145
IHR 145
IMNCI 132
Impact factor 280
Impaired glucose tolerance 225
Incidence 17
Indian diabetes risk score 228
Indian newborn action plan 153
Infant mortality rate 44
Injectable contraceptive 82
Injectable polio vaccine 84
Intermittent fever 169
Involution 182
Iodine testing kit 65

Iron deficiency anaemia 156, 157
Iron folic acid (IFA) tablet 103
Iron prophylaxis 161
Iron sucrose 159
IUGR 146

J

Jaggery 97
Janani shishu suraksha karyakram (JSSK) 188
Janani suraksha yojana (JSY) 186, 187
Japanese encephalitis 176
Jeliffe ratio 124
JNC 7 215
JNC 8 218, 219
Johari window 267
Joint family 114
Jowar 90
JSB stain 70, 71
Juvenile Justice Act 256

K

Kanawati and McLaren index 124
Kangaroo mother care 153
Kaplan-Meier curve 41
Kappa statistic 29
Kidney bean 92
Koilonychia 157
Kuppuswamy scale 115
Kwashiorkor 130

L

Lactational amenorrhoea 189
Lactometer 65
LADA 223
Ladyfinger 93
Leadership 275
Leishman stain 70
Lepra reaction 205
Lepromin test 206
Leptospirosis 123
Levothyroxine 186
Life table method 32
Lifetime risk 44
Likelihood ratio 39
Line graph 40
Lippies loop 79
LNG-20 80
Lochia 183
Louse 111
Lucio's phenomenon 208

M

Magnesium sulphate 184
Maize 90
Mala D 81
Mala N 80
Malaria 172–175
Male condom 78
Mango 97
Marasmus 130
Maternal mortality rate 44
Maternal mortality ratio 44
Maternity bill 256
Maximum and minimum thermometers 63
mDiabetes 229
MDR-TB 213
Mean 1
Measles vaccine 86
Measles-rubella vaccine 87, 254
Measures of
   dispersion 1
   variability 1
Median 1
Megaloblastic anaemia 157–158
Metabolic syndrome 223
Metoclopramide 187
MGNREGA 120
Mid upper arm circumference 128
Mid-day meal programme 257
Minimum wages 118
Mirena 80
Mode 1
MODY 223
Motivation 272
Mutton 94
Myocardial infraction 220

N

NACP 249, 250
Naegele's formula 178
National Food Security Act 120
National Iron Plus Initiative 161
National Leprosy Eradication Programme
   NLEP 208
NCDs 220, 221
Neonatal mortality rate 44
Net domestic product 275
Net national product 275
Net reproduction rate 44
New anti-tubercular treatment 100
Newborn care corner 149
Nobel prize winners 264

Normal foetal heart sound and foetal heart
   rate 181
Norplant 82
NPCDCS 226
Nuclear family 113
Nutritional anaemia 155–57
Nutritional rehabilitation centres 132
NVBDCP 251, 252

O

Oats 91
Odds ratio 27
Old anti-tubercular treatment 99
Oligohydramnios and polyhydramnios 183
Open vial policy 255
Operational research 275
Oral anti-diabetic drugs 227
Oral polio vaccine 84
Oral rehydration spot 103
ORS 141

P

Package of essential non-communicable (PEN)
   disease 220
Pallor 157
Paneer 96
Paradoxical hypertension 217
Parikh's formula 178
Partograph/prasavgraph 186
Pastry 98
PDCA cycle 273
Pearl index 43
Pearl millet 90
Peas 93
Pedagogy 276
Pentavalent vaccine 85
Performa-case 283
Personnel 279
PERT–CPM 268
Platelet infusion 178
PMSSY 283
Pneumococcal vaccine 138, 254
Pneumonia 134
Polio 247–249
Political science 276
Population attributable risk 26
Post-neonatal mortality rate 44
Postpartum haemorrhage 182, 185
Poverty line 276
P-P plot 40
Pradhan Mantri Surakshit Matritva
   Abhiyan 187

Precocious pregnancy 179
Predictive value 36
Pre-eclampsia 178, 179, 181, 183–186
Pregnancy Aid Yojana Scheme 187
Pregnancy-induced hypertension 183
Prevalence 17
Pritchard regimen 184
Probabilty proportion to sample size
      sampling 19
Problem-based learning 276
Problem family 114
Proportional mortality rate 15
Protein energy malnutrition 125
Pseudo hypertension 217
Pseudomonas aeruginosa colonies 74
Public health pioneers 263
PubMed 282
Puerperium 188
Purchasing power parity 276

Q

Quac stick 124
Quartan fever 170
Quickening 177, 178

R

Ragi 91
Range 2
Rao and Singh index 124
Rashtriya Kishor Swasthya Karyakram 161
Rat
    flea 111
    poision 106
Red gram 91
Referencing 281
Relative risk 26
ReSoMal 142
Rh blood group 179, 180, 185
Rice 90
RMNCH+A 161
RNTCP 245–247, 260
ROM strategy 206
Rotavirus vaccine 86
Rules of halves 217
RUTF 132

S

Saathiya salah mobile app 260
Salient features of placenta 183
Salmonella typhi colonies 74
Sample size calculation 24

Sandfly 110
Sanitary latrine 122
Scatter diagram 40
SDG 258
Sensitivity 36
Severe acute malnutrition 130
Shakir's tape 128
Shigella colonies 75
Sick neonate 145
Sickle cell anaemia 156
Skewed data 2
Skimmed milk 53
Skin fold thickness 128
Skin pinch 140
Sling psychrometer 64
Small for gestational age 146
Smoking cessation 278
Social defence 276
Social determinants: Marmot review 274
Social institution 276
Social security 118, 276
Social structure 276
Socialism 276
Socialization 276
Sociology 276
Soft tick 111
Soya bean 92
Specialised newborn care unit 149
Specific death rate 15
Specificity 36
Spinach 93
Spot map 41
Spring scale 127
Standard deviation 1
Standard error 1
Staphylococcus aureus colonies 73
Status epilepticus 167
Stem and leaf diagram 40
STEPS 220
STI kits 101
Streptococcus pyogenes colonies 74
Stridor 136
Stunting 123
Super super ORS 143
Survival analysis 31
Swachh Bharat Abhiyan 258
Syringe requirement 47

T

t-test 10
Target couple 42
Tertian fever 170

Test of significance 6
Tetanus vaccine 86
Thalassemia, alpha 156
Thalassemia, beta 156
Three delay model 188
Three generation family 114
Tinotometer 66
Tobbaco 278
Toned milk 53
Total fertility rate 44
Tree diagram 41
True labour, stages, prolong and normal
          labour 182
Tuber 94
Tuberculosis 253
Twin peak sign 184

U

Udai Pareek scale 116
Under-nutrition 123
Underweight 123
Unmet need 42
Urban area 276
Urban poor 115

V

Vaccine
   carrier 89
   requirement 45
   vial monitor 87
Vaginal contraceptive gel 79

Vaginal ring 83
VED analysis 271
Vibrio cholerae colonies 75, 76
Vital statistics 44
Vitamin A 88

W

Warning signs 181
Wasting 123
Wealth index 277
Weekly iron folic acid supplementation
          programme 161
Wheat 90
Wholesome water 60
Wright-Giemsa stain 69

X

XDR-TB 213

Y

Yasmini 81

Z

Z score 124
Zinc 103
ZN stain 67, 68
Zuspan regimen 184